Transformative
Nursing Education

Transformative Nursing Education

Edited by

Aby Mitchell

Barry Hill

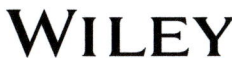

Registered Office(s)
John Wiley & Sons, Inc., 111 River Street, Hoboken, NJ 07030, USA
John Wiley & Sons Ltd, New Era House, 8 Oldlands Way, Bognor Regis, West Sussex, PO22 9NQ, UK
John Wiley & Sons Singapore Pte. Ltd, 134 Jurong Gateway Road, #04-307H, Singapore 600134
For details of our global editorial offices, customer services, and more information about Wiley products visit us at www.wiley.com.

The manufacturer's authorized representative according to the EU General Product Safety Regulation is Wiley-VCH GmbH, Boschstr. 12, 69469 Weinheim, Germany, e-mail: Product_Safety@wiley.com.

Library of Congress Cataloging-in-Publication Data has been applied for:

Paperback: 9781394324880
oBook: 9781394324934
ePub: 9781394324910
ePDF: 9781394324927

Cover Design: Wiley
Cover Image: © everythingpossible/stock.adobe.com

Typesetting: Set in 9.5/12pt STIXTwoText by Lumina Datamatics

Printed and bound by CPI Group (UK) Ltd, Croydon, CR0 4YY

C9781394324880_250326

Contents

List of Contributors   vi
Preface   vii
Acknowledgements   x

1 The Foundations of Transformative Nursing Education   1
   Barry Hill and Aby Mitchell

2 Critical Thinking and Reflective Practice   15
   Amsale Wamburu and Barry Hill

3 Leadership and Innovation in Nursing Education   32
   Melane Hayward and Karen Buckwell-Nutt

4 Ethical and Cultural Competence   52
   Luis Teixeira

5 Innovation and Practical Application in Nursing Education   68
   Sadie Diamond-Fox

6 Transformative Simulation   84
   Aby Mitchell

7 Digital and Immersive Technologies in Nursing Education   102
   Claire Ford and Behnam Jafari Salim

8 Embedding Global Health Perspectives in Nursing Education   115
   Jacqui Bolton

9 Sustainability   137
   Melanie Madison

10 Future Directions in Transformative Nursing Education   155
   Barry Hill and Aby Mitchell

Index   167

List of Contributors

Jacqui Bolton
Florence Nightingale Faculty of Nursing
Midwifery and Palliative Care
Department of Adult Nursing
King's College London
UK

Sadie Diamond-Fox
School of Healthcare and Nursing Sciences
Faculty of Health and Wellbeing
Northumbria University
UK

Claire Ford
School of Healthcare and Nursing Sciences
Northumbria University
Newcastle upon Tyne
UK

Melane Hayward
College of Health and Society
Buckinghamshire New University
UK

Karen Buckwell-Nutt
College of Health and Society
Buckinghamshire New University
UK

Barry Hill
School of Healthcare and Nursing Sciences (HNS)
Faculty of Health and Wellbeing
Northumbria University
UK

Melanie Madison
Florence Nightingale Faculty of Nursing
Midwifery and Palliative Care
Department of Adult Nursing
King's College London
UK

Aby Mitchell
Florence Nightingale Faculty for Nursing
Midwifery and Palliative care
King's College London
UK

Behnam Jafari Salim
King's College London
London
UK

Luis Teixeira
Florence Nightingale Faculty of Nursing
Midwifery and Palliative Care
Department of Adult Nursing
King's College London
UK

Amsale Wamburu
College of Health and Society
Buckinghamshire New University
UK

Preface

TRANSFORMING THE FUTURE OF NURSE EDUCATION

Barry Hill and Aby Mitchell

The future of nursing is closely tied to the quality and purpose of nursing education. In a world facing rapid social, environmental, and technological change, nurse education must respond to a wider range of challenges than ever before. These include global health inequalities, increasing demand for person-centred care, and a changing healthcare workforce. This book, *Transformative Nursing Education*, aims to support those tasked with preparing nurses for this evolving landscape. It brings together key topics and approaches that support the development of capable, reflective, and ethically responsible professionals.

This book has been developed for nurse educators working across higher education and clinical practice. It supports those designing, delivering, assessing, and leading nursing education programmes, and recognises the practical constraints and demands often experienced in these roles. Whether you are leading a module, supporting students in clinical settings, or influencing strategic decisions, the ideas and tools in this book aim to offer clarity, guidance, and encouragement.

RETHINKING THE PURPOSE OF NURSING EDUCATION

Traditional nursing education models have often focused on knowledge transfer, technical skill development, and professional behaviour. These remain essential. However, to prepare nurses who can navigate complexity, work collaboratively, respond to change, and uphold professional values in the face of pressure, we need education that also develops insight, judgement, and adaptability.

Transformative education places the learner at the centre of the process. It encourages them to examine their own assumptions, engage critically with practice, and recognise the social, political, and ethical dimensions of healthcare. It supports a shift from passive learning to active engagement and from surface understanding to meaningful learning that informs long-term professional identity.

This book is based on the belief that educators play a key role in shaping not just what students learn, but how they become nurses. This includes developing professional confidence, valuing person-centred care, and being willing to challenge unsafe or unequal practice. These attributes cannot be developed through content delivery alone; they require thoughtful teaching, reflection, and carefully designed learning environments.

OVERVIEW OF THE BOOK

The chapters that follow are organised thematically and written by educators and practitioners with direct experience in the areas they explore. Each chapter includes a clear aim and set of learning outcomes, alongside examples and practical suggestions to support implementation in teaching and curriculum planning. To encourage active engagement, every chapter contains a structured activity box and an innovation feature that introduces

applied ideas and real-world relevance. A bespoke figure or visual model is included to illustrate key concepts and support deeper understanding. Chapters conclude with Continuing Professional Development (CPD) reflective questions and a set of take-home points that reinforce the chapter's core messages and invite further reflection. This consistent format is intended to support both academic and practice-based educators, making each chapter accessible, engaging, and ready to apply within a range of learning and teaching contexts.

- **Chapter 1: The Foundations of Transformative Nursing Education**—*Barry Hill and Aby Mitchell*

  This chapter explores the historical development of nursing education, current professional expectations, and the educational theories that underpin transformative approaches to learning.

- **Chapter 2: Critical Thinking and Reflective Practice**—*Amsale Wamburu and Barry Hill*

  A practical exploration of how to support students to think critically, reflect meaningfully, and apply these skills in both academic and clinical learning environments.

- **Chapter 3: Leadership and Innovation in Nursing Education**—*Melane Hayward and Karen Buckwell-Nutt*

  This chapter considers a range of leadership approaches and how they influence innovation, curriculum design, and quality in nursing education.

- **Chapter 4: Ethical and Cultural Competence**—*Luis Teixeira*

  Focusing on embedding ethics and cultural sensitivity across programmes, this chapter supports educators to develop inclusive, respectful, and equitable learning environments.

- **Chapter 5: Innovation and Practical Application in Nursing Education**—*Sadie Diamond-Fox*

  Offers detailed examples of digital learning, technology-enhanced feedback, and flexible delivery models to meet contemporary student needs.

- **Chapter 6: Transformative Simulation**—*Aby Mitchell*

  This chapter positions simulation as more than a teaching technique—it is a tool for enhancing emotional, social, and cultural intelligence, as well as clinical judgement.

- **Chapter 7: Digital and Immersive Technologies in Nursing Education**—*Claire Ford and Behnam Jafari Salim*

  Explores virtual reality, artificial intelligence, and augmented reality, and their role in creating engaging, interactive learning environments.

- **Chapter 8: Embedding Global Health Perspectives in Nursing Education**—*Jacqui Bolton*

  This chapter places global health and interprofessional collaboration at the centre of curriculum thinking, supporting learners to understand the wider contexts of nursing.

- **Chapter 9: Sustainability**—*Melanie Maddison*

  Discusses how nursing education can align with sustainable development goals, promote wellbeing, and contribute to socially responsible teaching practices.

- **Chapter 10: Future Directions in Transformative Nursing Education**—*Barry Hill and Aby Mitchell*

  Reflects on what lies ahead for nursing education, considering policy developments, digital innovation, and the role of the nurse educator in shaping future practice.

SHARED COMMITMENTS

Although the chapters cover different topics, they are connected by shared commitments:

- A commitment to high-quality education that prepares students for the demands and responsibilities of contemporary practice.

- A belief in the importance of supporting students to become thoughtful, capable, and resilient professionals.

- A recognition that learning is shaped by relationships, context, and values—not just content.

- An awareness that education must support inclusion, equity, and fairness—for students, staff, and the populations we serve.

These principles are not limited to the classroom. They shape how we design assessment, select learning resources, develop faculty, and work with practice partners. Education that is transformative is not always about large-scale change. It can also be about careful adjustments, thoughtful conversations, or trying something different in response to student feedback. What matters is the intention: to improve learning and support professional growth.

A MESSAGE FROM THE COUNCIL OF DEANS OF HEALTH

Nurse education sits at the heart of a sustainable and high quality health and care system. Across the United Kingdom, higher education institutions are working within a complex and rapidly changing landscape, shaped by workforce pressures, financial constraints, evolving service needs and changing expectations of the professions. At the same time, there is a shared commitment across the Council of Deans of Health to ensure that nurse education remains rigorous, inclusive and responsive to the needs of patients, communities and the workforce.

Current challenges facing higher education and practice learning environments require continued collaboration between universities, health and care providers and national bodies. Recruitment, retention, placement capacity and the preparation of graduates for increasingly complex roles are all key areas of focus. Ensuring that nurse education continues to support professional identity, clinical excellence and leadership development is essential if we are to meet future population health needs.

The Council of Deans of Health continues to advocate for the value and impact of nurse education within higher education and across the wider health and care system. By working together across sectors, we can support innovation, maintain high standards and ensure that the next generation of nurses are prepared to deliver safe, compassionate and effective care in an increasingly complex world.

PROFESSOR ALISON I MACHIN
CHAIR OF THE COUNCIL OF DEANS OF HEALTH
PROFESSOR OF NURSING AND INTER-PROFESSIONAL
WORKFORCE DEVELOPMENT

Acknowledgements

We would like to express our sincere gratitude to all those who made *Transformative Nursing Education* possible.

First and foremost, we thank the contributing chapter authors, each of whom brought their insight, dedication, and experience to this book. Your commitment to nursing education, both in theory and in practice, is evident in every chapter. We are proud to have collaborated with such a knowledgeable and passionate group of educators and practitioners.

To our colleagues across higher education institutions and healthcare practice settings, thank you for your continued engagement, support, and collegiality. Your willingness to share ideas, challenge assumptions, and improve teaching through reflection and innovation has inspired much of the content in this book.

We also extend our appreciation to our students, past and present. Your questions, courage, and feedback continue to shape how we teach and why we remain committed to transforming the educational experience. You remind us daily of the importance of creating learning environments that are inclusive, reflective, and person-centred.

Thank you to the editorial and production team at Wiley, whose support and patience have guided us throughout the process. Your expertise has helped us shape a book that we hope will be practical, thought-provoking, and useful to nurse educators worldwide.

Finally, we would like to acknowledge our families, close friends and Professor Ian Peate OBE for their encouragement and support. Writing and editing a book of this nature is never done in isolation, and we are grateful for your continued support.

This book is the result of collaboration, shared purpose, and a belief in the power of education to shape the future of nursing. We hope it provides a useful companion for those seeking to lead, teach, and support the next generation of nursing professionals.

ABY MITCHELL AND BARRY HILL

The Foundations of Transformative Nursing Education

Barry Hill[1] and Aby Mitchell[2]

[1] *School of Healthcare and Nursing Sciences (HNS), Faculty of Health and Wellbeing, Northumbria University, UK*
[2] *Florence Nightingale Faculty for Nursing, Midwifery and Palliative care, King's College London, UK*

AIM

To explore the foundations, context, and theoretical frameworks of transformative education in UK nursing, enabling readers to understand its significance in shaping contemporary nursing curricula, teaching practice, and professional identity.

LEARNING OUTCOMES

By the end of this chapter, readers will be able to:

1. Describe the concept of transformative education and its relevance to nursing practice and policy.

2. Identify key historical developments and regulatory shifts that have influenced the evolution of nurse education in the UK.

3. Evaluate the educational and professional needs of contemporary nursing students considering current workforce challenges.

4. Apply core educational theories to the design and delivery of transformative learning experiences in nursing education.

CHAPTER INTRODUCTION

Nursing education is undergoing a profound transformation. In a healthcare system marked by rapid change, increasing complexity, and workforce pressures, there is a growing recognition that traditional models of teaching, rooted in transmission of technical knowledge and procedural skill, are no longer sufficient. Instead, a broader educational philosophy is needed, one that supports students not only to become competent practitioners but to develop as reflective, ethical, and engaged professionals.

Transformative education addresses this need. It challenges the notion of education as passive acquisition and instead presents learning as an active, relational process. It encourages students to question assumptions, engage in meaningful reflection, and develop a deeper understanding of their roles within health and care systems. This approach aligns closely with current expectations from the Nursing and Midwifery Council (2018), the NHS Long Term Plan (2019), and the NHS Long Term Workforce Plan (2023), which collectively highlight the need for compassionate, critical, and system-aware nurses.

This chapter provides a foundation for understanding transformative education in nursing. It explores the contemporary drivers for change, identifies current educational priorities, and reviews the evolution of nurse education in the UK. It also introduces the core theoretical frameworks that underpin this approach and considers how they inform curriculum, pedagogy, and assessment. In doing so, the chapter sets the stage for a wider conversation about how nurse education can be reimagined to support the professionals of tomorrow.

THE CONTEXT OF TRANSFORMATIVE EDUCATION

This section explores the rationale for adopting transformative approaches in nursing education. It discusses national policy drivers, workforce needs, regulatory standards, and the diversity of the student population, establishing why transformation is necessary in the current UK healthcare and educational landscape.

UNDERSTANDING TRANSFORMATIVE EDUCATION

Transformative education describes a process where learners critically examine their assumptions, develop new perspectives, and alter their understanding of the world and themselves. Mezirow's (1991) seminal theory of transformative learning positions critical reflection as the core of adult learning. In this model, individuals are encouraged to reconsider established beliefs, engage in dialogue, and reconstruct their frames of reference. This is particularly relevant in nursing, where learners must understand not only the science of care, but also the moral, emotional, and relational aspects of the profession.

Transformative education aligns with constructivist and humanistic educational theories. Knowles et al. (2015) described adult learners as autonomous, goal-oriented individuals who learn best through experience, relevance, and problem-solving. These principles underpin student-centred approaches in nurse education, including simulation, case-based learning, and reflective practice. The work of Freire (1970) is also influential. His critical pedagogy views education as a means of challenging inequality and enabling learners to become agents of change, an idea echoed in the values-based practice encouraged by the Nursing and Midwifery Council (NMC, 2018). This shift in educational philosophy can be clearly seen when comparing the features of transformative and traditional approaches to nurse education (see Table 1.1).

POLICY CONTEXT: NHS AND WORKFORCE TRANSFORMATION

The context for transformative education is shaped by major UK policy documents that outline how the healthcare workforce should evolve.

The NHS Long Term Plan (NHS England, 2019) highlights the need to integrate care across settings, improve health inequalities, and equip the workforce with the skills to deliver more personalised care. It stresses prevention, digital innovation, and the support of individuals with long-term conditions. These priorities require a nursing workforce that is not only clinically competent but capable of critical thinking, ethical decision-making, and leadership.

More recently, the NHS Long Term Workforce Plan (NHS England, 2023) has set out a strategic vision for growing and reforming the health and care workforce. It acknowledges current pressures on staffing and the need to expand training routes, embrace new technologies, and ensure that education prepares practitioners for multidisciplinary and patient-centred practice. The plan explicitly calls for education that develops staff to work with autonomy and professionalism, aligning closely with the aims of transformative education.

The plan also places significant emphasis on values, compassion, and retention, areas where transformative approaches can have real impact. By enabling learners to reflect on their motivations, develop a strong sense of professional identity, and feel connected to their learning journey, educators can contribute to both workforce resilience and quality of care.

REGULATORY AND INSTITUTIONAL EXPECTATIONS

The Nursing and Midwifery Council (NMC) (2018) standards for proficiency and education place high expectations on graduates. Nurses are expected to be critical

Table 1.1 Transformative Education vs. Traditional Education

Feature	Transformative education	Traditional education
Student Role	Active participant, critical thinker	Passive recipient, rule-follower
Educator Role	Facilitator, guide, reflective practitioner	Instructor, knowledge transmitter
Curriculum Focus	Values, identity, professional growth	Tasks, content, clinical competence
Assessment Approach	Reflective, developmental, portfolio-based	Exams, objective testing, skills checklists
Learning Environment	Inclusive, dialogic, psychologically safe	Hierarchical, compliance-focused
Core Values	Equity, compassion, critical consciousness	Discipline, obedience, standardisation

thinkers, emotionally aware, and capable of leading care across settings. These standards emphasise reflection, partnership working, professional accountability, and the ability to challenge poor practice, all of which benefit from transformative learning approaches.

The Quality Assurance Agency (QAA) subject benchmarks for nursing education also reference the development of independent learners with the capacity for analytical reasoning, ethical sensitivity, and evidence-informed practice (QAA, 2022). These benchmarks encourage curricula that are intellectually demanding and support personal development, again supporting the case for educational transformation.

At the institutional level, many universities are embedding teaching strategies that reflect these values. Flipped classrooms, digital portfolios, and authentic assessment methods are increasingly used to engage students as active participants in their education. Staff are also encouraged to develop relational approaches to teaching, which help build trust and engagement.

INNOVATION BOX

Title: *Flipped Classrooms in Pre-Registration Nursing: Enhancing Student Agency and Dialogue*

Innovation in Practice

At several UK universities, flipped classroom approaches are being embedded into pre-registration nursing modules. Instead of delivering core content during lectures, students engage with recorded lectures, reading packs, and interactive quizzes in advance. Class time is then used for case-based learning, structured dialogue, and collaborative problem-solving.

This shift supports transformative learning by encouraging students to come prepared with questions, engage in discussion, and reflect critically on real-world scenarios. For nurse educators, it offers an opportunity to act as facilitators rather than content deliverers, modelling inclusive and dialogic teaching practices that are central to contemporary HE.

Why It Matters

Flipped learning can enhance engagement, promote deeper thinking, and support the development of autonomy and critical enquiry in nursing students. It also aligns with the NMC's emphasis on professionalism, reflection, and person-centred thinking.

STUDENT DIVERSITY AND THE LEARNING ENVIRONMENT

UK nursing students come from diverse backgrounds. Many are mature learners, returners to education, carers, or first-generation university students. Others are international or multilingual learners. A one-size-fits-all approach to education no longer meets the needs of this varied student population.

Transformative education is well-suited to inclusive and differentiated teaching. It recognises and values the lived experience of learners, using it as a springboard for reflection and dialogue. Educators who apply a critical pedagogy approach (Freire, 1970) are better positioned to create respectful, participatory learning spaces. This enhances engagement, supports well-being, and helps address the awarding gaps and retention concerns highlighted across the sector (Thomas, 2022).

Importantly, transformative education makes space for students to reflect on their identity, values, and experiences of difference. This has particular value in preparing nurses to provide culturally sensitive care and to advocate for equity within their own practice.

SIMULATION, REFLECTION, AND PLACEMENT LEARNING

Experiential learning is a fundamental part of UK nursing curricula. Simulation offers students a safe environment in which to apply clinical knowledge, practise decision-making, and reflect on emotional responses. It aligns with Kolb's experiential learning theory (1984), which outlines the learning cycle as concrete experience, reflective observation, abstract conceptualisation, and active experimentation. When debriefed effectively, simulation supports the integration of theory and practice and contributes to confidence and preparedness for clinical placements.

Placements are a further site for transformative learning. Through direct engagement with patients, teams, and systems, students encounter both the complexity and the humanity of nursing. Critical incidents, emotionally charged experiences, and ethical dilemmas often serve as turning points in the development of professional identity (Taylor, 2017). When educators provide structured support, students can reflect on these moments and make sense of their growth.

Written and verbal reflection continues to be a requirement in practice assessment documentation. However, for this reflection to be transformative rather than transactional, educators must model openness and provide psychological safety. Transformative learning is more likely to occur when students feel valued, listened to, and able to take educational risks.

EMOTIONAL AWARENESS AND PROFESSIONAL FORMATION

Nursing education must account for the emotional and moral complexity of care. Nurses frequently encounter distressing situations, conflicting values, and organisational pressures. Helping students develop emotional literacy and ethical awareness is therefore essential.

Hochschild's (1983) concept of emotional labour is especially relevant in this context. Nurses are expected to manage their own emotional responses while supporting patients and relatives. Transformative education enables students to reflect on these demands, preparing them for professional resilience.

Identity formation is also key. Students must transition from being members of the public to healthcare professionals, and this requires not only knowledge and skill, but internalisation of professional values. Through mentorship, feedback, and opportunities for self-exploration, education can play a powerful role in shaping who students become.

CHALLENGES AND CONSIDERATIONS

While the value of transformative education is evident, there are barriers to its widespread implementation:

- Curriculum constraints and limited time for dialogue or reflection
- Inconsistent facilitation skills among educators
- An emphasis on measurable outcomes that can sideline personal development
- Variable quality and integration of placement learning experiences

Addressing these barriers requires leadership, curriculum redesign, and recognition of the value of personal development in regulatory and institutional priorities.

CONTEMPORARY NEEDS IN NURSING EDUCATION

This section focuses on the present-day demands of practice and education. This section identifies the knowledge, skills, values, and behaviours that modern nursing graduates require. Topics include digital innovation, inclusivity, interprofessional learning, well-being, research literacy, and career readiness.

The landscape of nursing education is constantly evolving in response to clinical, technological, and societal changes. Preparing students for registration is no longer only about ensuring competence in practical skills. Instead, it demands a holistic approach that equips graduates to manage uncertainty, work across disciplines, and care for increasingly diverse populations in complex environments. This section explores the current and emerging needs of nursing education in the UK, drawing on national priorities, workforce expectations, and student experience. It considers how curricula and teaching practices must adapt to ensure future nurses are well prepared, values-driven, and fit for contemporary practice.

COMPLEXITY AND UNCERTAINTY IN PRACTICE

The nature of nursing practice has changed significantly over the past two decades. Nurses now operate in highly pressurised environments, including acute care, community settings, and digital platforms. They are expected to make autonomous decisions, interpret complex clinical data, and manage escalating care demands across shifting systems. These realities were highlighted in the NHS Long Term Workforce Plan (NHS England, 2023), which highlighted the need to expand and reform nursing education to meet future workforce requirements. The plan emphasises developing staff who are confident, compassionate, and able to lead care delivery.

To meet these needs, education must move beyond basic clinical competence. Students require a deep understanding of systems, safety, and interprofessional dynamics. They also need to be prepared to work with ambiguity, recognising when to escalate care, adapt to change, and challenge practice where necessary. This has implications for curriculum design, which must embed real-world scenarios, critical incident analysis, and ethical reasoning as part of core learning.

PERSON-CENTRED AND INCLUSIVE PRACTICE

Central to contemporary nursing is the delivery of person-centred care. This principle is embedded within the NMC Standards of Proficiency for Registered Nurses and reflects a shift away from task-based nursing towards a holistic, values-led approach. Educators must support students to recognise patients as partners in care, drawing on lived experience and personalised goals.

In doing so, nursing curricula must engage with equality, diversity, and inclusion (EDI). The UK health and care system serves populations with varied needs, experiences, and histories of discrimination. Nurses must be equipped to understand the social determinants of health, challenge bias, and promote health equity. These expectations are mirrored in the NHS Long Term Plan (NHS England, 2019), which advocates for culturally appropriate care, prevention, and reducing health inequalities.

Education that reflects these aims should include case studies from a range of communities, opportunities for critical reflection on identity and power, and modules addressing public health, marginalisation, and patient advocacy. Inclusive teaching practice is essential for both learners and service users.

THE DIGITAL AND TECHNOLOGICAL AGENDA

The use of digital technology in healthcare has accelerated, with remote consultations, electronic records, and artificial intelligence becoming part of everyday care. Nursing education must therefore prepare students not only to use digital tools, but to evaluate their impact on patient experience, privacy, and quality.

The Topol Review (Topol, 2019) made clear recommendations for future training in digital healthcare, calling for digital professionalism, understanding of data ethics, and active participation in shaping technological change. While technical skills are essential, students must also develop a critical awareness of digital inequalities and their implications for access and outcomes.

Virtual learning environments, simulation, and augmented reality are increasingly used in nursing education itself. These tools offer opportunities for immersive learning, yet their use must be underpinned by pedagogical clarity and equity of access. Education providers must be mindful of digital exclusion and ensure that all students have the resources and support to engage effectively.

INTERPROFESSIONAL LEARNING AND TEAM-BASED CARE

Nurses rarely work in isolation. Healthcare is delivered by multidisciplinary teams that must collaborate to provide safe and effective care. The World Health Organization (WHO, 2010) defines interprofessional education as occasions where students from two or more professions learn about, from, and with each other to enable effective collaboration and improve health outcomes.

In the UK, the importance of interprofessional learning is recognised in NMC guidance and in institutional strategy. Opportunities for shared learning, including scenario-based teaching with other health students, can help break down professional silos, improve communication, and enhance understanding of roles. When managed well, these learning experiences contribute to safer and more coordinated patient care.

Embedding interprofessional learning in nursing curricula requires attention to timing, facilitation, and relevance. It also supports the wider development of teamwork, respect, and negotiation skills that are essential in today's health services.

ACADEMIC SKILLS AND RESEARCH LITERACY

Modern nursing requires an ability to understand, appraise, and apply evidence in practice. Students must be introduced early to principles of evidence-based practice and taught how to locate, interpret, and apply research findings in real-world contexts.

The QAA (2022) subject benchmark for nursing education highlights research literacy as a key graduate outcome. This includes critical reading, data interpretation, and understanding methodology. Embedding these skills throughout the curriculum, not just in final-year dissertations, helps students recognise the value of research and prepares them to contribute to service improvement.

In parallel, education should promote academic integrity, writing skills, and critical engagement. These are essential for success in higher education and for developing professional accountability. Students should feel confident navigating both the clinical and academic demands of their role.

WELL-BEING AND RETENTION

Supporting student well-being is increasingly seen as a key responsibility of nursing education. Attrition rates remain a concern, particularly for students in the early stages of training. Pre-registration nursing programmes are demanding, with placement pressures, shift work, academic assessments, and financial stress all contributing to student fatigue and dropout.

A recent report by the Council of Deans of Health (2016) reiterated the importance of psychological support, inclusive learning communities, and responsive curriculum design. Educators play a vital role in noticing signs of distress, providing appropriate signposting, and encouraging open dialogue around mental health.

Nursing education must also prepare students for the emotional aspects of practice. Developing emotional resilience, moral sensitivity, and peer support skills should be seen as part of the curriculum, not an optional extra. Reflective spaces, supervision models, and values-based discussion groups can all contribute to better preparation and retention.

CAREER READINESS AND PROFESSIONAL IDENTITY

Graduates need to enter the workforce with a strong sense of professional identity and confidence in their ability to contribute. This involves understanding the values of nursing, recognising their own strengths, and feeling prepared for transition to practice.

Personal tutoring, mentorship, and exposure to role models are key strategies. So too are assessment methods that require students to articulate their decision-making, values, and learning journey. Simulation and practice-based learning continue to offer important experiences in this regard, especially when supported by feedback that encourages self-awareness and goal setting.

There is increasing interest in tracking outcomes beyond graduation, including employability, career progression, and advanced practice development. Education providers should consider how they support alumni, maintain connections with service providers, and prepare students for longer-term career development.

FLEXIBLE AND SUSTAINABLE EDUCATION MODELS

Finally, there is growing recognition that education delivery must itself be flexible, inclusive, and sustainable. Many nursing students balance learning with employment, caring responsibilities, or health needs. Offering multiple modes of learning, such as hybrid, online, or asynchronous content, can enhance access and engagement. However, this must be balanced with the need for connection, community, and experiential learning.

Sustainability is also a growing concern. The Florence Nightingale Foundation and others have called for the integration of environmental awareness into nursing curricula, recognising the climate crisis as a public health issue. Students should understand the principles of sustainable healthcare and be encouraged to reflect on their role in supporting environmental stewardship in clinical practice.

HISTORICAL PERSPECTIVES AND EVOLUTION OF NURSING EDUCATION

This section provides an overview of the key milestones and reforms in UK nursing education. It traces the shift from apprenticeship to university-based learning, the influence of policy reports and professional regulation, and the changing nature of curriculum and pedagogy over time.

Understanding the historical development of nursing education provides essential context for its current form and direction. The evolution from apprenticeship-style training to university-based education reflects broader shifts in societal values, professional expectations, and healthcare delivery models. This section examines key milestones in the development of nursing education in the UK, the influence of pivotal individuals and policy drivers, and the implications of these developments for contemporary curriculum and pedagogy.

EARLY MODELS OF NURSE TRAINING

Modern nursing education in the UK can trace its roots to the late nineteenth century, with the establishment of formal training schools influenced by Florence Nightingale.

Nightingale's approach, shaped by her experiences in the Crimean War, placed emphasis on discipline, observation, and sanitation (McDonald, 2010). The Nightingale Training School for Nurses, opened at St Thomas' Hospital in London in 1860, became a model for nurse education worldwide. Training was largely hospital-based, with nurses learning by observing and performing tasks under supervision. The emphasis was on character, obedience, and practical skill rather than academic study.

Although Nightingale supported the professionalisation of nursing, she was sceptical of over-academic models. This early ambivalence between practical experience and theoretical knowledge has remained a tension in nurse education. Nevertheless, Nightingale's influence on structured, purpose-driven education is widely acknowledged.

TWENTIETH CENTURY: GRADUAL REFORM

The early twentieth century saw incremental reform in nurse education. The Nurses Registration Act of 1919 introduced a professional register and acknowledged nursing as a regulated occupation. This formalised entry standards and signalled a shift toward professional autonomy. However, education remained hospital-based, and training continued to be controlled by the medical profession.

Significant change occurred in the post-war years, driven in part by the creation of the National Health Service (NHS) in 1948. The growing demand for healthcare required a reliable nursing workforce, and there was increased recognition of the need for systematic training. Nurse tutors emerged as a distinct group, and the General Nursing Council introduced standardised syllabuses and examinations.

By the 1970s, criticisms of the apprenticeship model were growing. Concerns included lack of educational coherence, inadequate preparation for complex care, and limited opportunities for critical thinking or leadership. A number of influential reports began to challenge the status quo.

THE BRIGGS REPORT AND THE PUSH FOR REFORM

A major turning point came with the Briggs Report (DHSS, 1972), which reviewed nursing education in the UK and advocated for a shift towards academic integration. The report called for nursing to become a fully recognised profession, with an emphasis on the development of knowledge, judgement, and research literacy. Briggs identified that nursing was 'at a crossroads' and that continued reliance on hospital training was unsustainable.

Despite its significance, implementation of the Briggs recommendations was slow and uneven. Nevertheless, it set the tone for future reforms and contributed to the recognition that nursing required a broader educational foundation, including behavioural and social sciences, ethics, and communication.

PROJECT 2000 AND UNIVERSITY INTEGRATION

A pivotal moment came in the late 1980s with the introduction of Project 2000, a national initiative that aimed to relocate pre-registration nurse education into higher education institutions (UKCC, 1986). This marked the transition from training to education and formally established nursing as a university-level discipline. Project 2000 aimed to prepare nurses with a balance of academic and clinical learning, supporting the development of critical thinking and professional autonomy.

Students now enter nursing as full-time undergraduates, with a greater emphasis on theoretical knowledge and reflective practice. Academic staff with nursing backgrounds became embedded within universities, and nursing research began to develop as a specialty. Although the shift was not without criticism, particularly from those who feared a loss of clinical emphasis, it significantly elevated the status of the profession and aligned nursing with other health disciplines.

Following Project 2000, the UK Central Council for Nursing, Midwifery and Health Visiting (UKCC) introduced further reforms, including the move from diploma-level training to all-degree programmes by 2013. This change further consolidated nursing's position within higher education and aligned with the broader agenda of professionalisation.

BOLOGNA PROCESS AND EUROPEAN INFLUENCE

The Bologna Process, initiated in 1999 to standardise higher education across Europe, had a direct impact on UK nursing education by promoting comparability of qualifications, learning outcomes, and academic credit. This process contributed to the widespread adoption of degree-level education for nurses and supported mobility across countries.

In the UK context, it also encouraged clearer curriculum frameworks, quality assurance mechanisms, and student-centred pedagogies. Nursing education increasingly came to reflect the higher education values of academic rigour, inclusivity, and research-led teaching.

DEVELOPMENT OF ADVANCED AND SPECIALIST ROLES

As the scope of nursing practice expanded, new educational pathways were required to prepare nurses for advanced, extended, and specialist roles. From the 1990s onwards, postgraduate education grew significantly, with the introduction of Specialist Practitioner Qualifications, Nurse Prescribing, and Advanced Clinical Practice (ACP) programmes.

These roles required nurses to undertake complex assessments, make diagnostic decisions, and lead service development. Education for these roles necessitated a strong academic foundation, including knowledge of pathophysiology, pharmacology, and systems leadership. Universities responded by designing master's level qualifications aligned with national competency frameworks such as the Multi-professional Framework for Advanced Clinical Practice in England (Health Education England, 2017).

This expansion of roles reinforced the importance of academic credibility and flexibility in nursing education and contributed to the development of career pathways that support progression, retention, and leadership.

SHIFTS IN CURRICULUM AND PEDAGOGY

Alongside structural changes, there have been important pedagogical shifts in nursing education. Historically, the emphasis was on passive learning, memorisation, and repetition. Over time, this has given way to student-centred approaches that value critical thinking, reflection, and dialogue.

Transformative learning theory (Mezirow, 1991) and experiential learning theory (Kolb, 1984) have become influential in informing curriculum design. The use of simulation, reflective writing, and problem-based learning has increased, helping students to apply knowledge and develop professional judgement.

Technological advances have further reshaped delivery. Online learning platforms, digital assessment, and virtual simulation are now common components of nurse education. The COVID-19 pandemic accelerated this trend, prompting rapid adaptation and reflection on how best to balance accessibility, engagement, and quality.

THE CURRENT ERA: REGULATION AND QUALITY ASSURANCE

The NMC introduced new standards in 2018 that revised the expectations for pre-registration education. These standards place greater emphasis on critical reflection, person-centred care, leadership, and evidence-informed practice. They also reflect contemporary values around equality, inclusion, and partnership working.

Education providers must now demonstrate not only that students can perform skills, but that they can apply knowledge ethically, communicate effectively, and respond to changing needs. The NMC also requires that student learning be supported through collaboration with practice partners, integrated assessment, and supervision models that encourage professional development.

The QAA continues to influence education through its subject benchmark statements, which articulate the academic and professional expectations for nursing graduates (QAA, 2022). These benchmarks reinforce the academic legitimacy of nursing and help ensure that education remains current and responsive.

ONGOING TENSIONS AND AREAS FOR DEVELOPMENT

Despite progress, some tensions persist. These include balancing academic content with clinical experience, ensuring that education remains inclusive and accessible, and addressing concerns around student preparedness for practice. There are also debates about the status of nursing knowledge, with calls for greater recognition of nursing theory, research, and epistemology within curricula (McEwen & Wills, 2023).

In addition, educators must now prepare students not only for current practice but for future systems shaped by digital innovation, integrated care, and sustainability. This requires a future-facing curriculum that is both flexible and grounded in the core values of the profession.

THEORIES UNDERPINNING TRANSFORMATIVE EDUCATION

This section introduces the major theoretical frameworks that inform transformative education. These include Mezirow's transformative learning theory, Freire's critical pedagogy, experiential learning (Kolb), adult learning (Knowles), constructivism, reflective practice, and related concepts such as emotional intelligence and threshold concepts.

Transformative education is shaped by a range of theoretical frameworks that support learner engagement, critical reflection, identity development, and meaningful change. In nursing education, these theories provide the foundation for creating learning environments that go beyond knowledge transfer, encouraging students to challenge assumptions, develop insight, and respond compassionately to complex practice situations. This section explores the key theories that underpin transformative education, with a focus on those most relevant to nurse education. It includes seminal contributions such as Mezirow's transformative learning theory

and Freire's critical pedagogy, as well as adult learning, constructivism, and experiential learning.

TRANSFORMATIVE LEARNING THEORY (MEZIROW)

The concept of transformative learning was developed by Jack Mezirow (1991), whose seminal work examined how adults make meaning of their experiences. According to Mezirow, transformation occurs when learners critically reflect on their assumptions, leading to a shift in their frame of reference. This type of learning involves questioning established beliefs, engaging in rational discourse, and developing more inclusive and integrated perspectives.

In nursing education, this is highly relevant. Students frequently encounter emotionally charged situations, ethical dilemmas, and professional tensions. Mezirow's theory provides a structure through which these experiences can be examined and understood. Through guided reflection, dialogue, and critical engagement, students are supported to make sense of their roles and responsibilities in practice.

Mezirow distinguished between instrumental learning (focused on tasks and problem-solving) and communicative learning (focused on understanding others' perspectives and forming judgements). Both are necessary in nursing, but transformative learning is more aligned with the latter. It encourages practitioners to reflect not just on what they do, but why they do it and what it means in a broader social context.

CRITICAL PEDAGOGY (FREIRE)

Paulo Freire's work on education as a practice of freedom (1970) is another foundational influence. Freire criticised traditional models of education in which knowledge is 'deposited' into passive learners, a process he termed the 'banking model'. Instead, he advocated for dialogical education, where learners and teachers work in partnership to explore issues of power, justice, and meaning.

In nursing education, Freire's critical pedagogy can be used to empower students to question inequity in health systems, reflect on their position in care relationships, and explore their responsibilities as advocates. This aligns closely with the Nursing and Midwifery Council's (2018) emphasis on partnership working, person-centred care, and moral agency.

Critical pedagogy invites learners to become conscious of their social, cultural, and political contexts and to see themselves as agents of change. This is especially important in preparing nurses who work in diverse communities, often with limited resources or within systems marked by structural inequality.

ADULT LEARNING THEORY (KNOWLES)

Malcolm Knowles' adult learning theory, or andragogy, provides another key framework for transformative education. Knowles et al. (2015) described adult learners as self-directed, motivated by relevance, and capable of drawing on life experience to inform new learning. These assumptions underpin many features of contemporary nurse education, including portfolio-based assessment, experiential learning, and reflective practice.

Knowles highlighted six core principles of adult learning: the need to know, the learner's self-concept, prior experience, readiness to learn, orientation to learning, and motivation. These principles support the design of curricula that are practice-focused, personalised, and responsive to student goals.

In the nursing context, adult learning theory is particularly useful when working with mature students, career changers, and those entering nursing through apprenticeship or return-to-practice routes. It supports the idea that learners bring valuable insight to the classroom and should be treated as partners in their development.

EXPERIENTIAL LEARNING (KOLB)

David Kolb's experiential learning theory (1984) presents learning as a continuous cycle involving four stages: concrete experience, reflective observation, abstract conceptualisation, and active experimentation. This model underpins much of the reflective practice and simulation activity in nurse education.

In practice, a student might participate in a clinical experience (concrete experience), reflect on what happened and how they felt (reflective observation), draw conclusions or identify areas for improvement (abstract conceptualisation), and then apply their learning in a future situation (active experimentation). When facilitated well, this cycle deepens learning and builds confidence.

Simulation-based education, debriefing sessions, and critical incident analysis all draw on Kolb's model. They allow students to test ideas, develop insight, and prepare for real-world care delivery. The model supports the development of clinical reasoning and professional judgement, both of which are essential for safe practice.

CONSTRUCTIVISM

Constructivist theories view learning as an active, social process in which knowledge is constructed through interaction and reflection. Influenced by theorists such as Vygotsky and Piaget, constructivism sees the learner as central to meaning-making. Educators act as facilitators, helping learners to build understanding through engagement with ideas, peers, and real-world problems (Fosnot, 2013).

Constructivism underpins many modern teaching methods, including problem-based learning, enquiry-based learning, and case study approaches. These methods support the development of critical thinking and encourage students to apply concepts rather than memorise facts.

In nursing, constructivist pedagogy aligns with the emphasis on practice application, professional values, and collaborative learning. It supports students to connect theory and practice, consider multiple perspectives, and reflect on how knowledge is shaped by context.

COMMUNITIES OF PRACTICE (LAVE AND WENGER)

The theory of communities of practice, developed by Lave and Wenger (1991), emphasises the social nature of learning. According to this model, individuals learn by participating in shared activities and gradually moving from peripheral to full participation in a community. In nurse education, this is reflected in the journey from student to registered professional.

Communities of practice exist in clinical placements, interprofessional teams, and academic groups. Learning is shaped by interaction, mentorship, and shared goals. The concept helps explain how identity and competence are developed not just through instruction, but through meaningful engagement in professional life.

This theory supports the value of collaborative placement learning, peer learning groups, and longitudinal relationships with practice supervisors. It also highlights the need for inclusive and supportive learning environments that allow students to contribute and grow.

REFLECTIVE PRACTICE

Reflective practice is both a pedagogical strategy and a theoretical orientation in nurse education. The works of Schön (1983) and Gibbs (1988) have been particularly influential. Schön introduced the concept of reflection-in-action (thinking during the event) and reflection-on-action (thinking after the event), both of which are essential for professional learning.

Reflection enables students to process complex experiences, develop insight, and improve future performance. It is embedded in the Nursing and Midwifery Council's (2018) standards and widely used in assessment, portfolio development, and supervision.

While models such as Gibbs' reflective cycle are often used as frameworks, educators must ensure that reflection is meaningful and supported. Reflection should move beyond description and encourage critical engagement with values, power, and impact.

THRESHOLD CONCEPTS

Another useful framework is the theory of threshold concepts (Meyer & Land, 2003). These are core ideas that, once understood, transform perception of a subject. They are often difficult to grasp initially but result in significant shifts in understanding.

In nursing, threshold concepts might include person-centred care, evidence-based practice, or clinical reasoning. Teaching should anticipate these moments of transformation and support students through the discomfort and uncertainty that often precede insight. Threshold concepts are important in designing curricula that support deep and lasting learning.

EMOTIONAL INTELLIGENCE AND AFFECTIVE LEARNING

Transformative education also draws on ideas from emotional intelligence and affective learning theories. Goleman's (1995) work on emotional intelligence highlights the importance of self-awareness, empathy, and emotional regulation in professional practice. In nursing, these attributes support compassionate care, ethical decision-making, and team relationships.

Learning in the affective domain, feelings, attitudes, and values, requires intentional teaching. This might include structured reflection, values clarification exercises, or narrative pedagogy. These methods allow students to explore the emotional dimensions of nursing and develop the resilience needed for practice.

INTEGRATING THEORIES INTO PRACTICE

Nurse educators are tasked with drawing on these theories in ways that are relevant, inclusive, and aligned with professional standards. This means choosing methods that allow students to engage with uncertainty, explore their identities, and develop practical and ethical judgement. It also requires educators to develop their own skills in facilitation, supervision, and emotional support.

Transformative education is not tied to a single theory. Rather, it emerges from the integration of multiple perspectives that value criticality, connection, and change. Educators must be reflexive in their own practice, continually adapting approaches in response to learner needs, evidence, and evolving contexts. Table 1.2 summarises the key theoretical models that underpin transformative education and their core concepts, offering a concise reference for educators designing or evaluating nurse education programmes.

Table 1.2   Theoretical Frameworks in Transformative Nursing Education

Theory/model	Key concepts
Transformative Learning (Mezirow)	Critical reflection, perspective transformation, communicative learning
Critical Pedagogy (Freire)	Dialogue, empowerment, social justice, learner agency
Experiential Learning (Kolb)	Learning cycle: experience, reflection, conceptualisation, experimentation
Adult Learning Theory (Knowles)	Self-directed learning, readiness, relevance, motivation
Constructivism	Active construction of knowledge through experience and interaction
Communities of Practice (Lave & Wenger)	Situated learning, legitimate peripheral participation, identity formation
Reflective Practice (Schön)	Reflection-in-action and reflection-on-action for learning from experience
Emotional Intelligence (Goleman)	Self-awareness, emotional regulation, empathy in practice
Threshold Concepts (Meyer & Land)	Transformative ideas that change understanding and are often irreversible once grasped

ACTIVITY BOX

Title: *Mapping Your Teaching Philosophy: A Reflective Activity for Nurse Educators*

Activity

As an emerging nurse academic, consider the educational values and experiences that shape your teaching practice. Use the prompts below to develop or revise your personal teaching philosophy statement (around 300–400 words).

- What do I believe about how nursing students learn best?
- How do my experiences as a nurse inform the way I approach teaching?

- Which educational theories resonate most with my current or aspirational practice, and why?
- How do I aim to create inclusive, engaging, and transformative learning experiences?

Facilitator Note: This activity can be followed by peer dialogue, group discussion, or formative feedback to deepen self-awareness and link personal values to pedagogical frameworks.

REIMAGINING NURSING EDUCATION THROUGH TRANSFORMATION

Nursing education in the United Kingdom stands at a critical juncture. In the face of growing complexity in clinical practice, the evolving needs of diverse populations, rapid digital transformation, and the demand for moral and professional leadership, nurse educators must ensure that programmes are fit not only for present challenges but for an uncertain and changing future. This chapter has examined how transformative education offers a compelling and necessary response to these demands.

Transformative education represents more than a pedagogical approach, it is a philosophical stance that values reflection, critical consciousness, inclusivity, and personal and professional growth. It supports students to become active participants in their learning, encouraging

them to challenge assumptions, navigate ambiguity, and develop their own professional identities. At its core, transformative education prepares nurses not only to do things right, but to do the right things.

Figure 1.1 presents the Hill and Mitchell Model of Transformative Practice in Higher Education, a conceptual framework designed to support nurse academics as they navigate and develop their teaching identity. The model illustrates the integration of three foundational domains that shape transformative practice within higher education:

1. **Pedagogical Theory**

   This domain draws on established educational frameworks, including Mezirow's transformative learning, Freire's critical pedagogy, Kolb's experiential learning, and Knowles' adult learning theory. These

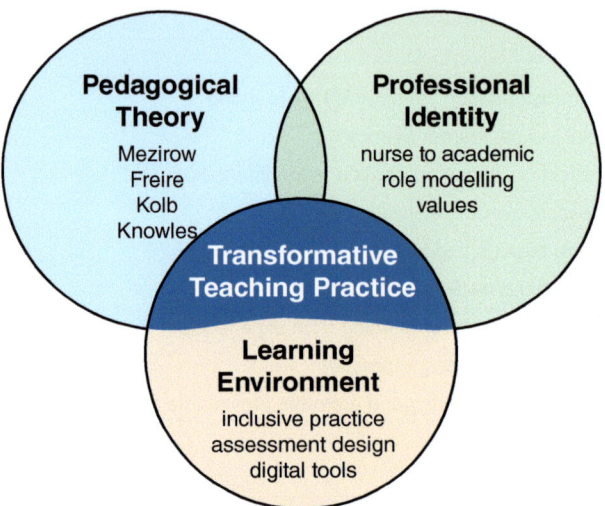

FIGURE 1.1 The Hill and Mitchell model of transformative practice in higher education

approaches offer the theoretical grounding needed to develop inclusive, reflective, and student-focused teaching practices in nurse education.

2. **Professional Identity**

    This domain recognises the diverse routes into academia taken by nurse educators, including those transitioning from clinical practice, research roles, leadership positions, or other areas of professional nursing. It encompasses the ongoing development of academic identity, informed by prior experience, values, and the evolving role of the nurse educator in higher education.

3. **Learning Environment**

    This domain addresses the design and facilitation of inclusive, psychologically safe, and digitally enhanced learning spaces. It includes assessment strategies, student engagement, and the use of educational technologies, all of which contribute to the conditions in which transformative learning can occur.

At the intersection of these three domains lies transformative teaching practice, the space where theory, identity, and context converge to support critical, adaptive, and relational approaches to education. This centre point reflects the aspiration for nurse academics to teach in ways that are not only informed and inclusive, but also reflexive and future-facing.

For nurses entering or progressing within academic roles, whether as educators, researchers, or clinical-academic hybrids, this model provides a framework for integrating educational theory, lived professional experience, and student-centred values into effective and personally meaningful teaching practice. It also acknowledges that transformation is not only a pedagogical goal, but a professional journey for the educators themselves.

CHAPTER SUMMARY

In exploring the context of transformative education, the chapter highlighted the importance of responding to health system pressures, regulatory expectations, and global agendas. The NHS Long Term Plan (NHS England, 2019) and NHS Long Term Workforce Plan (NHS England, 2023) both articulate a vision of a more adaptable, compassionate, and skilled workforce. The Nursing and Midwifery Council's (2018) standards echo these priorities, calling for reflective, person-centred professionals who can work in partnership and lead in practice.

Transformative education is ideally placed to meet these aims. It supports development not only of knowledge and skills, but of values, confidence, and identity. It places relationships, dialogue, and critical enquiry at the heart of learning and fosters the kind of resilient, reflective graduate the NHS and wider society now require.

The section on contemporary needs in nursing education examined the growing complexity of practice environments, including digital innovation, interprofessional working, and rising health inequalities. Students must be prepared to manage complexity, act with cultural humility, engage with evidence, and maintain emotional resilience. They must also be supported to transition into professional roles with clarity and confidence.

Transformative education addresses these needs by embedding inclusive pedagogy, experiential learning, and critical reflection into curriculum design. It ensures students are not only assessed on clinical competence, but also supported to make meaning of their experiences and to understand their wider responsibilities as practitioners in a publicly accountable profession.

The historical perspective provided important context for understanding the shifts that have shaped nursing education over the past century. From the apprenticeship models of the Nightingale era, through the reforms of the Briggs Report, to the university integration of Project 2000, the evolution of nursing education reflects broader societal changes in how the profession is understood and valued. Each reform was, in its own way, a step towards transformation, moving from obedience to autonomy, from doing to knowing, and now towards questioning and leading.

This history also reveals enduring tensions: the balance between academic learning and clinical immersion, the value of tacit knowledge alongside evidence-based practice, and the challenge of keeping education aligned with workforce realities. Understanding these tensions helps educators remain grounded and strategic as they continue to innovate.

Finally, the chapter explored the theories that underpin transformative education. Mezirow's (1991) transformative learning theory, Freire's (1970) critical pedagogy, and Kolb's (1984) experiential learning model offer robust and well-established foundations. Constructivism, adult learning theory, and the concept of communities of practice provide further frameworks to support curriculum design, teaching methods, and assessment strategies. These theories promote reflective, relational, and socially aware learning. They also remind educators of the emotional and moral dimensions of nursing, which cannot be reduced to competencies or learning outcomes alone.

The theoretical landscape supports an integrated, dialogical, and inclusive vision of nurse education. It also encourages educators to adopt a critical lens—on power, privilege, and systems, and to create space for students to do the same.

IMPLICATIONS FOR PRACTICE

The implications of this chapter are clear. If the aim of nursing education is to develop practitioners who are safe, effective, and ethical, then transformation must be built into every aspect of the educational experience. This includes:

- Programmes should go beyond technical knowledge to include ethics, equity, leadership, and digital literacy. Global and environmental issues should be incorporated as part of preparing nurses for the future.

- Methods should encourage dialogue, critical enquiry, and reflection. Simulation, case-based learning, flipped classrooms, and co-created learning materials can all support deeper engagement.

- Tools should measure not only what students know, but how they apply that knowledge, how they reflect on their actions, and how they make decisions. Portfolios, reflective accounts, and viva-based assessments may be used to support this.

- Clinical settings should be viewed as spaces for learning, not just service delivery. Students should be encouraged to reflect, question, and be supported by educators who understand the value of guided transformation.

- Academics and Clinical Educators themselves must be supported to understand and apply transformative principles. This includes developing skills in facilitation, supervision, and inclusive practice.

It also requires institutional commitment to inclusivity, student well-being, and valuing education as a process of personal development, not just professional qualification.

CHALLENGES AND CONSIDERATIONS

Implementing a transformative approach is not without challenges. Curriculum overcrowding, workforce shortages, and performance-driven metrics can limit opportunities for critical and reflective learning. Educators may face pressure to prioritise efficiency over engagement. Moreover, students may need support in developing the emotional and intellectual maturity required for transformation.

Despite these pressures, the argument remains that a transactional, competency-only approach to nurse education is no longer sufficient. The context of modern healthcare demands practitioners who are flexible, questioning, and aware of their values and impact. The challenge for educators is to hold space for this kind of development, despite constraints, and to advocate for the time, resources, and pedagogical freedom required to do so.

TAKE-HOME POINTS

1. Transformative education is essential for preparing nurses who can think critically, lead ethically, and adapt to the complexities of modern healthcare. It moves beyond technical skill acquisition and focuses on identity, values, and professional judgement.

2. Nursing education is shaped by a unique interplay of historical evolution, regulatory standards, and workforce expectations. Understanding this context is crucial for developing curricula that are relevant, inclusive, and contemporary.

3. A range of educational theories, such as Mezirow's transformative learning, Kolb's experiential learning, and Freire's critical pedagogy, provide a strong foundation for curriculum design and reflective teaching practice. These models support learners in becoming engaged, resilient, and socially aware professionals.

CPD REFLECTIVE QUESTIONS

1. How does my current approach to teaching or supervision create opportunities for students to reflect critically on their assumptions and values?

2. In what ways do I actively consider student diversity, lived experience, and emotional development when designing or delivering learning activities?

3. How can I better integrate the principles of transformative education into assessment, feedback, or placement support within my educational or clinical role?

REFERENCES

Council of Deans of Health. (2016). *Educating the future nurse: a paper for discussion*. London: Council of Deans of Health. https://www.councilofdeans.org.uk/wp-content/uploads/2016/08/Educating-the-Future-Nurse-FINAL-1.pdf?utm_source=chatgpt.com. Accessed: (9 December 2025).

Department of Health and Social Security (1972). *Report of the Committee on Nursing (Briggs Report)*. London: HMSO.

Fosnot, C. T. (2013). *Constructivism: Theory, Perspectives, and Practice* (2nd ed.). Teachers College Press.

Freire, P. (1970). *Pedagogy of the Oppressed*. New York: Herder and Herder.

Gibbs, G. (1988). *Learning by Doing: A Guide to Teaching and Learning Methods*. Oxford: Oxford Polytechnic.

Goleman, D. (1995). *Emotional Intelligence: Why It Can Matter More than IQ*. New York: Bantam Books.

Health Education England. (2017). *Multi-professional framework for advanced clinical practice in England*. https://www.hee.nhs.uk/sites/default/files/documents/multi-professionalframeworkforadvanced-clinicalpracticeinengland.pdf. Accessed: (9 December 2025).

Hochschild, A. R. (1983). *The Managed Heart: Commercialisation of Human Feeling*. Berkeley: University of California Press.

Knowles, M. S., Holton, E. F., & Swanson, R. A. (2015). *The Adult Learner: The Definitive Classic in Adult Education and Human Resource Development* (8th ed.). Routledge.

Kolb, D. A. (1984). *Experiential Learning: Experience as the Source of Learning and Development*. Englewood Cliffs, NJ: Prentice Hall.

Lave, J., & Wenger, E. (1991). *Situated Learning: Legitimate Peripheral Participation*. Cambridge University Press.

McDonald, L. (2010). *Florence Nightingale at First Hand: Vision, Power, Legacy*. London: Continuum.

McEwen, M., & Wills, E. M. (2023). *Theoretical Basis for Nursing* (6th ed.). Wolters Kluwer.

Meyer, J. H. F., & Land, R. (2003). Threshold concepts and troublesome knowledge: Linkages to ways of thinking and practising. In C. Rust (Ed.), *Improving Student Learning – Ten Years On* (pp. 412–424). Oxford Centre for Staff and Learning Development.

Mezirow, J. (1991). *Transformative Dimensions of Adult Learning*. San Francisco: Jossey-Bass.

NHS England (2019). *The NHS long term plan*. https://www.kingsfund.org.uk/insight-and-analysis/blogs/the-nhs-long-term-plan-2019-five-things. Accessed: (9 December 2025).

NHS England (2023). *NHS long term workforce plan*. https://www.england.nhs.uk/publication/nhs-long-term-workforce-plan/. Accessed: (9 December 2025).

Nursing and Midwifery Council (2018). *Future nurse: standards of proficiency for registered nurses*. https://www.nmc.org.uk

Quality Assurance Agency for Higher Education (2022). *Subject benchmark statement: Nursing*. https://www.qaa.ac.uk

Schön, D. A. (1983). *The Reflective Practitioner: How Professionals Think in Action*. Basic Books.

Taylor, C. (2017). Learning to be a nurse: constructing professional identity in nurse education. *International Journal of Nursing Education Scholarship*, 14(1), 1–10. https://doi.org/10.1515/ijnes-2016-0029.

Thomas, L. (2022). *Belonging in Higher Education: Policy and Practice*. Higher Education Policy Institute.

Topol, E. (2019). *Preparing the healthcare workforce to deliver the digital future: the Topol review*. NHS Health Education England. https://www.hee.nhs.uk/sites/default/files/documents/Topol%20Review%20interim%20report_0.pdf. Accessed: (9 December 2025).

UK Central Council for Nursing, Midwifery and Health Visiting (1986). *Project 2000: A New Preparation for Practice*. London: UKCC.

World Health Organization (2010). *Framework for action on interprofessional education and collaborative practice*. https://www.who.int/publications/i/item/framework-for-action-on-interprofessional-education-collaborative-practice. Accessed: (9 December 2025).

Critical Thinking and Reflective Practice

CHAPTER 2

Amsale Wamburu[1] and Barry Hill[2]

[1] *College of Health and Society, Buckinghamshire New University, UK*
[2] *School of Healthcare and Nursing Sciences (HNS), Faculty of Health and Wellbeing, Northumbria University, UK*

AIM

To explore the interrelationship between critical thinking and reflective practice in nursing, highlighting their role in professional judgement, decision-making, and clinical reasoning within person-centred care.

LEARNING OUTCOMES

By the end of this chapter, readers will be able to:

1. Define critical thinking and explain its role in effective nursing practice.

2. Evaluate models of reflective practice and how they enhance clinical decision-making.

3. Apply reflective tools to analyse real-life clinical situations.

4. Integrate critical thinking and reflective strategies into personal and professional development.

CHAPTER INTRODUCTION

Nursing practice is complex, requiring the ability to interpret dynamic clinical data, assess patient needs, prioritise interventions, and evaluate outcomes—all while maintaining empathy and professional accountability. To navigate these demands, nurses must engage in both critical thinking and reflective practice. These two concepts, while distinct, are interconnected and mutually reinforcing. Critical thinking allows nurses to question assumptions, evaluate evidence, and reach sound clinical decisions, while reflective practice encourages continual learning from experience. Together, they promote safe, ethical, and person-centred care. This chapter explores how critical thinking and reflection contribute to the development of autonomous, competent nursing professionals capable of responding to the evolving needs of healthcare systems.

THE IMPORTANCE OF CRITICAL THINKING IN NURSING

Critical thinking is the cognitive process that enables nurses to interpret information, make clinical judgments, and solve problems in real time. Facione (1990) defines critical thinking as 'purposeful, self-regulatory judgment which results in interpretation, analysis, evaluation, and inference'. In nursing, this translates into the ability to assess complex clinical presentations, weigh options, and act in the patient's best interest.

The Nursing and Midwifery Council (NMC, 2018) emphasises the importance of critical thinking in the standards for proficiency for registered nurses, noting that nurses must use evidence-based reasoning to assess and manage risk while providing safe, person-centred care. In a landscape of increasing acuity and patient complexity, critical thinking is essential to ensure sound clinical reasoning and avoid errors.

CHARACTERISTICS OF CRITICAL THINKERS IN NURSING

According to Alfaro-LeFevre (2020), critical thinking in nursing includes intellectual traits such as (Table 2.1).

These intellectual traits form the foundation of effective critical thinking in nursing, enabling practitioners to respond thoughtfully and safely in complex and unpredictable environments. Their application extends beyond theoretical constructs into the realities of clinical care, where nurses must often make rapid decisions with incomplete information, under time pressure, and within ethically charged contexts.

APPLYING TRAITS IN CLINICAL PRACTICE

Curiosity drives inquiry and a desire to understand the 'why' behind clinical presentations, guidelines, and patient behaviours. A curious nurse may question why a patient is not responding to a treatment as expected, prompting a review of medication interactions or alternative diagnoses. This mindset fosters a culture of continual learning and guards against complacency.

Open-mindedness ensures nurses consider the values, beliefs, and preferences of each patient, particularly in culturally diverse care settings. For example, when managing a patient who declines a certain intervention on religious grounds, the open-minded nurse seeks to understand and explore acceptable alternatives rather than dismissing the patient's concerns.

Analytical thinking enables nurses to deconstruct complex clinical situations into manageable components. In a patient with multiple comorbidities presenting with non-specific symptoms, the ability to logically process assessment findings, laboratory data, and patient history is essential for identifying priorities and planning safe care.

Systematic thinking supports consistency and thoroughness in nursing assessment and care delivery. Nurses who follow structured approaches—such as the ABCDE method in acute care or SBAR in communication—are more likely to identify deteriorating patients early and ensure critical information is conveyed accurately to the wider team.

Self-reflection plays a critical role in evaluating personal biases, emotional responses, and habitual ways of thinking. A reflective nurse who recognises they responded abruptly to a patient's question due to stress or fatigue is more likely to seek support, adapt their approach, and learn from the encounter. This trait is also foundational to professional integrity and accountability.

SUPPORTING STUDENTS TO DEVELOP CRITICAL THINKING TRAITS

In nurse education, these traits should be explicitly introduced and embedded throughout the curriculum. Educators can foster their development through:

- **Clinical questioning** that prompts analysis and reflection: 'What assumptions are we making about this patient's condition'?

- **Scenario-based learning** that challenges students to apply systematic reasoning and defend their decisions.

- **Debrief sessions** that create space for self-reflection and peer discussion about differing perspectives and clinical reasoning.

- **Journalling and portfolios** that encourage students to explore how their thinking evolves across placements and in response to feedback.

Table 2.1 Characteristics of Critical Thinkers in Nursing

Trait	Description
Curiosity	A desire to learn more, ask questions, and explore alternatives
Open-mindedness	Willingness to consider different perspectives without bias
Analytical Thinking	Ability to break down complex information logically and identify patterns
Systematic Thinking	Approaching problems in a methodical, organised way
Self-reflection	Recognising one's own assumptions and how they influence decisions

Furthermore, assessment strategies should move beyond content recall to evaluate students' reasoning processes, openness to multiple perspectives, and ability to integrate theory with practice. This ensures that learners are not only knowledgeable but also capable of adapting, analysing, and reflecting on the realities of care delivery.

Ultimately, critical thinking traits are not static qualities but develop through experience, reflection, and educational support. By intentionally nurturing these capacities, nurse educators help students become thoughtful, adaptable, and ethically grounded practitioners—essential qualities for delivering safe and person-centred care.

CLINICAL REASONING AND JUDGEMENT

Tanner's (2006) Clinical Judgement Model provides a useful framework for understanding how critical thinking is operationalised in practice. It includes four stages:

1. **Noticing**—Recognising signs and symptoms.

2. **Interpreting**—Making sense of the data.

3. **Responding**—Implementing interventions.

4. **Reflecting**—Evaluating the effectiveness of actions.

In this model, critical thinking underpins each phase, enabling nurses to draw from their experience, apply theoretical knowledge, and act decisively. For example, recognising subtle cues of sepsis in an older adult requires the nurse to notice deviations from baseline, interpret clinical signs, and respond with urgency, all of which require analytical and evaluative thinking.

RELEVANCE TO EVIDENCE-BASED PRACTICE

Critical thinking is essential to implementing evidence-based practice (EBP). Nurses must appraise research, consider its relevance, and determine its applicability to specific patients.

This critical appraisal process ensures that care is grounded in the best available evidence, tailored to the patient's needs and preferences (Melnyk & Fineout-Overholt, 2019).

STRATEGIES FOR DEVELOPING REFLECTIVE PRACTICE

Reflective practice is widely recognised as a fundamental component of professional nursing development, underpinning safe and effective care. As Schön (1983) described in his seminal work, reflective practice bridges the gap between theory and practice by encouraging practitioners to

examine their experiences critically and constructively. Developing reflective capacity in student nurses involves more than encouraging journal writing or portfolio compilation; it requires a deliberate pedagogical approach supported by theory, feedback, and practice.

INTRODUCING REFLECTION IN NURSE EDUCATION

Reflection should be introduced early in pre-registration programmes to encourage habitual critical thinking and personal insight. Structured sessions using real-life scenarios, peer discussions, and case-based learning allow students to explore clinical decision-making in a supported environment. Introducing reflective frameworks (Table 2.2) such as Gibbs' Reflective Cycle (1988), Johns' Model for Structured

Reflection (1995), or Rolfe's Reflective Model (2001) can guide students through structured reflection.

When embedding reflection, educators should clarify that the goal is not just a description of events, but a critical engagement with them. This includes recognising biases, evaluating actions, understanding ethical dilemmas, and considering alternative responses (Moon, 2004).

Table 2.2 Summary of Common Reflective Models in Nursing

Model	Key components	Strengths
Gibbs (1988)	Description, Feelings, Evaluation, Analysis, Conclusion, Action Plan	Widely used, easy to apply, encourages emotional awareness
Johns (1995)	Based on Carper's ways of knowing: Empirical, Aesthetic, Personal, Ethical	Deeply analytical, suitable for complex practice situations
Rolfe et al. (2001)	What? So what? Now what?	Simple and versatile, useful in time-limited settings

Title: *Exploring the Educator's Lens: Critical Thinking or Reflective Practice?*

Activity

In pairs or small groups, explore and compare the concepts of critical thinking and reflective practice in your own teaching experience. Use the prompts below:

- Which approach do you feel more confident applying: critical thinking or reflective practice? Why?

- Can you think of a recent teaching or marking experience where you used one or both?

- Are these approaches always complementary, or can they pull in different directions?

Extension

Write a short (250 word) reflective commentary on how you might more intentionally integrate both approaches into a specific element of your teaching, such as feedback, facilitation, or assessment.

CREATING A SAFE REFLECTIVE ENVIRONMENT

Psychological safety is critical when encouraging reflection, particularly when discussing challenging or emotional experiences. Learners must feel confident that their insights and vulnerabilities will not be judged harshly. Facilitators can foster this by modelling reflective thinking themselves, responding supportively to learners' disclosures, and allowing time for reflection without forcing immediate answers (Levett-Jones et al., 2009).

Simulation-based education provides a powerful opportunity for reflective learning. Following a simulation exercise, structured debriefs using models such as PEARLS (Cheng et al., 2016) can be used to support reflection-in-action and reflection-on-action. These sessions not only help learners make sense of their performance but also help them build confidence and resilience for future practice.

ENCOURAGING REFLECTIVE DIALOGUE

Reflective dialogue can be a highly effective method for enhancing critical thinking, particularly when facilitated in group settings such as seminars, skills debriefs, or interprofessional learning activities. Dialogues can include peer feedback, Socratic questioning, or guided reflection prompts, helping students explore multiple perspectives and navigate uncertainty. This approach aligns with Vygotsky's (1978) social constructivist theory, which emphasises the importance of social interaction in cognitive development.

Supervised reflection in clinical practice, supported by practice assessors, supervisors, or academic link lecturers, further reinforces classroom-based learning. These opportunities are vital in supporting learners to make sense of emotionally charged or ethically complex scenarios encountered during placement.

INTEGRATING REFLECTIVE WRITING

Reflective writing is a common strategy to foster critical thinking, but it must be supported with clear expectations and feedback. Students should be guided to move beyond descriptive accounts toward analytical and evaluative reflections. Educators can use annotated exemplars, feedback rubrics, and scaffolded writing activities to gradually build students' confidence and capability.

Technology-enhanced learning can also support reflection. E-portfolios, digital journals, or video reflections enable students to document experiences and receive feedback. Some universities incorporate structured tools such as PebblePad or Mahara to facilitate this. Using audio-visual reflection (e.g. recording a summary of key learning points after simulation) can be particularly effective for learners who struggle with written expression.

ALIGNING REFLECTION WITH ASSESSMENT

Assessment of reflective practice remains contentious, as grading a student's introspective process can risk inauthentic responses. However, assessment can focus on the demonstration of reflective thinking rather than the personal content itself. Rubrics can assess critical thinking, ethical awareness, evidence of development, and application of theory to practice (Table 2.3).

It is essential to ensure that students understand the criteria and purpose of reflection-related assessments and that reflection is not treated as a mere tick-box exercise. Embedding reflective activities throughout a programme in both formative and summative forms helps reinforce its importance in professional practice.

Table 2.3 Sample Reflective Assessment Rubric

Criterion	Developing	Proficient	Advanced
Describes experience	Lists basic facts	Includes context and personal response	Critically engages with complex details
Analyses situation	Limited interpretation	Demonstrates awareness of issues	Demonstrates multiple perspectives
Links to theory	Rarely references theory	Applies theory appropriately	Integrates theory with insight
Action planning	No future plan	General ideas for improvement	Clear, specific, and feasible actions

SUPPORTING NOVICE REFLECTORS

First-year students may struggle to engage with reflection, especially if they are unfamiliar with nursing culture or lack clinical exposure. Support should include:

- Introducing reflection through discussion and story-telling before written tasks

- Providing sentence starters or reflective prompts

- Encouraging personal journaling without assessment

- Using peer-supported reflection circles

As confidence grows, more structured activities can be introduced, such as case discussions using ethical frameworks, critical incident analysis, or debriefs following placements. Reflective skills can be tracked through learning contracts, supervision meetings, and personal development plans.

THE ROLE OF EDUCATORS AND PRACTICE PARTNERS

Educators must model reflective practice themselves, demonstrating openness to feedback and willingness to learn from their own experiences. This modelling helps normalise reflection and reinforces its value. Practice assessors and supervisors should be prepared to support learners' reflection in placements, using coaching strategies and collaborative goal-setting.

Academic institutions can support this by providing training in reflective facilitation for staff, creating structured placement activities, and embedding reflection in curriculum documentation. Engaging with learners regularly about their reflective progress fosters a culture of self-awareness and professional growth.

THE IMPORTANCE OF CRITICAL THINKING IN NURSING

In the dynamic and unpredictable environment of healthcare, critical thinking is not a luxury; it is a necessity. Nurses must synthesise complex information, recognise deteriorating conditions, advocate for patients, and make evidence-informed decisions, often under time pressure. Critical thinking supports nurses in avoiding errors, anticipating complications, and delivering safe and ethical care. It is foundational to clinical judgement, problem-solving, and professional accountability (Benner et al., 2010).

DEFINING CRITICAL THINKING

Critical thinking in nursing refers to the ability to think in a systematic and logical manner, while remaining open to questioning and reflecting on the reasoning process used to ensure safe nursing practice and quality care (Facione, 2011). It involves cognitive skills such as interpretation, analysis, evaluation, inference, explanation, and self-regulation. Paul

and Elder (2006) further argue that critical thinking is based on universal intellectual values such as clarity, accuracy, precision, relevance, depth, breadth, and fairness.

In nursing, critical thinking is embedded in daily tasks—from prioritising care to interpreting diagnostic results and evaluating treatment options. Importantly, it also includes ethical reasoning, cultural sensitivity, and emotional intelligence (Alfaro-LeFevre, 2019).

CHARACTERISTICS OF A CRITICAL THINKER

Critical thinkers in nursing typically exhibit the following characteristics:

- **Inquisitiveness:** They are curious and seek to understand rather than accept things at face value.

- **Systematic Thinking:** They follow a logical, step-by-step approach to decision-making.

- **Open-Mindedness:** They consider a range of perspectives and recognise their own biases.
- **Analytical Thinking:** They can break down complex information into smaller components.

- **Confidence in Reasoning:** They trust evidence and logic to guide their conclusions.
- **Reflectiveness:** They learn from experiences and evaluate outcomes for improvement.

EMBEDDING CRITICAL THINKING IN CURRICULA

To foster critical thinking, nurse educators must go beyond content delivery and instead focus on developing reasoning skills. Strategies include (Table 2.4):

- **Problem-based Learning (PBL):** Students are presented with a clinical scenario and must identify the problem, research evidence, and propose a solution collaboratively.
- **Case-based Discussions:** Real or simulated patient cases are used to promote application of theory to practice.

- **Concept Mapping:** Students visually link clinical signs, diagnostics, and interventions to support reasoning.
- **Debates and Ethical Dilemmas:** Exploring complex moral issues develops reasoning and argumentation skills.
- **Clinical Questioning:** The use of open-ended and Socratic questioning during skill sessions or placements can stimulate deeper thinking.

CRITICAL THINKING IN CLINICAL PRACTICE

In clinical settings, the application of critical thinking is particularly important. Nurses must assess patients holistically, anticipate risks, and make judgements that may have life-altering implications. The NMC (2018) Future Nurse Standards explicitly include critical thinking as a key requirement, stating that nurses must 'demonstrate the ability to think critically when applying knowledge and evidence to make decisions'.

Critical thinking is developed over time through exposure to increasingly complex clinical situations. Benner's (1984) Novice to Expert model highlights how critical thinking evolves through clinical experience. Novices may rely heavily on rules and guidelines, while experts use intuition shaped by deep contextual understanding.

DEVELOPING CLINICAL REASONING

Critical thinking and clinical reasoning are closely linked but not identical (Table 2.5). Clinical reasoning refers to the cognitive processes used to assess a clinical situation, interpret data, make diagnoses, and decide on interventions

(Levett-Jones et al., 2010). Educators can support its development through strategies such as:

- **Think-Alouds:** Encouraging students to verbalise their thought process during tasks.
- **Reflection-on-Action:** Reviewing decisions made during simulations or clinical practice.
- **Decision Trees:** Helping students structure their thinking around key signs and decision points.

SUPPORTING EDUCATORS AND PRACTICE PARTNERS

Educators and clinical supervisors must be supported to model and scaffold critical thinking. This includes:

- Training in questioning techniques and feedback strategies
- Using structured observation tools to assess thinking
- Building critical thinking into supervision forms and assessment criteria

Table 2.4   Sample Socratic Questions for Nursing Students

Focus area	Example question
Clarification	What do you mean by that? Can you give me an example?
Assumptions	What are you assuming here? Why do you think that is true?
Evidence	What evidence supports this? Is there any contradictory evidence?
Implications	What might happen if we take this course of action? What are the consequences?
Alternatives	What else could we consider? What are the pros and cons of another approach?

Table 2.5   Comparing Critical Thinking and Clinical Reasoning

Aspect	Critical thinking	Clinical reasoning
Focus	Broad, includes logic, ethics, and judgement	Patient-focused decision-making
Application	Across learning, ethical, and clinical areas	Clinical assessment and planning
Outcome	Reasoned judgement	Clinical decisions and action planning

Interprofessional learning also plays a key role, as it encourages students to consider alternative perspectives and challenge their own thinking. Simulation-based education provides safe spaces for testing decisions, experiencing complexity, and debriefing rationales.

INTEGRATING CRITICAL THINKING AND REFLECTION INTO PROFESSIONAL IDENTITY AND PERSON-CENTRED CARE

The development of critical thinking and reflective practice in nursing is not an isolated academic exercise but a core part of professional identity formation. Both are essential in cultivating nurses who are not only clinically competent but also self-aware, ethically grounded, and person-centred in their approach. This section explores how the integration of these capabilities supports nurses' professional growth, enhances person-centred care, and aligns with regulatory expectations across the UK healthcare landscape.

CRITICAL THINKING AND REFLECTIVE PRACTICE AS FOUNDATIONS OF PROFESSIONAL IDENTITY

Professional identity in nursing is shaped through a combination of education, clinical experience, personal values, and socialisation into the profession. Critical thinking and reflective practice underpin this development, offering tools for nurses to evaluate their actions, understand their decisions, and construct meaning from practice experiences.

The formation of a strong professional identity enables nurses to internalise professional standards, navigate complex ethical situations, and adapt to the demands of multi-disciplinary teams. Reflection allows nurses to question their assumptions, understand their responses to challenging scenarios, and align their practice with core nursing values such as compassion, respect, and dignity.

Through critical thinking, nurses gain the capacity to interrogate evidence, resist ritualistic practice, and ensure that their interventions are not only technically proficient but also appropriate for everyone. This process is essential in building confidence and autonomy, especially in early-career practitioners transitioning from the 'student' to the 'registered nurse' identity.

ENHANCING PERSON-CENTRED CARE THROUGH REFLECTIVE THINKING

Person-centred care is a core principle of nursing, endorsed by the NMC (2018) and central to policy frameworks such as the NHS Long Term Plan. It requires a commitment to recognising the person behind the diagnosis and tailoring care to their unique preferences, values, and lived experiences.

Critical thinking ensures that person-centred care is not reduced to a set of standardised gestures, but remains responsive, respectful, and informed. For instance, a nurse critically appraising a discharge plan must evaluate not only the clinical stability of the patient but also their social circumstances, understanding of medications, and access to follow-up care. Reflective practice further supports this by enabling nurses to learn from prior interactions, consider their communication styles, and evaluate whether care truly met the patient's needs.

Reflecting on interactions, both successful and challenging, allows nurses to explore how their own beliefs, emotions, and cultural backgrounds influence care delivery. This is particularly important in culturally diverse healthcare settings where sensitivity, adaptability, and humility are key components of equitable care (Papadopoulos, 2021).

CASE STUDY: REFLECTIVE PRACTICE IN END-OF-LIFE DECISION-MAKING

A newly qualified nurse, Amira, is caring for an older patient with advanced chronic obstructive pulmonary disease (COPD) who has been admitted multiple times over the past year. During handover, it is suggested that the patient be referred for a palliative care review, but Amira feels uncertain, shouldn't everything be done to prolong life?

After the shift, she reflects using Rolfe's model:

- **What?** The patient expressed exhaustion and a wish not to return to hospital again. Amira felt conflicted.

- **So what?** She recognised her instinct to focus on cure rather than comfort and questioned whether she truly heard the patient's perspective.

- **Now what?** She plans to explore palliative approaches and engage in conversations with her mentor about end-of-life care preferences.

This reflective process allows Amira to challenge assumptions, realign her actions with the patient's values, and grow her understanding of holistic care. In this way, reflection complements critical thinking by embedding empathy, self-awareness, and ethical reasoning into decision-making.

ALIGNMENT WITH NMC STANDARDS AND REGULATORY EXPECTATIONS

The NMC's Future Nurse Standards (2018) position critical thinking and reflection as key proficiencies for safe and effective practice. Specific domains, such as Domain 1: Being an accountable professional, and Domain 3: Assessing needs and planning care, require the application of sound judgement, evidence appraisal, and learning from experience.

Additionally, reflective practice is central to the NMC's revalidation process. Nurses are required to maintain a record of reflective accounts that demonstrate how they have met the Code's four themes: prioritise people, practise effectively, preserve safety, and promote professionalism and trust. These accounts must be discussed with a professional colleague, embedding reflection as a shared, dialogical process rather than a private activity.

Educators must prepare students for these professional expectations by embedding critical reflection into both academic and clinical learning. For example, formative reflection tasks can be aligned with the four pillars of the NMC Code (Table 2.6), helping students to see how their experiences contribute to professional development and public accountability.

PROMOTING PSYCHOLOGICAL SAFETY IN CLINICAL LEARNING ENVIRONMENTS

Critical thinking thrives in environments where learners are encouraged to question, challenge, and explore uncertainty. In clinical placements, however, students may hesitate to speak up due to hierarchical structures, fear of judgement, or a perceived expectation to conform.

Promoting psychological safety, defined by Edmondson (1999) as a climate in which people feel safe to take interpersonal risks, is essential to nurturing both criticality and reflection. Educators and clinical partners must consciously create space for students to share concerns, explore doubts, and reflect without fear of punitive responses. Approaches include:

- Encouraging debriefs after difficult situations.

- Modelling vulnerability and openness by educators and supervisors.

- Framing mistakes as learning opportunities rather than personal failings.

Creating this environment is a collective responsibility, with benefits extending to better teamwork, reduced errors, and improved patient outcomes (NHS Improvement, 2019).

SUPPORTING TRANSITION TO REGISTERED PRACTICE THROUGH CRITICAL REFLECTION

The transition from student to registered nurse is marked by increased responsibility, complex decision-making, and emotional adjustment. Reflection and critical thinking play a crucial role in supporting this transition, helping new registrants process their experiences, identify knowledge gaps, and develop resilience.

Structured transition programmes, such as preceptorship schemes, can embed reflective sessions where nurses analyse key clinical encounters, review their decision-making processes, and link learning to future practice. Using a consistent model (e.g. Gibbs or Johns) provides a common language across the preceptorship experience.

Table 2.6 Linking Reflection and Critical Thinking to NMC Code Domains

NMC code domain	Reflective prompt example
Prioritise people	Did my care reflect the person's wishes and dignity?
Practise effectively	How did I use evidence to guide my decision?
Preserve safety	What risks did I identify, and how did I respond?
Promote professionalism and trust	How did I represent nursing values in this situation?

Mentors and preceptors can also model critical questioning, prompting reflection through discussions such as:

- 'What evidence supported that intervention'?
- 'What other actions could you have taken'?
- 'How might your values have influenced your response'?

These questions reinforce reflection-in-action, helping new nurses internalise clinical reasoning patterns that will sustain their growth across the career trajectory.

EMBEDDING INTERPROFESSIONAL PERSPECTIVES IN CRITICAL REFLECTION

Modern nursing practice occurs in diverse teams comprising doctors, physiotherapists, social workers, pharmacists, and others. Reflecting across disciplinary boundaries can strengthen critical thinking by exposing students to varied approaches and values.

For instance, a debrief following a multi-agency safeguarding meeting could prompt reflection on:

- Differing interpretations of risk.
- Ethical tensions between autonomy and protection.
- Communication styles across professions.

Interprofessional education (IPE) should include joint simulation activities, collaborative case reviews, and shared reflective writing tasks. These foster mutual understanding and prepare nurses for complex team-based decision-making in practice.

TEACHING AND ASSESSING CRITICAL THINKING AND REFLECTIVE PRACTICE IN NURSE EDUCATION

INTRODUCTION

For educators delivering pre-registration nursing programmes or clinical education, developing learners' critical thinking and reflective practice is a central goal. These capabilities do not develop in isolation; they require intentional, scaffolded teaching and a supportive environment where reasoning, reflection, and self-awareness are regularly practised. This section provides practical, evidence-informed strategies for educators to embed critical thinking and reflection across the curriculum, aligned with the NMC (2018) standards and the expectations of academic teaching at Levels 6 and 7.

PEDAGOGICAL APPROACHES TO TEACHING CRITICAL THINKING

Teaching critical thinking involves more than encouraging students to 'think critically'; it requires structuring learning to challenge assumptions, promote analysis, and encourage evidence-informed decisions. The following approaches support this.

Problem-based Learning

Problem-based learning (PBL) places students in complex, often ambiguous clinical scenarios requiring collaborative reasoning and evidence appraisal. The facilitator's role is not to provide answers, but to guide learners in identifying what they know, what they need to learn, and how to apply knowledge in context (Barrows, 1986). PBL develops not only critical thinking but also self-direction, teamwork, and clinical confidence.

Case-based Learning

Case-based learning (CBL) uses real or simulated cases to encourage application of theory to practice. It is especially effective when linked to learning outcomes related to clinical reasoning, decision-making, and risk management. Educators should include prompts such as 'What is the priority here'?, 'What else should you consider'?, and 'What are the ethical implications'?

Concept Mapping

Concept mapping encourages students to visually link patient signs, nursing assessments, interventions, and rationales. This helps in organising knowledge hierarchically and making reasoning visible. When used during skills sessions or after simulations, it promotes diagnostic reasoning and care planning.

Socratic Questioning and Dialogic Teaching

Using Socratic questioning in teaching prompts students to interrogate their assumptions and consider multiple perspectives (Table 2.7). This approach requires planning and practice by the educator and is particularly effective during seminar discussions, simulation debriefs, and interprofessional learning sessions. It also helps scaffold students' academic writing, especially in constructing arguments or justifying clinical decisions.

Table 2.7 Sample Questions to Promote Critical Thinking During Teaching

Type of question	Example
Clarifying thinking	'Can you explain that idea further?'
Challenging assumptions	'What are you basing that on?'
Exploring evidence	'What sources support this view?'
Considering alternatives	'What might be another way to approach this situation?'
Reflecting on impact	'What might the consequence be for the patient or family?'

TEACHING REFLECTIVE PRACTICE: INTENTIONAL SCAFFOLDING

While reflection is often introduced in pre-registration programmes, the depth and quality of student reflection vary greatly. This variability often results from a lack of scaffolding and unclear expectations. To address this, educators should adopt a developmental approach to teaching reflection.

Stepwise Progression of Reflective Tasks

1. **Initial Familiarisation**: Begin with storytelling, discussion, and shared narratives to help students understand what reflection is and why it matters.

2. **Model Use of Frameworks**: Introduce simple models such as Rolfe's (2001) before progressing to more analytical frameworks like Johns' (1995).

3. **Link Reflection to Real-time Practice**: Encourage reflection-on-action during placement debriefs and reflection-in-action during simulations.

4. **Provide Scaffolded Writing Support**: Use exemplars, reflective prompts, and structured templates. Avoid assuming that students inherently know how to reflect critically.

ROLE OF FEEDBACK IN DEVELOPING REFLECTIVE SKILLS

Constructive feedback is essential to deepen reflective ability. Educators should avoid simply commenting on whether reflection is 'good' or 'weak' and instead give targeted feedback related to depth of analysis, ethical awareness, linkage to theory, and personal insight. Examples of helpful feedback comments:

- 'You have clearly described the situation. Can you explore what influenced your response further?'

- 'How might this situation have unfolded differently if another approach was taken?'

- 'What have you learned that could change your practice in future?'

Feedback should also validate emotional responses, especially in ethically or emotionally charged reflections, while guiding students to make sense of those emotions within their professional role.

USING SIMULATION AND DEBRIEF TO FOSTER CRITICAL THINKING AND REFLECTION

Simulation is a high-impact method for engaging students in critical thinking and reflection. Scenarios should be designed to include uncertainty, ethical tensions, or deteriorating patient conditions that require prioritisation and justification of actions. Simulation is most effective when followed by a structured debrief.

The Pearls Framework for Debriefing

- **Reactions**—Allow learners to express emotional responses.

- **Description**—Clarify what happened without judgement.

- **Analysis**—Explore thought processes, decision-making, and team dynamics.

- **Summary**—Reinforce key learning and strategies for future practice.

Educators should facilitate debriefs with openness and curiosity, avoiding punitive or overly corrective tones. Encouraging self-assessment before peer or educator feedback can also help promote self-regulation and deeper insight **(Cheng et al., 2016)**.

ASSESSMENT OF CRITICAL THINKING AND REFLECTIVE PRACTICE

Assessment of critical thinking and reflection presents challenges. It is possible to assess outcomes (e.g. the application of theory to a case) but assessing internal processes

Table 2.8 Example Reflection Assessment Criteria

Area	Developing	Competent	Advanced
Description of event	Minimal context	Clear, structured narrative	Rich context, identifies complexity
Depth of analysis	Surface-level observations	Evidence of critical analysis	Explores multiple influences and dynamics
Integration of theory	Limited or missing	Links to relevant theory	Integrates multiple theories with insight
Future planning	Vague ideas	Clear actions proposed	Specific, realistic, and proactive plans

(e.g. personal insight) must be approached carefully to avoid reducing reflection to a performative task.

Designing Assessment for Critical Thinking

Assessment tasks that support critical thinking include:

- Structured case analyses with evidence justification.
- Written debates or position statements on ethical dilemmas.
- Simulation-based OSCEs requiring decision-making and rationale.
- Viva examinations requiring verbal articulation of clinical reasoning.

Rubrics should include criteria such as logical coherence, use of evidence, awareness of bias, and the ability to consider alternatives.

Assessing Reflective Practice

When assessing reflective writing, clarity must be given to students on what is being assessed. This may include:

- Demonstrated learning from experience.
- Application of a reflective model or theoretical lens.
- Integration of feedback into future action.
- Depth of personal insight while maintaining professional boundaries.

Where possible, reflection should be used formatively, with summative use limited to less emotionally charged topics. Feedback remains the most valuable tool for supporting reflection development (Table 2.8).

DEVELOPING EDUCATORS' CAPACITY TO TEACH CRITICAL THINKING AND REFLECTIVE PRACTICE

Teaching critical thinking and reflective practice effectively requires educators to model these capabilities themselves. Whether in university classrooms or clinical settings, nurse educators must continuously reflect on their own practice, assess the impact of their teaching strategies, and remain open to feedback. This section explores how educators can evaluate and enhance their own pedagogical approaches using structured reflection, peer observation, educator-specific reflective tools, and collaborative learning models such as communities of practice.

INNOVATION BOX

Title: *Using Collaborative Writing to Develop Critical Thinking and Reflection in Student Nurses*

Innovation in Practice

Collaborative writing projects, where small groups of students co-author reflective blogs or clinical case commentaries, have been shown to enhance critical thinking and reflection. Each student contributes a section that incorporates evidence, critical questioning, and personal insight. The group then collectively reflects on the process and explores the diversity of their perspectives.

This approach promotes deeper engagement with clinical decision-making, builds academic confidence, and fosters mutual learning. It also provides educators with valuable insight into how students negotiate different viewpoints and justify their reasoning, offering rich opportunities for formative feedback.

Why It Matters

Collaborative writing encourages students to move beyond descriptive accounts to critically examine the complexity of nursing practice and professional judgement. It supports inclusive pedagogy by recognising and valuing the varied experiences, cultural perspectives, and voices that students bring to the learning environment.

REFLECTIVE PRACTICE FOR EDUCATORS

Just as reflection is encouraged in students, it must also be embedded in the professional routines of educators. Reflective teaching involves examining one's own pedagogical decisions, lesson design, facilitation skills, and interactions with learners. This self-inquiry helps educators remain responsive to student needs, curriculum shifts, and regulatory expectations.

USING STRUCTURED REFLECTION TOOLS

Educators may benefit from adapting models such as Brookfield's Four Lenses (2017), which encourages reflection through multiple perspectives:

1. **Self-reflection**—What do I believe about teaching and learning?

2. **Student Feedback**—What do learners say about their experiences?

3. **Colleague Input**—What can peers observe or share about my teaching?

4. **Scholarly Literature**—What evidence-based practices inform this work?

Combining these lenses enables educators to interrogate their assumptions, address bias, and strengthen evidence-informed teaching (Table 2.9).

PEER OBSERVATION AND COLLABORATIVE FEEDBACK

Peer observation schemes offer a supportive, developmental opportunity for educators to receive constructive feedback on their teaching practice. When focused on areas such as critical thinking facilitation or reflective writing support, observations can yield highly targeted insights.

Educators can request feedback on:

• How questioning was used to stimulate critical thought.

• Whether learners were encouraged to challenge assumptions.

• How reflection was introduced, supported, and debriefed.

• The clarity of language when explaining complex or sensitive concepts.

Reciprocal observation, where both parties benefit from observation and feedback, promotes mutual growth and normalises continuous development. Institutions delivering PGCAP programmes may consider incorporating peer observation logs and joint reflection activities into modules, reinforcing their role in practice-based pedagogy.

EDUCATOR SELF-ASSESSMENT AND REFLECTION TOOLS

A range of tools are available or adaptable for nurse educators to self-assess their teaching of critical thinking and reflection. These may include:

• **Educator Reflective Diaries**—Structured templates guiding reflection after each session.

• **Critical Incident Logs**—Short analyses of unexpected teaching moments that prompted reflection or change.

• **Teaching Inventories**—Tools such as the Critical Thinking Teaching Inventory (Behar-Horenstein & Niu, 2011) help map educator behaviours to critical thinking pedagogy.

• **360° Feedback Tools**—Collect input from students, peers, and supervisors to form a holistic view of teaching impact.

Institutions may also encourage educators to include these reflections in academic portfolios, professional development reviews, or revalidation submissions (for those with dual clinical roles).

COMMUNITIES OF PRACTICE AND PROFESSIONAL DIALOGUE

Communities of practice (CoPs) offer an effective model for developing critical teaching capacity, particularly when formed around shared challenges such as developing

Table 2.9 Example Reflective Prompts for Educators

Lens	Reflective question
Self	How did I adapt my teaching when the session wasn't going as planned?
Student	What feedback have I received about my use of reflective models?
Colleague	What did my peer observation reveal about student engagement or clarity?
Scholarship	Which learning theory underpins my simulation debrief strategy?

students' reflective writing or embedding clinical reasoning in simulation. A CoP involves a group of practitioners who share a domain of interest, engage in joint activities, and build a repertoire of resources, language, and approaches (Wenger, 1998).

Examples of activities within educator-focused CoPs might include:

- Sharing and discussing annotated examples of student reflections.

- Joint development of marking rubrics for reflective assignments.

- Exploring dilemmas in assessment of critical thinking.

- Co-designing interdisciplinary simulation scenarios that foster decision-making.

These forums allow clinical and academic educators to align practice, discuss the challenges of teaching in regulatory contexts, and reduce variability across placements and campuses. In dual-role contexts (e.g. practice educators or university-based clinical lecturers), CoPs also support consistency in student experience.

MENTORSHIP AND LEADERSHIP IN DEVELOPING TEACHING PRACTICE

Experienced nurse educators should also consider their role in mentoring junior colleagues and contributing to a culture of teaching excellence. Opportunities include:

- Leading workshops on using reflective models or critical thinking techniques.

- Supporting others in curriculum design with a focus on decision-making and judgment.

- Acting as peer reviewers for assessment tasks or student feedback approaches.

- Contributing to internal or external panels for programme validation, ensuring reflection and reasoning are explicitly integrated into programme learning outcomes and assessments.

This work supports the development of scholarly teaching and can contribute to recognition pathways such as Advance HE Fellowships, senior educator awards, or university teaching fellow schemes.

EMBEDDING CRITICAL THINKING AND REFLECTIVE PRACTICE ACROSS THE CURRICULUM

INTRODUCTION

Embedding critical thinking and reflective practice into the nursing curriculum requires strategic alignment of learning outcomes, teaching methods, assessment, and learning environments. These elements must work together to ensure learners encounter repeated, meaningful opportunities to practise decision-making, engage in self-reflection, and apply theory to practice. This section offers practical guidance for curriculum teams, module leaders, and clinical educators involved in designing, delivering, or quality-assuring nursing education at undergraduate and postgraduate levels.

CURRICULUM DESIGN CONSIDERATIONS

Critical thinking and reflection should not be confined to isolated modules or occasional portfolio tasks; rather, they should be introduced early, developed progressively, and assessed appropriately throughout the programme. This can be achieved through vertical and horizontal integration:

- **Vertical Integration**: Ensures that reflective and critical capabilities are revisited and deepened year-on-year (e.g. from describing practice in Year 1 to analysing ethical dilemmas in Year 3).

- **Horizontal Integration**: Embeds reflection and reasoning across modules within a level (e.g. in clinical skills, biosciences, communication, and leadership).

The Nursing and Midwifery Council (NMC, 2018) proficiencies, particularly those in Domains 1 (Accountability), 3 (Assessment and Planning), and 6 (Improving Safety and Quality), support the inclusion of these themes (Table 2.10).

LINKING LEARNING OUTCOMES TO REFLECTIVE AND CRITICAL THINKING CAPABILITIES

When developing or reviewing modules, module learning outcomes (MLOs) should explicitly state expectations for critical engagement and reflective reasoning. Clear verbs from Bloom's taxonomy or similar frameworks can support this.

Table 2.10 Curriculum Design Alignment Example

Year	Module	Example outcome or activity	Focus
1	Fundamentals of Nursing Practice	Reflect on the first clinical encounter using Rolfe's model	Fundamental reflective skills
1	Biosciences	Use a concept map to explain physiological changes in sepsis	Structured critical thinking
2	Assessing Needs and Planning Care	Analyse a case study using Tanner's Clinical Judgement Model	Clinical reasoning
2	Communication and Ethics	Reflect on an ethical scenario using Johns' model	Ethical reasoning and reflection
3	Leadership in Practice	Defend a care plan using evidence and ethical frameworks	Advanced decision-making
3	Practice Portfolio	Submit a critical reflection on managing a challenging patient episode	Consolidation of reflective practice

Examples of Well-aligned MLOs:

- 'Critically evaluate clinical decision-making strategies in relation to patient safety and evidence-based practice'.

- 'Reflect analytically on clinical experience using a recognised reflective framework to inform future learning'.

- 'Apply theoretical models to justify person-centred interventions in complex care scenarios'.

Outcomes should then be mapped to assessment and teaching activities to ensure constructive alignment.

TEACHING STRATEGIES AT MODULE LEVEL

To embed critical thinking and reflection consistently, module leaders and teaching teams can:

- Include regular case-based seminars and debriefs across all modules—not just practice-focused ones.

- Use digital tools (e.g. Padlet, discussion boards) to allow students to post short reflections linked to weekly topics.

- Provide scaffolded reflective tasks—starting with structured templates and moving toward independent journaling.

- Offer low-stakes critical appraisal tasks that ask students to evaluate short clinical guidelines or articles.

- Introduce 'ethics corners' or 'reflection spots' in lectures to pause and analyse key decisions or events.

Educators should model critical and reflective behaviours by thinking aloud, sharing practice dilemmas, and exploring uncertainty rather than promoting definitive answers.

ASSESSMENT STRATEGIES AND CURRICULUM MAPPING

Critical thinking and reflective practice should be visible in assessment strategies across a programme, not restricted to practice portfolios or academic essays. Consider:

- Embedding reflection within OSCE stations (e.g. ask for rationale and post-scenario reflection).

- Using online discussion forums for collaborative reflection, assessed using rubrics.

- Designing group debates or care planning tasks that assess justification and reasoning.

- Including reflective elements in summative case studies or quality improvement proposals.

Assessment maps (Table 2.11) can be used to check whether critical and reflective learning is:

- Introduced, reinforced, and mastered across the programme.

- Assessed in varied formats (written, oral, group, individual).

- Represented in both academic and practice-based modules.

Table 2.11 Assessment Map Example

Module	Assessment type	Skill assessed
Foundations of Nursing	Reflective log (formative)	Personal insight and application
Ethics and Law	Group debate	Ethical reasoning and articulation
Long-Term Conditions	Case study analysis	Clinical reasoning and justification
Practice Learning	Supervisor feedback on reflection	Real-time reflective discussion
Final Leadership Module	Critical incident report	Advanced reflective synthesis

QUALITY ASSURANCE AND PROGRAMME REVIEW

To ensure that critical thinking and reflection remain core components of the curriculum:

- **Include these elements in validation documentation**—linking them to NMC proficiency statements.

- **Use student feedback** to evaluate whether learners feel able to think critically and reflect meaningfully.

- **Engage external examiners** in reviewing reflective and reasoning-related assessment criteria.

- **Review samples of student work** across levels to evaluate progression in depth and complexity.

For PGCAP participants, curriculum mapping exercises can be used in assignments to demonstrate how teaching and assessment approaches promote these higher-order skills.

Figure 2.1 is 'The Hill and Wamburu Model of Purposeful Pedagogy in Nurse Education' and presents a visual representation of the dynamic relationship between critical thinking and reflective practice in nurse education. While distinct in their purposes and processes, both approaches are essential to the development of thoughtful, responsive teaching. Critical thinking invites educators to examine assumptions, use evidence rigorously, and engage in systematic reasoning. Reflective practice draws attention to emotion, context, values, and meaning, enabling a deeper connection to the human elements of education.

For nurse academics, the integration of these domains is not a simple task but a continual balancing

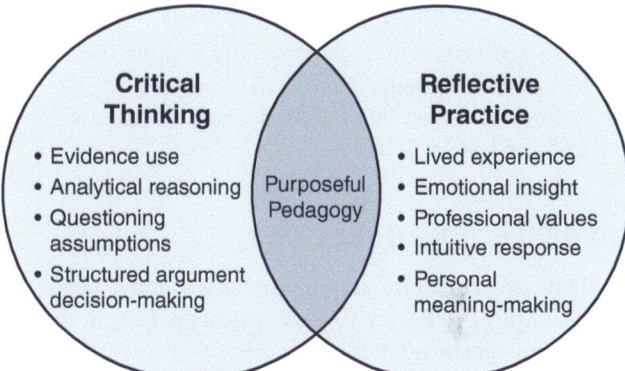

The nurse academic draws on both criticality and reflection to teach with integrity, insight, and intent.

FIGURE 2.1 The Hill and Wamburu model of purposeful pedagogy in nurse education

act. The central space in the model, Purposeful Pedagogy, represents the aim of using both modes of thinking to shape inclusive, meaningful, and developmentally appropriate learning environments. Whether designing assessments, providing feedback, or navigating complex teaching moments, the most impactful teaching emerges when educators apply both criticality and reflection with intent.

The Hill and Wamburu Model of Purposeful Pedagogy in Nurse Education reinforces the idea that effective nurse education requires more than technical skill or subject knowledge. It calls for intellectual curiosity, emotional awareness, and an ongoing commitment to professional growth through integrated thinking.

RECOMMENDATIONS FOR PRACTICE

To develop confident, safe, and critically engaged nursing professionals, nurse educators and practice supervisors must embed critical thinking and reflective practice into all aspects of teaching, assessment, and clinical support. This involves modelling thoughtful decision-making, encouraging reflective dialogue, using structured frameworks, and providing consistent feedback. Both academic and practice settings should offer psychologically safe spaces for learners to question, analyse, and reflect on their experiences. Curricula should be mapped to ensure progressive development of these skills, with assessment tasks that go beyond recall and require students to justify their actions and evaluate outcomes. These approaches prepare future nurses not only to meet regulatory standards but to respond ethically, analytically, and compassionately to the evolving needs of healthcare.

TAKE-HOME POINTS

1. Critical thinking and reflective practice are interdependent skills essential to nursing professionalism, safe care, and lifelong learning.

2. Nurse educators must purposefully scaffold these skills using strategies such as case-based learning, structured reflection models, Socratic questioning, and simulation debriefs.

3. Assessment should focus on students' ability to justify decisions, demonstrate ethical awareness, and apply learning to future practice—not just describe experiences.

CPD REFLECTIVE QUESTIONS

1. How do I currently support students to move beyond descriptive reflection toward critical analysis in their clinical learning?

2. In what ways does my teaching encourage students to justify their clinical decisions using evidence and theory?

3. How might I use peer feedback, simulation debriefs, or interdisciplinary dialogue to enhance my own teaching practice in this area?

REFERENCES

Alfaro-LeFevre, R. (2019). *Critical thinking, clinical reasoning, and clinical judgment* (7th ed.). Elsevier.

Alfaro-LeFevre, R. (2020). *Critical Thinking, Clinical Reasoning, and Clinical Judgement: A Practical Approach to Outcome-focused Thinking* (7th ed.). Elsevier.

Barrows, H. S. (1986). A taxonomy of problem-based learning methods. *Medical Education*, 20(6), 481–486. https://doi.org/10.1111/j.1365-2923.1986.tb01386.x.

Behar-Horenstein, L. S., & Niu, L. (2011). Teaching critical thinking skills in higher education: a review of the literature. *Journal of College Teaching & Learning*, 8(2), 25–41. https://doi.org/10.19030/tlc.v8i2.3554.

Benner, P. (1984). *From Novice to Expert: Excellence and Power in Clinical Nursing Practice*. Addison-Wesley.

Benner, P., Sutphen, M., Leonard, V., & Day, L. (2010). *Educating Nurses: A Call for Radical Transformation*. Jossey-Bass.

Brookfield, S. D. (2017). *Becoming a Critically Reflective Teacher* (2nd ed.). Jossey-Bass.

Cheng, A., Eppich, W., Grant, V., Sherbino, J., Zendejas, B., & Cook, D. A. (2016). Debriefing for technology-enhanced simulation: a systematic review and meta-analysis. *Medical Education*, 48(7), 657–666. https://doi.org/10.1111/medu.12961.

Edmondson, A. (1999). Psychological safety and learning behavior in work teams. *Administrative Science Quarterly*, 44(2), 350–383. https://doi.org/10.2307/2666999.

Facione, P. A. (1990). Critical thinking: a statement of expert consensus for purposes of educational assessment and instruction. Research Findings and Recommendations. 315.

Facione, P. A. (2011). *Critical thinking: what it is and why it counts* (2011 update). Insight Assessment. https://www.insightassessment.com/resources/critical-thinking-what-it-is-and-why-it-counts/

Gibbs, G. (1988). *Learning by Doing: A Guide to Teaching and Learning Methods*. Oxford Polytechnic.

Johns, C. (1995). The value of reflective practice for nursing. *Journal of Clinical Nursing*, 4(1), 23–30. https://doi.org/10.1111/j.1365-2702.1995.tb00003.x.

Levett-Jones, T., Hoffman, K., Dempsey, J., Jeong, S. Y. S., Noble, D., Norton, C. A., Roche, J., & Hickey, N. (2010). The 'five rights' of clinical reasoning: an educational model to enhance nursing students' ability to identify and manage clinically 'at risk' patients. *Nurse Education Today*, 30(6), 515–520. https://doi.org/10.1016/j.nedt.2009.10.020.

Levett-Jones, T., Pitt, V., Courtney-Pratt, H., Harbrow, G., & Rossiter, R. (2009). What are the primary concerns of nursing students as they prepare for and contemplate their first clinical placement experience? *Nurse Education in Practice*, 9(6), 371–377. https://doi.org/10.1016/j.nepr.2008.08.003.

Melnyk, B. M., & Fineout-Overholt, E. (2019). *Evidence-Based Practice in Nursing and Healthcare: A Guide to Best Practice* (4th ed.). Wolters Kluwer.

Moon, J. A. (2004). *A Handbook of Reflective and Experiential Learning: Theory and Practice*. RoutledgeFalmer.

NHS Improvement (2019). *A just culture guide* https://www.england.nhs.uk/patient-safety/patient-safety-culture/being-fair-tool/. Accessed: (9 December 2025).

Nursing and Midwifery Council (2018). *Future nurse: standards of proficiency for registered nurses*. https://www.nmc.org.uk/standards/standards-for-nurses/

Papadopoulos, I. (2021). *Culturally Competent Compassion: A Guide for Healthcare Students and Practitioners*. Routledge.

Paul, R., & Elder, L. (2006). *The Miniature Guide to Critical Thinking: Concepts and Tools*. Foundation for Critical Thinking Press.

Rolfe, G., Freshwater, D., & Jasper, M. (2001). *Critical Reflection in Nursing and the Helping Professions: A User's Guide*. Palgrave Macmillan.

Schön, D. A. (1983). *The Reflective Practitioner: How Professionals Think in Action*. Basic Books.

Tanner, C. A. (2006). Thinking like a nurse: a research-based model of clinical judgment in nursing. *Journal of Nursing Education*, 45(6), 204–211. https://doi.org/10.3928/01484834-20060601-04.

Vygotsky, L. S. (1978). *Mind in Society: The Development of Higher Psychological Processes*. Harvard University Press.

Wenger, E. (1998). *Communities of Practice: Learning, Meaning, and Identity*. Cambridge University Press.

CHAPTER 3

Leadership and Innovation in Nursing Education

Melane Hayward and Karen Buckwell-Nutt

College of Health and Society, Buckinghamshire New University, UK

AIM

To explore how different leadership styles and innovative practices influence nursing education, with a focus on promoting inclusive learning environments, supporting educator development, and ensuring regulatory quality.

LEARNING OUTCOMES

After reading this chapter, readers will be able to:

1. Differentiate between transformational, servant, democratic, and autocratic leadership styles and their application in nursing education settings.

2. Understand the role of innovative leadership in embedding creativity, digital pedagogy, and evidence-based strategies in nurse education.

3. Examine the concept of learnership and its relevance to both nursing students and educators in supporting clinical competence and teaching capability.

4. Evaluate quality assurance mechanisms and accreditation processes in upholding standards in nursing education and supporting continuous improvement.

CHAPTER INTRODUCTION

Leadership and innovation are pivotal in shaping the future of nursing education. This chapter explores various leadership styles and their impact on nursing education, focusing on transformational, servant, democratic, and autocratic leadership. Each leadership style is explored in terms of its principles, implementation, benefits, and challenges within the context of nursing education. Additionally, the chapter highlights the importance of innovative leadership in fostering a culture of creativity, critical thinking, and evidence-based practice.

Transformational leadership is emphasised for its role in inspiring and motivating educators and students to achieve excellence through vision, trust, and empowerment. Servant leadership is discussed for its focus on serving others, fostering a nurturing learning environment, and promoting ethical and holistic care. Democratic leadership is highlighted for its participatory approach, encouraging collaboration, inclusivity, and shared decision-making. Autocratic leadership, while less favoured, is examined for its effectiveness in specific contexts requiring quick decision-making and strict adherence to protocols.

The chapter also explores the concept of learnership, which integrates theoretical education with practical experience, ensuring that nursing students develop essential clinical competencies and professional conduct. Learnership also applies to the nursing educators, as they need to learn the craft of teaching. The importance of quality assurance, regulation, and accreditation in maintaining high standards in nursing education is underscored, with a focus on continuous quality improvement and stakeholder coproduction.

By the end of this chapter, readers will gain a comprehensive understanding of various leadership styles and their application in nursing education, the significance of innovation in fostering a dynamic learning environment, and the critical role of quality assurance in ensuring educational excellence.

TRANSFORMATIONAL LEADERSHIP

DEFINITION AND PRINCIPLES

Transformational leadership is an approach that emphasises vision, trust, and empowerment in achieving shared objectives. For nursing educators, this style translates to creating an environment where educators and students are inspired to innovate and excel. The transformational leader promotes a culture of collaboration, guiding their team to align individual and institutional goals while addressing challenges in creative and sustainable ways. Central principles include promoting shared values, nurturing professional growth, and championing a vision of excellence in professional and educational practice.

Seminal work by Bass (1985) outlines transformational leadership characterised by four key 'I behaviours': idealised influence, inspirational motivation, intellectual stimulation, and individualised consideration. Idealised influence involves role-modelling ethical behaviour and professionalism, earning trust and respect from students and colleagues. Inspirational motivation is the ability to

articulate a compelling vision that energises and unites a team. Intellectual stimulation encourages critical thinking and creativity, challenging traditional methods and fostering a culture of inquiry. Lastly, individualised consideration ensures personalised mentorship and support, recognising the unique needs and potential of everyone. These behaviours are crucial in holistically supporting educators and preparing future nurses for the complexities of modern higher education and healthcare, empowering them to become competent, ethical, and compassionate professionals (Boamah, 2022). Table 3.1 highlights how transformational leadership's 'I behaviours' can apply both to student and staff engagement and development within UK nursing education.

Transformational leadership fundamentally influences both the theoretical and practical aspects of nursing education, cultivating an environment conducive to learning and self-improvement (Kim et al., 2022). The transformational framework not only equips educators

Table 3.1   Transformational Leadership Behaviours in Nursing Education

I Behaviour	Example related to students	Example in education teams/staff
Idealised Influence	A clinical skills tutor actively engages in professional development, staying updated with the latest research in nursing education and clinical practice. By consistently sharing their learning and demonstrating a commitment to evidence-based practice, they inspire students to value lifelong learning	A department head models integrity, ethical decision-making, transparency, and accountability, encouraging a culture of respect, trust, and professionalism within the education team
Inspirational Motivation	A nurse researcher develops a student-led patient advocacy project, encouraging students to collaborate with healthcare providers to improve patient-centred care in local NHS trusts	A programme lead articulates a strategic contemporary vision for postgraduate pre-registration nursing education, inspiring staff and partners to collaborate on curriculum enhancements
Intellectual Stimulation	A nursing lecturer integrates virtual reality simulations into their module to develop critical thinking, problem-solving, and enhance clinical reasoning skills, enabling students to practice responding to emergency scenarios in a safe learning environment	A senior lecturer organises interprofessional learning workshops amongst health and social care educators to promote research-led teaching, challenging colleagues to integrate multiprofessional evidence-based innovations into their teaching
Individualised Consideration	A nursing apprenticeship personal tutor conducts one-to-one coaching sessions with struggling apprentices, identifying individual learning preferences and needs, creating tailored study plans, and signposting to other services to support their success	A senior nurse educator supports early-career nurse educators by offering mentorship and career guidance, helping them develop teaching strategies, research skills, and confidence

with the tools needed to inspire their students but also creates pathways for nurturing resilient, compassionate, and ethical professionals within the field.

IMPACT ON NURSING EDUCATION

Transformational leadership positively influences nursing and its education by encouraging an inclusive and empowering culture. This style enables educators to motivate students to embrace lifelong learning and critical thinking. For example, educators can role model transformational behaviours by encouraging interprofessional collaboration, engaging in reflective practice, and developing curricula that challenge traditional pedagogies. These efforts cultivate resilient students and registrants equipped to navigate the complexities of healthcare systems. Moreover, transformational leadership can address systemic challenges by developing a shared commitment to excellence. In education settings, this might involve creating mentorship programmes where senior educators support new educators, ensuring alignment with institutional goals and student success. Initiatives using peer learning models that pair experienced educators with early-career educators ensure that institutional knowledge is preserved while adapting to contemporary demands.

By championing professional development opportunities and facilitating open dialogue, transformational leaders enable education teams to innovate while maintaining alignment with regulatory standards. Boamah (2022) found that transformational leadership significantly improves workplace culture, job satisfaction, and reduces burnout among nursing educators. This leadership style creates a supportive environment that enhances staff retention and well-being. Delgado and Mitchell (2016) also highlighted the challenges faced by academic nurse leaders, such as finding and retaining qualified educators, obtaining resources, and team building. Transformational leaders can address these challenges by nurturing a supportive and collaborative environment, ensuring that resources are effectively utilised, and building strong, cohesive teams.

Enhancing Education Satisfaction and Reducing Burnout

Transformational leadership has been shown to have a strong positive impact on satisfaction and a negative impact on burnout. Boamah (2022) highlights that transformational leaders create a supportive workplace culture that mediates the relationship between leadership and job satisfaction. This supportive culture includes open communication, trust, and respect, which are essential for educator engagement and retention. During the COVID-19 pandemic, transformational leadership proved particularly effective in mitigating the risks of burnout and improving job satisfaction. Transformational leaders were able to adjust to the rapidly changing environment, providing the necessary support and resources to their teams. This adaptability and support helped staff navigate the challenges posed by the pandemic, maintaining their well-being and commitment to their roles (Boamah, 2022).

Promoting a Positive Workplace Culture

A positive workplace culture is crucial for the success of transformational leadership. Transformational leaders promote and develop inclusivity and empowerment, where staff feel valued and supported. This culture advances professional growth, collaboration, and innovation, which are essential for achieving excellence in nursing education. Shaping a supportive workplace culture is created by role modelling positive behaviours, providing constructive feedback, and creating opportunities for professional development. By prioritising the well-being of their teams, transformational leaders ensure motivation and engagement, leading to better outcomes for both educators and students. Delgado and Mitchell (2016) identified integrity, communication clarity, and problem-solving ability as top-valued leadership qualities for educational leaders. These qualities align with the principles of transformational leadership, emphasising the importance of ethical behaviour, and contributing to creating a positive workplace culture where staff feel respected, understood, and supported. Figure 3.1 outlines the key components to create and maintain a supportive and empowering work environment. It highlights the essential elements that contribute to a positive workplace culture, which is crucial for job satisfaction, retention, and overall success in nursing education.

Addressing Incivility and Enhancing Teamwork

Transformational leadership is also pivotal in addressing issues of incivility and promoting teamwork within nursing education. Fischer (2016) highlights that transformational leadership can counter alienating behaviours such as incivility by fostering a culture of respect and collaboration. Leaders who model professional conduct, nurture an environment where unprofessional behaviours are actively challenged and discouraged, consequently building a cohesive and supportive learning community. Encouraging open communication, collaboration, and mutual support among staff leaders can lead their teams in a manner that positively impacts both the work environment and student

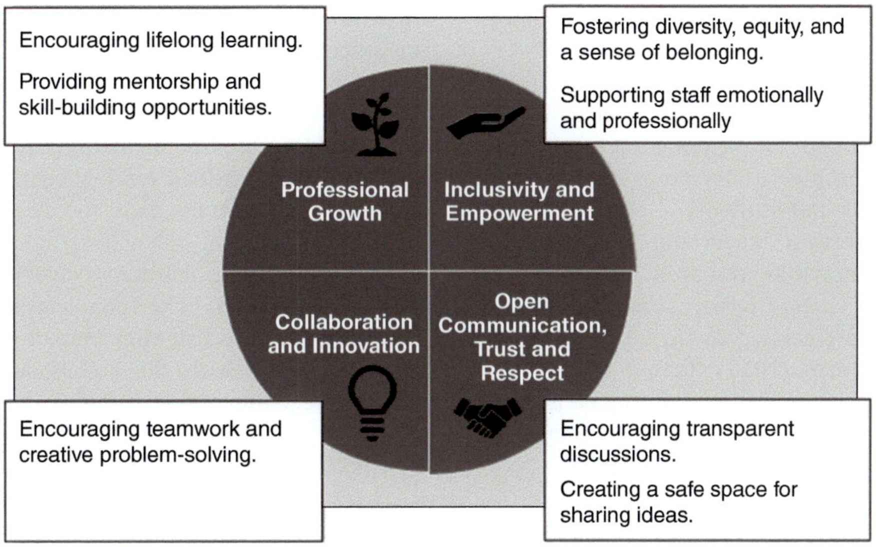

FIGURE 3.1   Key components of a positive workplace culture

outcomes. They establish a culture of mutual respect that further enhances collaborative practices among educators, accordingly, reinforcing the importance of teamwork in nursing education.

Role in Development and Mentorship

Transformational leadership also plays a critical role in staff development and mentorship. Greenway and Acai (2024) emphasise that effective nursing education leaders who master the roles of manager, mentor, educator, and nurse promote a culture of growth and professional development. Transformational leaders invest in staff growth and development, promoting research and success, and prioritise supportive workplaces. They provide individual support and guidance, helping educators and students develop to their full potential. Mentorship

is a key component of transformational leadership, as it supports scholarly achievements while cultivating a sense of community. Transformational leaders use their skills to invest in staff development, promote work-life balance, and offer continuing education opportunities. This approach not only enhances job satisfaction but also improves staff retention and the overall quality of nursing education (Greenway & Acai, 2024). Delgado and Mitchell (2016) found that mentoring is a crucial aspect of leadership preparation, with many respondents highlighting the importance of mentoring in their own leadership development. Leveraging a nurturing approach facilitates a supportive environment where staff can thrive, consequently reinforcing their commitment to the discipline and enhancing their leadership capabilities (Afsar & Masood, 2018).

SERVANT LEADERSHIP

CONCEPT AND CHARACTERISTICS

Servant leadership, like transformational leadership, empowers followers but also recognises the importance of leaders being followers. It emphasises the philosophy of 'serving first' to lead effectively, challenging traditional notions of leadership by placing the success of the team above individual accolades. The servant leader's role is to empower team members, providing them with the tools, motivation, and environment they need to excel. In nursing education, servant leaders act as facilitators, encouraging a nurturing space that values empathy, active listening, and the development of others.

Neville et al. (2021) highlight the deep connections between servant leadership and caring theories in nursing, arguing that servant leadership's focus on altruism and holistic care makes it particularly relevant to nursing education. This perspective is reinforced by Tropello and DeFazio (2014), who describe servant leadership as essential for fostering respect, trust, and collaboration in education settings. Jackson (2008) further expands this perspective by linking servant leadership to the development of research capacity, highlighting its role in adopting mentorship networks and reducing isolation. Sherman (2019) builds on these ideas, emphasising that servant leadership fosters psychological safety, which enhances educator and student engagement while mitigating burnout.

Servant leaders recognise that success in education stems from a sense of shared purpose, collective effort, akin to the idea that 'managers don't win games: teams do.' This philosophy underscores the need to support both educators and students to achieve shared goals. Additionally, servant leadership facilitates the development of sustainable research communities, ensuring that early career researchers receive the mentorship and support needed to thrive in academia (Jackson, 2008). Sherman (2019) further argues that persuasion rather than coercion is a defining element of servant leadership, reinforcing its ability to encourage trust and autonomy in educational environments.

CHARACTERISTICS OF SERVANT LEADERSHIP IN NURSING EDUCATION

The concept of servant leadership was first articulated by Greenleaf's (2002) foundational work in the 1970s. In his seminal essay, *The Servant as Leader*, Greenleaf (2002) outlined the philosophy of servant leadership, which emphasises prioritising the needs of others and empowering them to achieve their potential. Greenleaf's (2002) work has since become a cornerstone in leadership theory, particularly in education and healthcare, where the principles of service and care are paramount.

Building on Greenleaf's (2002) foundational ideas, Spears (1996) identified ten key characteristics of servant leadership. These traits distil the essence of servant leadership into practical behaviours, making the philosophy accessible and applicable across diverse contexts, including nursing education. The characteristics Spears (1996) identified—such as listening, empathy, and stewardship—resonate deeply with the collaborative and supportive nature of teaching and learning.

Connecting Framework and Practice

In nursing education, these characteristics guide educators in creating environments where students and colleagues can thrive. To provide clarity and relevance for educators, Table 3.2 reframes Spears' (1996) original characteristics, aligning them with key elements of leadership in higher education. This adaptation forms the acronym 'LEADERSHIP,' reflecting the multifaceted role of servant leaders in cultivating growth and resilience among students and colleagues.

Table 3.2   Characteristics of Servant Leadership in Nursing Education

Characteristic	Description
L – Listening	Actively listen to team members' concerns and ideas, fostering trust and ensuring their voices are heard. In the classroom, this might involve giving students the opportunity to express their learning needs and adapting teaching strategies accordingly
E – Empathy	Understand students' perspectives and emotions, creating a supportive environment where students feel valued and understood
A – Awareness	Have a heightened sense of awareness to perceive challenges and opportunities clearly, adapting their approach to meet evolving educational needs
D – Development (Commitment to Growth)	Encourage personal and professional development, mentoring students and colleagues to reach their full potential and enhance resilience
E – Ethics (Stewardship)	Take responsibility for the growth and well-being of their team, ensuring resources are used effectively to benefit all. This trait aligns closely with nursing's commitment to ethical care. Stewardship as a moral responsibility
R – Resilience (Healing)	Support the emotional and personal well-being of students, helping them overcome challenges and build their confidence. This links to the transformative potential of caring theories in nursing and can be an antidote to burnout, promoting well-being
S – Support (Building Community)	Encourage a sense of community within educational settings, promoting and strengthening collaboration, meaningful engagement, trust, and shared purpose
H – Holistic Vision (Conceptualisation)	Articulate a clear vision for the future, helping students and colleagues understand how their efforts contribute to broader goals. This may include interdisciplinary research and knowledge-sharing initiatives
I – Influence (Persuasion)	Use influence rather than authority to inspire and guide their teams, encouraging collaboration, mutual respect, and building consensus
P – Planning (Foresight)	Anticipate future challenges and opportunities, preparing their teams for success by planning curricula that address emerging healthcare trends

This framework not only encapsulates the theoretical foundations of servant leadership but also provides a practical roadmap for nursing educators to implement these principles effectively. By embracing these characteristics, educators can build resilient and collaborative learning communities that prioritise student success and professional growth.

HUMILITY: THE CORE OF SERVANT LEADERSHIP

Humility is a defining trait of servant leadership, setting it apart from other leadership styles. It is the ability to prioritise the needs of others, acknowledge one's limitations, and remain open to learning and growth, where team members feel valued and empowered, contributing to a culture of collaboration and mutual respect.

Mrayyan and Al-Rjoub (2024) emphasise that humility in servant leadership enhances ethical decision-making, as leaders are more likely to consider the collective good over personal gain. This alignment with nursing's professional values reinforces the relevance of humility in education settings.

Humility also supports the development of resilience among students and staff. Leaders who model humility encourage open communication and create a safe space for individuals to express concerns and share ideas without fear of judgement. Such an approach is essential in higher education, where cultivating psychological safety can enhance learning outcomes.

Furthermore, humility bridges the gap between leadership and followership. By recognising their role as part of a larger team, servant leaders demonstrate that leadership is not about authority but about service and shared success. This perspective resonates strongly in nursing education, where collaboration and teamwork are integral to professional practice. Figure 3.2 summarises the role of humility in servant leadership. By integrating humility into their leadership approach, nursing educators can promote an inclusive and empowering environment that benefits both students and colleagues.

THE ROLE OF THE SERVANT LEADER ACROSS TEAM STAGES

Building on the foundational work of Greenleaf (2002) and the practical insights provided by Spears (1996), servant leadership demonstrates its adaptability across different team development stages. Tuckman's (1965) model of team development—forming, storming, norming, and performing—offers a useful framework to illustrate how servant leaders adjust their approach to meet evolving team needs in educational contexts.

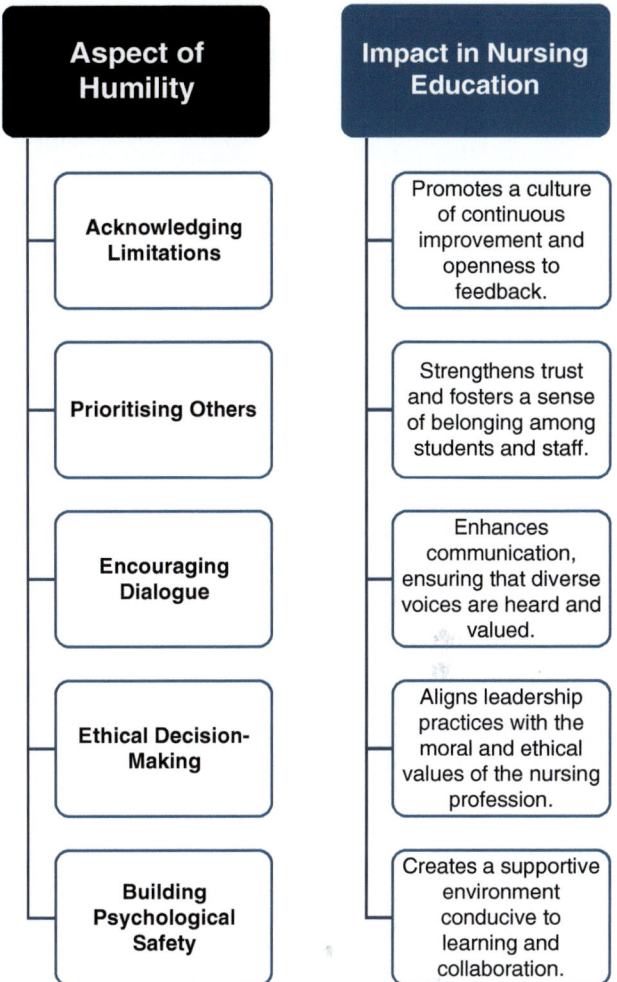

FIGURE 3.2 Humility in servant leadership

Connecting Framework and Practice

In nursing education, these stages reflect the dynamic nature of staff teams and student cohorts.

Table 3.3 provides a detailed breakdown of how servant leaders align their roles and actions with each stage, fostering team cohesion and productivity. This approach ensures that both educators and students thrive, supported by a leadership style that prioritises collaboration, trust, and shared goals.

Servant leadership's emphasis on serving others resonates strongly with the collaborative and people-centric nature of Tuckman's (1965) stages. However, situational leadership's flexibility in adapting leadership styles to the needs of the team also aligns with this framework. For example, in the forming stage, the directive approach typical of situational leadership could resemble a servant leader's provision of clarity and structure.

Table 3.3   Role of Servant Leaders Across Team Stages

Team stage	Role of the servant leader	Actions
Forming (New Teams)	Providing clarity and building confidence	Clearly defining roles and creating a safe environment to enable team members to get acquainted and begin collaborating effectively
Storming (Conflict and Challenge)	Addressing and resolving tensions promptly	Promoting trust and maintaining focus on shared goals. Demonstrating confidence and fairness, understanding conflicts are a natural part of team growth
Norming (Established Teams)	Implementing systems and practices that enhance efficiency	Connecting team members with additional resources or colleagues to optimise unity through collaboration
Performing (Autonomous Teams)	Adopting a light touch	Providing essential resources while shielding the team from external distractions, enabling teams to perform independently while feeling supported in achieving peak productivity

Similarly, adaptive leadership, which focuses on navigating complex challenges and enabling teams to adapt, could intersect with servant leadership in the storming stage. Here, the adaptive leader's capacity to address resistance and build resilience complements the servant leader's emphasis on empathy and conflict resolution. However, the distinction lies in the servant leader's intrinsic motivation to prioritise the team's development over task accomplishment alone.

Tuckman's (1965) performing stage particularly underscores the unique aspects of servant leadership. Unlike situational or adaptive leadership, which may pivot towards strategic goals, servant leadership maintains its focus on supporting autonomy and growth. This enduring commitment to cultivating a thriving community aligns closely with Greenleaf's (2002) foundational philosophy.

Nurse academics who adopt servant or transformational leadership styles often serve as powerful role models for their students and teams. Through consistent modelling of empathy, active listening, and professional integrity, these leaders create a culture of learning that shapes both attitudes and behaviours. This dynamic can be understood through Bandura's Social Learning Theory, which highlights how individuals learn by observing others and internalising those behaviours (see Figure 3.3). Attention, retention, reproduction, and motivation are key elements in this process, each influenced by the credibility, visibility, and approachability of the leader. In the context of nurse education, students are more likely to adopt collaborative, ethical, and person-centred practices when they consistently see these values demonstrated by educators in both academic and clinical environments.

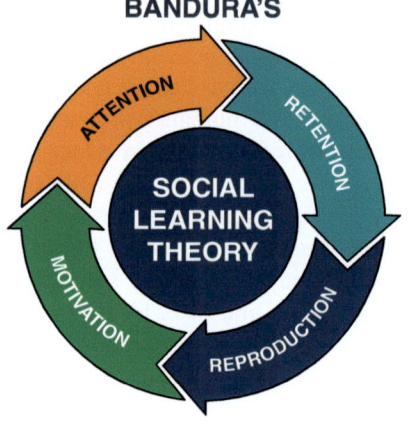

FIGURE 3.3
Modelling leadership through Bandura's social learning theory in nursing education

APPLICATION IN NURSING EDUCATION

Servant leadership is particularly relevant for educators working with diverse student populations. By prioritising personal tutoring and addressing individual learning needs, servant leaders create an environment where students feel supported to achieve their potential. This approach also extends to modules, programmes, and other types of educator teams.

The holistic approach championed by Neville et al. (2021), Todt and Covington (2023), and Tropello and DeFazio (2014) highlights how servant leadership supports student-centred approaches, such as tailored learning pathways for non-traditional students. Educators who adopt this style often establish open-door policies and create platforms for students to voice their concerns, ensuring that their unique needs are met. Servant leaders also frequently engage in reflective practices that allow them to adapt their teaching methods to better serve their students and colleagues.

- *Cultural Competency* is an essential aspect of servant leadership in the diverse landscape of UK higher education. Servant leaders demonstrate cultural sensitivity by recognising and valuing the unique backgrounds, experiences, and perspectives of their students and colleagues. Neville et al. (2021) argue that servant leadership's emphasis on empathy and community building is instrumental in addressing cultural diversity effectively.

- *Interdisciplinary Collaboration* in nursing education is uniquely suited to servant leadership. By prioritising shared goals and mutual respect, servant leaders create an environment where educators from various disciplines can work together to develop integrated curricula and collaborative teaching strategies. Tropello and DeFazio (2014) highlight how servant leadership can bridge gaps between disciplines, ensuring that nursing students receive a holistic education that prepares them for the complexities of modern healthcare environments.

- *Building Resilience* among students is a critical component of servant leadership. By providing emotional support, encouraging self-efficacy and adaptive thinking, servant leaders help students navigate the challenges of nursing education. Neville et al. (2021) link this to the broader framework of caring theories, which emphasise holistic student development. For example, servant leaders might implement mentorship programmes that pair students with experienced practitioners, creating a supportive network that bolsters resilience.

- *Ethics* are central to servant leadership, particularly in nursing education, where moral responsibility is a core professional value. Neville et al. (2021) emphasise that servant leadership aligns closely with nursing's commitment to integrity, accountability, and advocacy. By modelling ethical behaviour, servant leaders inspire their teams to uphold the highest standards of professional conduct.

BENEFITS AND CHALLENGES

Despite its philosophical appeal, implementing servant leadership in academia requires practical strategies. Tropello and DeFazio (2014) suggest that institutions should provide professional development programmes that equip education leaders with the skills to practise servant leadership effectively. Additionally, embedding servant leadership principles into organisational policies and performance development activities and reviews can help institutionalise this approach. For nursing educators, this might involve adopting reflective practices, collaborative decision-making, and prioritising the professional growth of team members.

The benefits of servant leadership in academia include improved staff morale, enhanced student satisfaction, and stronger community ties. However, challenges such as balancing individual and organisational priorities or maintaining clear boundaries between support and accountability require careful navigation.

Despite its potential, servant leadership faces criticism for its lack of operationalisation and empirical evidence (Neville et al., 2021; Todt & Covington, 2023). Tropello and DeFazio (2014) further note that while servant leadership principles are highly relevant, their implementation requires sustained effort and a supportive organisational culture.

DEMOCRATIC LEADERSHIP

OVERVIEW

Democratic leadership is a participatory style of leadership that emphasises collaboration, inclusivity, and shared decision-making. Within nursing education, democratic leadership plays a crucial role in fostering an environment where students, educators, and practice learning partners feel valued and empowered to contribute to the educational process. By incorporating democratic principles, nursing education programmes can enhance learning outcomes, professional development, and the overall quality of care provided by future nurses.

Democratic leadership is characterised by its focus on participation, open communication, and mutual respect. This in turn fosters an environment where key stakeholders can openly discuss and resolve issues. For instance, open communication ensures that concerns such as assignment workload imbalances or curriculum gaps are brought to light and collaboratively addressed.

Mutual respect between students, educators, and practice learning partners builds a foundation for trust, enabling more effective mentorship and reducing the hierarchical barriers that can stifle innovation and learning. In nursing education, this style of leadership prioritises the involvement of all stakeholders, inclusive of people who use services and carers. The following principles underpin democratic leadership:

- *Inclusivity*: Democratic leaders in nursing education actively seek input from diverse perspectives. This inclusivity ensures that decisions are well-informed and reflect the needs and aspirations of the entire educational community (Huber, 2018).

- *Collaboration*: Teamwork and collaboration are central to democratic leadership. Educators work closely with students to identify challenges and develop solutions, fostering a sense of shared responsibility (Huston & Marquis, 2024).

- *Empowerment:* By involving students, educators, and people who use services and carers in decision-making, democratic leaders empower individuals to take ownership of their roles and responsibilities. This empowerment enhances motivation, confidence, and a sense of agency (Northouse, 2021).

- Transparency: Open communication and transparency in decision-making processes build trust and accountability within the educational community.

- Flexibility: Democratic leaders are adaptable and responsive to feedback, allowing them to address emerging needs and challenges effectively (Yoder-Wise & Sportsman, 2023).

IMPLEMENTATION OF DEMOCRATIC LEADERSHIP IN NURSING EDUCATION

Curriculum Development

Professional, statutory, and regulatory bodies (PSRBs) often require wide stakeholder engagement in curriculum development. Utilising democratic leadership in curriculum design and evaluation, educators can involve students, practice learning partners, and people who provide services and carers in the development of course content, objectives, and assessment methods. Students and people who provide services and carers' feedback solicited through surveys, focus groups, or open forums ensure that the curriculum remains relevant and aligned with the needs of learners and the healthcare industry (Billings & Halstead, 2024). This participatory approach not only enhances the quality of the curriculum but also fosters a sense of ownership among students. When students feel that their input is valued, they are more likely to engage actively in their education and strive for excellence (Svinicki & McKeachie, 2014).

Classroom Environment

In the classroom, democratic leadership manifests through interactive teaching strategies that encourage active student participation. For example, nursing educators may implement simulated role-playing exercises where students take on various healthcare roles to solve patient care scenarios, promoting teamwork and practical application of knowledge. Similarly, incorporating peer-led discussions enables students to share insights and learn collaboratively, fostering a deeper understanding of complex topics. Using case-based learning allows students to openly debate and propose solutions, leading to more engaged and reflective learners. These examples demonstrate how democratic teaching methods can effectively bridge theoretical concepts with real-world applications. By engaging students in meaningful discussions about ethical dilemmas, patient care scenarios, and healthcare policies, they encourage learners to develop their analytical skills and consider multiple perspectives. Nursing educators who adopt a democratic leadership style also emphasise critical thinking and self-reflection.

Leadership Development

One of the primary goals of democratic leadership in nursing education is to prepare students for leadership roles within the healthcare system. By modelling democratic principles, nursing educators instil values such as collaboration, ethical decision-making, and inclusivity in their students. Leadership development programmes, workshops, and simulation exercises can further enhance students' ability to lead effectively in clinical and organisational settings (Grossman & Valiga, 2021).

BENEFITS AND CHALLENGES OF DEMOCRATIC LEADERSHIP IN NURSING EDUCATION

Students' learning can benefit from democratic leadership as it creates an engaging and interactive learning environment that promotes critical thinking, problem-solving, and knowledge retention. When students actively participate in their education, they are more likely to internalise concepts and apply them effectively in clinical practice. By involving students in decision-making, democratic leadership empowers them to take an active role in their learning journey. This empowerment fosters independence, self-confidence, and a sense of responsibility, which are essential attributes for successful nursing professionals.

While democratic leadership offers some benefits, it also presents certain challenges. For example, the participatory nature of this leadership style can sometimes lead to delays in decision-making as consensus-building requires significant time and effort. Additionally, some students or novice educators may feel hesitant to voice their opinions due to fear of judgment or lack of confidence in their contributions. Nursing educators have addressed these issues by establishing clear guidelines for discussions and encouraging a culture of psychological safety and inclusivity where all perspectives are respected. The use of anonymous time-sensitive surveys can also mitigate delays while ensuring inclusive participation (Huber, 2018).

Democratic leadership is an approach that has significant implications for nursing education. By prioritising collaboration, inclusivity, and empowerment, this leadership style enhances student learning, fosters professional development, and prepares students for leadership roles in healthcare. Despite its challenges, the benefits of democratic leadership far outweigh the drawbacks, making it an essential component of modern nursing education. By embracing democratic principles, nursing educators can cultivate a new generation of compassionate, competent, and collaborative nursing professionals who are well-equipped to meet the demands of a dynamic and evolving healthcare system.

AUTOCRATIC LEADERSHIP

DEFINITION AND FEATURES

Autocratic leadership, sometimes known as authoritarian leadership, is a style characterised by centralised decision-making, strict control, and a clear hierarchy. In this approach, leaders maintain significant authority and typically do not involve junior staff, students, or wider stakeholders in decision-making processes. While often viewed critically, autocratic leadership has specific contexts where it can be effective, particularly in settings requiring quick decision-making or adherence to strict protocols or compliance requirements. While PSRBs require observance of standards of education and proficiency/competency attainment, the curriculum design can be interpreted by the educational institution for necessary approval. The autocratic approach would typically utilise senior educators experienced in curriculum development to design the curriculum with minimal collaboration. In nursing education, this style of leadership does not require the involvement of stakeholders, which could be contradictory to most PSRB guidance.

An autocratic teaching approach is more teacher-expert-led and would rely less on student participation unless they were instructed to do so. There is also likely to be a more hierarchical or power dynamic between the educator and student, which could result in more passive learning.

The following key features are evident in autocratic leadership:

- *Centralised Authority:* Decision-making is concentrated in the faculty or school leadership team. The institution's administration teams follow clear protocols.

- *Limited Collaboration*: Junior faculty or school staff and students are typically not involved in discussions or decisions. Some evaluative feedback might be sought as part of centralised quality assurance processes (Northouse, 2021).

- *Clear Expectations:* Leaders set precise objectives, instructions, policies, and procedures that must be followed.

- *Strict Supervision:* Close monitoring of tasks and performance is a hallmark of this leadership approach (Cherry & Jacob, 2023).

- *Focus on Efficiency:* Autocratic leadership prioritises achieving goals quickly and effectively, often at the expense of inclusivity.

IMPLEMENTATION OF AUTOCRATIC LEADERSHIP IN NURSING EDUCATION

The effective use of autocratic leadership in nursing education largely depends on the context and the way it is implemented.

Curriculum Enforcement

An autocratic leadership style might be observed in cases where nursing education institutions implement new policies or curriculum changes. For example, during the adoption of stricter accreditation standards, the faculty or school leadership team may adopt an authoritarian approach to ensure compliance. By clearly outlining requirements and enforcing adherence, leaders can successfully transition the institution to meet new benchmarks, albeit with limited input from faculty or school staff, students, and practice partners.

Clinical Simulation or Emergency Protocol Training

In a clinical simulation setting, an autocratic approach may be necessary to ensure safety and order. For instance, a nursing educator may take full control during a high-fidelity simulation exercise involving a medical emergency. By issuing clear commands and supervising closely, the nursing educator ensures that the simulation progresses smoothly and that students learn to respond promptly to critical situations. During emergency protocol training, an autocratic leadership style can prove effective in teaching students how to handle real-world crises. A nursing educator might use direct commands to instruct students on performing tasks such as CPR or managing patient triage. This strict approach ensures that students understand the critical importance of following established protocols accurately and efficiently.

BENEFITS AND CHALLENGES OF AUTOCRATIC LEADERSHIP IN NURSING EDUCATION

The key benefits of autocratic leadership are clarity of roles, responsibilities, and expectations of educators and students. Junior staff will be led and guided by more experienced senior staff, and students will be given instruction and direction throughout their course of study. Autocratic leadership enables swift and decisive action, and this, coupled with strict oversight, can ensure consistent clinical standards and compliance with protocols and PSRB requirements.

Table 3.4   Democratic Leadership vs. Autocratic Leadership

Principles of democratic leadership	Features of autocratic leadership
Inclusivity	Focus on efficiency
Collaboration	Limited collaboration
Empowerment	Strict supervision
Transparency	Clearly set expectations
Flexibility	Centralised authority

While autocratic leadership offers some benefits, it also presents certain challenges. The exclusion of junior educators and students from decision-making practices can lead to disengagement, resistance, and a lack of ownership over educational processes. It can also reduce teaching creativity and innovation and limit critical thinking, an essential component of nursing education.

While there is a place for autocratic leadership in nursing education, teams should consider integrating elements of other leadership approaches to foster a more balanced and adaptive learning environment. For example, after a clinical simulated autocratic session, the nursing educator could encourage a reflective discussion to analyse the experience and gather student feedback. This hybrid approach combines the efficiency of autocratic leadership with the inclusivity of democratic practices. See Table 3.4 which outlines the differences between democratic and autocratic leadership styles. By understanding the appropriate contexts and complementing the autocratic leadership approach with more inclusive leadership styles, nursing educators can utilise the strengths of autocratic leadership without compromising the quality of the student experience.

LEADERSHIP IN INNOVATION

INNOVATIVE LEADERSHIP

Innovative leadership in nursing education refers to the ability of leaders to foster an environment that encourages creativity, challenges traditional norms, critical thinking, and seeks evidence-based developments to improve the quality and effectiveness of nursing education. This type of leadership is not just about managing resources and staff but about envisioning new possibilities, using creativity to address complex challenges, and inspiring others to contribute to transformative change. An innovative leader in nursing education actively supports a culture of continuous learning, collaboration, and adaptability, all while prioritising patient-centred care and improving nursing practice.

Key traits of innovative leaders in nursing education include:

- *Visionary Thinking:* They look beyond the current state of nursing education and anticipate future trends.

- *Flexibility:* They adapt to changes in the healthcare environment, curriculum, pedagogic practices, and technology.

- *Collaboration:* They work with staff, students, healthcare professionals, and other stakeholders to generate new ideas and solutions.

- *Empowerment:* They encourage staff and students to take risks, challenge assumptions, and experiment with novel approaches.

STRATEGIES FOR INNOVATION IN NURSING EDUCATION

To foster innovation in nursing education, leaders can employ various strategies:

- *Encourage Creative Thinking:* Leaders can create a culture that values creative problem-solving by providing an open and inclusive space where staff, stakeholders, and students feel able to share ideas and even trial new pedagogical approaches to teaching and learning. Impact evaluation, using a model such as the Kirkpatrick Framework, should be conducted (Heydari et al., 2019; Lee et al., 2024).

- *Assist Development of Teaching Approaches:* Leaders can support staff in learning how to effectively use a range of pedagogic approaches and new teaching tools. These could include simulation-based, virtual reality (VR) and augmented reality (AR) learning. The promotion of interprofessional learning between nursing students and other healthcare professionals not only cultivates an interdisciplinary perspective on patient-centred healthcare, but it can also enhance knowledge and skills, improve communication, teamwork, and collaborative practices.

- *Build a Collaborative Environment:* Leaders can facilitate collaboration and create opportunities for partnership working among staff, students, and healthcare professionals to co-design curriculum. The engagement of technology companies and research institutions would drive innovation and the integration of real-world advancements into nursing curricula.

- *Advocate Evidence-based Practice:* Leaders can encourage staff and students to engage with and participate in nursing education practice research to enable practices to develop. Staff will need support for ongoing professional development.

- *Incorporate Advanced Technologies:* Leaders can promote the use of digital advances and technology in teaching practices. Delivery of teaching through online learning platforms for flexibility, integration of artificial intelligence (AI) for personalised learning, and use of data analytics for insights into curriculum effectiveness and student progression.

EXAMPLES OF INNOVATION IN NURSING EDUCATION

Simulation-based Learning

Nursing programmes have increasingly adopted simulation methods that mirror authentic clinical scenarios. The simulated environment can include high-fidelity manikins or the use of actors or people who use services and carers in role-play scenarios. This approach allows students to practice skills in a safe and controlled environment (Dolan et al., 2021). They may be core clinical skills or complex multidimensional healthcare scenarios. Preparation needs to include scenario planning, equipment set-up, and clear learning objectives. Complex and challenging scenarios must include debrief approaches. Effective simulations promote decision-making, teamwork and clinical judgment, and opportunity to reflect on learning (Alshehri et al., 2023).

Interprofessional Learning

Leaders can encourage interprofessional learning (IPL) opportunities to prepare nursing students for the variety of settings they will encounter throughout their professional practice. A key benefit of IPL is that it fosters collaboration between nursing students and students from other healthcare disciplines (allied health, medicine, pharmacy, and social work).

Use of Digital Technologies

Virtual reality (VR) and augmented reality (AR) approaches are being used to create immersive clinical learning experiences (Foronda et al., 2020). This digital approach has the flexibility to transport students to different healthcare settings without the need for physical resources such as simulation suites. They can be pre-programmed to include biological data, the latest care interventions, a range of medications, and authentic responses to interventions, i.e. positive response to medications or if deteriorating vital sign data is not responded to effectively, the patient could collapse.

Gamification

The use of interactive platforms and audience response systems like Kahoot!, Slido, and Mentimeter, that incorporate game-based learning strategies, can make education more interactive and engaging. Similarly, serious gaming applications are being used to reinforce nursing concepts (Tavares, 2022).

Leaders who utilise these strategies and implement these types of examples into nursing education can help promote a culture of innovation that leads to better-quality learning for students, improved healthcare outcomes, and enhanced patient care practices.

INNOVATION BOX

Title: *Embedding Collaborative Innovation: The Curriculum Sprint Approach*

A growing number of nursing faculties are adopting the 'Curriculum Sprint' model to co-create innovative educational content quickly and collaboratively. Inspired by agile design methods, this approach brings together educators, students, people who use services, and practice partners for short, intensive design workshops focused on a specific learning challenge. For example, one sprint at a UK university brought together mental health nurses and people with lived experience to co-develop a new interprofessional teaching resource on trauma-informed care. Feedback was instantly incorporated, and the tool was piloted within six weeks. This model promotes distributed leadership, inclusive innovation, and rapid curriculum enhancement grounded in real-world need.

A good example is -

Donaghy, P., Gillies, C., & McCann, N. (2023). Using a digital escape room to engage first-year pre-registration nursing students in evidence-based practice learning: a case study. *Journal of Learning Development in Higher Education*, (27). https://journal.aldinhe.ac.uk/index.php/jldhe/article/view/1003/737

THE CONCEPT OF LEARNERSHIP IN NURSING EDUCATION

DEFINITION AND IMPORTANCE

Learnership is a concept that encompasses the diverse ways students can acquire knowledge, skills, and behaviours emphasised through the integration of theoretical education with practical experience into a cohesive educational framework resulting in qualification. In the context of nursing education, this approach ensures that nursing students develop essential clinical competencies, critical thinking abilities, and the professional conduct necessary for safe and effective practice (Hays & Reinders, 2018). Learnership not only facilitates knowledge acquisition but also aids the development of crucial personal skills, such as adaptability, reflective practice, problem solving, compassion, and interpersonal communication. Given the ever-evolving landscape of health and social care, it is particularly important that nurses be proficient in clinical skills, underpinned by an understanding of the ethical, cultural, and social dimensions of care and its leadership. By focusing on creating compassionate and reflective practitioners, learnership supports the development of nursing professionals capable of critical analysis and ethical decision-making in complex health and social care environments.

LEARNERSHIP PATHWAYS IN UK NURSING EDUCATION

By integrating theoretical learning with experiential learning through placements or work-based learning via apprenticeships, nursing education ensures that students can apply theoretical knowledge to real-world scenarios, facilitating deeper understanding and retention of essential skills (Mills et al., 2020). Nursing and Midwifery Council (NMC) education programmes are mandated to combine theoretical learning with diverse practice-based experiences, ensuring that students acquire both the knowledge and practical expertise needed for professional registration (NMC, 2025a). The concept of learnership is particularly relevant in this context, as it aligns with the competency-based approach underpinning UK nursing education. There are three main nursing learnership pathways in the UK:

1. *Pre-registration Direct Entry*

   Pre-registration direct entry programmes are designed for individuals who wish to become registered nurses. These programmes involve a 50/50 split between theoretical learning and practice. Students spend half of their time in academic settings, learning for example, nursing theory, professionalism, ethics, public health, care delivery, research, leadership, collaborative practice, and healthcare technologies, and the other half in various healthcare environments, applying the knowledge and skills and gaining hands-on experience through placements (NMC, 2025a).

2. *Post-registration Direct Entry*

   Post-registration programmes are designed for registered nurses who wish to specialise further. NMC programmes include Specialist Community Public Health Nursing (SCPHN), Specialist Practice Qualifications (SPQ), and prescribing qualifications, but there are also others such as General Practice Nursing, Advanced Nurse Practitioners (ANPs) as well as CPD opportunities. Students in these programmes are employed in healthcare settings and undertake practical and/or theoretical components to enhance their expertise in specific areas of nursing practice.

3. *Apprenticeships for Pre- and Post-registration*

   In England, apprenticeships are the most recent introduction within the healthcare education system. Programmes remain compliant to relevant education standards such as those by the NMC, like direct entry, but as employer-led programmes, they allow non-registrants to train as nurses, and registrants to train in specialist practice (e.g. district nurses, health visitors) or advanced practice (e.g. ANPs) while working in clinical or community settings, with study components provided by a partner higher education institution. This model ensures that apprentices develop both academic knowledge and practical skills simultaneously, like direct entry courses, but with several key benefits:

   o Employer sponsorship reduces financial barriers for learners
   o A focus on workforce development allows employers to address staffing and skills shortages while supporting career progression for their staff; and
   o Apprentices are more likely to be loyal to the organisation that invested in them, resulting in improved staff satisfaction and retention.

DEVELOPING A CULTURE OF LEARNERSHIP IN NURSING EDUCATION

To develop a culture of learnership, nursing curricula must be designed to integrate both theoretical and practice-based learning while ensuring high-quality support mechanisms. Collaborative learning environments that promote peer interaction, mentorship, and high-quality practice supervision alongside academic personal tutorship are essential for fostering a sense of belonging, confidence, and competence among nursing students (Dowling et al., 2021; Flott et al., 2022; Hill, 2024). These environments enable greater engagement and collaboration, significantly enhancing the educational experience by providing support systems that encourage safe exploration and critical reflection on learning and practice.

Moreover, integrating diverse practice experiences, such as hub and spoke or elective placements as well as service-learning opportunities, such as observational placements or volunteering has been shown to improve not only clinical competence but also social justice awareness among students (Scheffer et al., 2019; Emrani et al., 2024). By learning or volunteering in community and PIVO services that address health disparities and societal challenges, nursing students can develop a more empathetic approach to patient care, reinforcing the ethical dimensions of their profession.

Additionally, nursing programmes that focus on innovative teaching methodologies, including simulation-based, digital, immersive, and interprofessional learning, are essential for enhancing the pedagogical skills of nursing educators (Felton & Wright, 2017; Semple & Currie, 2022; Donaghy et al., 2023; Bruce et al., 2024). By equipping nursing educators with the tools to facilitate enhanced active learning, institutions can create a more dynamic and responsive learning environment that aligns with the principles of transformative education. This, in turn, can foster a stronger culture of learnership among nursing students who will benefit from increased engagement and more meaningful educational experiences.

IMPACT OF LEARNERSHIP ON LEARNING OUTCOMES AND PROFESSIONAL DEVELOPMENT

Effective implementation of learnership leads to improved learning outcomes for nursing students, including enhanced critical thinking skills, greater clinical judgment, and increased readiness for practice. Students exposed to high-quality learnership opportunities report higher levels of satisfaction with their education, which correlates with better emotional and psychological well-being during their studies (Dursun Ergezen et al., 2022; Cant et al., 2023). By promoting a holistic approach that encompasses both cognitive and emotional growth, learnership supports the formation of well-rounded nursing professionals who are prepared to tackle the complexities of contemporary health and social care. The broader implications of learnership extend beyond individual student success to the nursing profession. Enhanced competencies and leadership abilities among nursing graduates contribute to improved patient care outcomes and foster a culture of continual practice improvement (Mills et al., 2020). As nursing roles become more multidisciplinary and integrated into broader health and social care systems, the ability to navigate complex interactions and contribute to team-based care becomes paramount (Hays & Reinders, 2018).

LEARNERSHIP OF EDUCATORS

Nursing educators typically transition from clinical practice, bringing with them a wealth of professional experience. However, adapting to academia often presents challenges related to role identity and the acquisition of new educative skills (Cantillon et al., 2019; Halton et al., 2024). Many new nursing educators in higher education report feeling unprepared for aspects of their academic role, including classroom management, student engagement, and assessment (Wilkinson, 2020). These challenges can contribute to imposter syndrome, impacting confidence and professional development.

Supporting the transition into academia requires both formal and informal mechanisms (Dickinson & Griffiths, 2022). Structured induction programmes, mentoring, and peer support networks help early-career academics navigate the complexities of their new roles. Additionally, professional development programmes, such as Postgraduate Certificates in Academic Practice, provide educators with pedagogical training and opportunities to engage in Communities of Practice (CoPs), which foster collaboration and peer support (Mulholland et al., 2023). The formal Post-Graduate Certificate in Academic Practice enables pedagogic knowledge and skills, and the opportunity to develop COP.

Developing nursing educators who are not only knowledgeable but also passionate about teaching and learning is crucial. When nursing educators actively engage in reflective practice and continuous professional development, they serve as role models for students, instilling a commitment to lifelong learning and professional growth. By embedding learnership principles within academic development strategies, institutions can ensure that both students and educators thrive in an ever-evolving healthcare education landscape.

ENSURING QUALITY, REGULATION, AND ACCREDITATION IN NURSING EDUCATION

QUALITY ASSURANCE

Ensuring quality in nursing education is fundamental to producing competent and confident practitioners. For nursing academics, quality assurance involves aligning and maintaining curricula with professional standards, such as those set by the Nursing and Midwifery Council (NMC), and cultivating an environment that supports academic excellence. This includes regular curriculum reviews, learning environment audits, peer evaluations, scrutiny of data, and integrating stakeholder feedback to continuously improve teaching and learning outcomes.

A good place to start with enhancing quality assurance practice is through collaborative staff workshops focused on evidence-based teaching and learning strategies. These workshops promote shared understanding of quality standards and benchmarks and encourage innovative approaches to curriculum design. Moreover, establishing clear metrics for assessing academic rigor, such as alignment with evidence-based practices and measurable student outcomes, ensures that both academics and students are consistently achieving high standards of performance. This integration of rigorous standards directly supports the development of resilient, practice-ready graduates who excel in diverse healthcare settings (Abou Hashish et al., 2025).

REGULATORY AND ACCREDITATION REQUIREMENTS

Programme regulatory approval or professional accreditation ensures nursing programmes meet established benchmarks for quality and rigor. Educator leaders play a crucial role in preparing for regulatory and accreditation processes, which involve coordinating documentation, ensuring staff development, and demonstrating the programme's alignment with relevant standards. Developing and securing approval for regulated nursing programmes in the UK requires strict adherence to the Nursing and Midwifery Council (NMC) (2025a) standards and the Quality Assurance Agency (QAA) for Higher Education (2025) framework. Both accreditation and regulation ensure that nursing programmes produce professionals who are professionally confident and competent, ethically sound, and equipped to deliver safe, evidence-based, and compassionate care across a variety of settings.

Each NMC programme must align with its specific NMC standard education framework and standard of proficiencies to ensure graduates meet the required competencies, professional values, and patient safety expectations (Nursing and Midwifery Council, 2025b). The NMC updates from 2018 through to 2024 introduced revised competency requirements for Registered Nurses (Nursing and Midwifery Council, 2018a), Nursing Associates (Nursing and Midwifery Council, 2018b), Specialist Community Public Health Nurses (SCPHNs) (Nursing and Midwifery Council, 2022b) and Specialist Practitioner Qualifications (SPQs) (Nursing and Midwifery Council, 2022a), alongside updated prescribing education guidelines (Nursing and Midwifery Council, 2021). These changes reflect the evolving healthcare landscape, with a stronger emphasis on public health, digital literacy, interprofessional education, and safeguarding policies.

The NMC's programme approval and monitoring processes ensure that nursing education remains consistent, high-quality, and aligned with professional standards. Programme approval is not just a regulatory requirement but a mechanism for safeguarding educational quality, cultivating a culture of excellence, and promoting continuous enhancement (Abou Hashish et al., 2025). Modification also plays a vital role in supporting innovation and continuous quality improvement. Beyond meeting minimum standards, institutions should use modification as an opportunity to enhance curriculum design, integrate emerging technologies, and strengthen clinical partnerships (Halstead, 2020). By embedding a culture of quality enhancement, nursing programmes can remain agile, evidence-informed, and future-ready.

Performance Review

Quality assurance in regulated nursing education extends beyond programme approval to ongoing performance review processes that ensure continued alignment with NMC standards. The NMC Annual Self-Assessment Report (ASAR) is a key component of this review, requiring higher education institutions (HEIs) to evaluate their programmes' effectiveness, regulatory compliance, and student outcomes. The ASAR provides an opportunity to assess programme performance against key indicators such as retention rates, student feedback, practice placement evaluations, and graduate employment outcomes. This process enables institutions to identify strengths, address areas for improvement, and implement evidence-based enhancements.

In addition to annual self-assessment, Exceptional Reporting is required when significant issues arise that may impact programme quality or student experience. This may include concerns related to the practice learning environment, regulatory non-compliance, or significant changes to faculty staffing. Institutions must report these concerns to the NMC promptly and outline action plans for resolution. Exceptional reporting ensures transparency and enables proactive intervention to maintain programme integrity and student safety.

Stakeholder Coproduction in Nursing Education

Effective programme coproduction requires early and ongoing engagement with learners, alumni, practice learning and employer partners, people who use services and carers, academic and professional services staff, and wider professional networks. This collaborative approach ensures programmes are transparent, practice-relevant and aligned with both academic and patient needs while also meeting professional standards such as NMC (Kang et al., 2018; Sezer & Şahin, 2021).

Establishing a Programme Advisory Panel (PAP) with key representatives from each group structures stakeholder involvement. At a minimum, this should occur at three key stages:

1. *Initial Consultation:* A stakeholder event should establish the programme vision, key learning outcomes, and workforce needs. Expectations should be clearly defined, and any standards reviewed to ensure alignment with professional, regulatory, and/or accreditation requirements.

2. *Midway Review:* Stakeholders should review draft curriculum content, assessment models, and any work-based learning and/or placement structures. Pilot-testing new elements with existing learners, such as digital learning tools and simulation-based assessments, can help refine the programme before finalisation.

3. *Pre-approval Review:* Before formal validation, approval, or accreditation, a final review session should take place to secure stakeholder agreement with the final programme. This process ensures the programme remains aligned with workforce demands and evolving healthcare priorities.

Stakeholder coproduction is equally vital in performance review activities, particularly in the NMC Annual Self-Assessment Report (ASAR) process. Engaging students, employers and practice learning partners, people who use services and carers, and academic colleagues in reflective reviews of programme effectiveness strengthens the accuracy and relevance of self-assessment reporting. This participatory approach ensures that performance reviews are not merely compliance exercises but opportunities for genuine quality enhancement. Additionally, stakeholders can contribute to exceptional reporting by identifying risks early and collaboratively designing intervention strategies. By embedding structured feedback loops, such as student evaluation panels, practice placement advisory boards, and employer roundtables, HEIs can proactively identify and address challenges before they escalate to formal exceptional reports.

Diverse stakeholder coproduction also plays a vital role in fostering equity, diversity, and inclusion (EDI). Nursing curricula must integrate learning in cultural safety, unconscious bias awareness, and inclusive healthcare (Kang et al., 2018). Ensuring the curriculum explicitly addresses health disparities, social determinants of health, and cultural competence training strengthens the profession's ability to deliver equitable care.

ACTIVITY BOX

Title: *Leadership Style Self-Audit and Peer Dialogue*

Activity: Mapping Your Leadership Identity in Education
Reflect on your own educational leadership practices. Using the four leadership styles discussed in this chapter, complete the following:

- Which leadership style do you most naturally adopt in your teaching, programme design, or team interactions?

- Identify a real example where this style was effective and another where it presented challenges.

- What style do you least identify with, and why?

- In pairs or small groups, discuss how blending elements of multiple styles may offer a more flexible and context-sensitive leadership approach.

Extension
Map your leadership evolution over the past 12 months using a reflective timeline. What changed, and why? What impact did this have on your students or team?

CONTINUOUS QUALITY IMPROVEMENT

Maintaining the integrity and reputation of nursing education institutions requires a strong commitment to accountability and continuous improvement. Regulation and accreditation serve as critical drivers of ongoing evaluation and enhancement in nursing education, ensuring that programmes align with professional standards and remain responsive to the evolving healthcare landscape (Abou Hashish et al., 2025). One effective strategy for achieving this is conducting internal mock approval or validation events. Engaging external reviewers, practice learning partners, employer representatives, and academic quality assurance teams in these events helps identify areas for refinement before formal submission, strengthening the programme's compliance and quality (Halstead, 2020).

To ensure continued relevance and compliance, all approved and validated programmes must undergo regular review processes. Continuous Quality Improvement (CQI) mechanisms integrate real-time stakeholder feedback, address changes in healthcare practice, and help maintain curricula that are responsive to workforce needs (Ard et al., 2017b). A key component of this process is curriculum mapping, which systematically identifies course redundancy, curriculum creep, knowledge gaps, and areas requiring enhancement (Neville-Norton & Cantwell, 2019). Effective curriculum mapping ensures that all learning outcomes are explicitly aligned with mandated proficiencies, competencies, and essential subject content. The use of curriculum mapping tools allows programme teams to maintain coherence and alignment across courses, assessments

and practice expectations, and supports a structured and evidence-based educational approach.

Reflective practice is central to both nursing education and academic professional growth. Just as structured reflective assessments and debriefing strategies in placements encourage students to engage in continuous self-evaluation, critical thinking, and decision-making, similar reflective practices enhance the quality assurance processes of educator staff. Embedding self-assessment, structured debriefing, and peer feedback mechanisms allows educators to critically evaluate their quality assurance experiences and refine their approaches (Sezer & Şahin, 2021).

Additionally, given the increasing demand for placements and the pressures on the healthcare workforce, it is essential that nursing programmes establish strong, long-term agreements with their practice learning partners such as NHS Trusts, social care providers, and community health services (Ard et al., 2017a). Formalising Memorandums of Understanding (MOUs) or Practice Placement Agreements (PPAs) with providers ensures access to sustainable, high-quality placements. These agreements not only reinforce strong industry partnerships but also contribute to the long-term success of nursing programmes by ensuring students receive diverse, high-quality experiential learning opportunities.

By embedding rigorous quality assurance mechanisms, fostering collaborative stakeholder engagement, and maintaining robust monitoring and improvement processes, nursing education programmes can uphold excellence and remain fit for purpose within an evolving healthcare landscape.

KEY TAKE-HOME POINTS

1. Leadership styles such as transformational and servant leadership can create supportive and empowering educational environments that promote resilience, inclusivity, and innovation.

2. Innovative practices, including simulation, VR, and interprofessional learning, enhance engagement and support preparation for complex healthcare environments.

3. Quality assurance, accreditation, and learnership are central to ensuring that both nursing students and educators develop the competencies needed to meet evolving healthcare demands.

CPD REFLECTIVE QUESTIONS

1. How can I apply transformational or servant leadership principles in my teaching or team leadership role?

2. In what ways does my current practice support or limit innovation in nursing education, and what changes could I implement?

3. How do I contribute to quality assurance or regulatory processes, and how could I further enhance these contributions in my academic role?

REFERENCES

Abou Hashish, E. A., Alnajjar, H., & Rawas, H. (2025). Voices on academic accreditation: lived experiences of nurse educators, administrators, students, and alumni in nursing education. *BMC Medical Education*, 25(1), 64. https://doi.org/10.1186/s12909-025-06657-2.

Afsar, B., & Masood, M. (2018). Transformational leadership, creative self-efficacy, trust in supervisor, uncertainty avoidance, and innovative work behavior of nurses. *The Journal of Applied Behavioral Science*, 54(1), 36–61. https://doi.org/10.1177/0021886317711891.

Alshehri, F. D., Jones, S., & Harrison, D. (2023). The effectiveness of high-fidelity simulation on undergraduate nursing students' clinical reasoning-related skills: a systematic review. *Nurse Education Today*, 121, 105679. https://doi.org/10.1016/j.nedt.2022.105679.

Ard, N., Beasley, S., & Nunn-Ellison, K. (2017a). Accreditation commission for education in nursing: your supportive partner in successful nursing accreditation. *Teaching and Learning in Nursing*, 12(4), 234–236. https://doi.org/10.1016/j.teln.2017.06.002.

Ard, N., Beasley, S., & Nunn-Ellison, K. (2017b). Quality education through accreditation. *Teaching and Learning in Nursing*, 12(2), 85–87. https://doi.org/10.1016/j.teln.2017.01.007.

Bass, B. M. (1985). *Leadership and Performance Beyond Expectations.* New York: Free Press.

Billings, D. M., & Halstead, J. A. (2024). *Teaching in Nursing: A Guide for Faculty* (7th ed.). St. Louis: Elsevier.

Boamah, S. A. (2022). The impact of transformational leadership on nurse faculty satisfaction and burnout during the COVID-19 pandemic: a moderated mediated analysis. *Journal of Advanced Nursing*, 78(9), 2815–2826. https://doi.org/10.1111/jan.15198.

Bruce, T. A., Flynn, D., Simpson, D., Peat, A., & Hill, B. (2024). Innovations in nurse education: creating the multisensory learning approach of The WISE Room. *British Journal of Nursing*, 33(15), 726–733. https://doi.org/10.12968/bjon.2024.0103.

Cant, R., Gazula, S., & Ryan, C. (2023). Predictors of nursing student satisfaction as a key quality indicator of tertiary students' education experience: an integrative review. *Nurse Education Today*, 126, 105806. https://doi.org/10.1016/j.nedt.2023.105806.

Cantillon, P., Dornan, T., & De Grave, W. (2019). Becoming a clinical teacher: identity formation in context. *Academic Medicine: Journal of the Association of American Medical Colleges*, 94(10), 1610–1618. https://doi.org/10.1097/ACM.0000000000002403.

Cherry, B., & Jacob, S. R. (eds.) (2023). *Contemporary Nursing: Issues, Trends, & Management* (9th ed.). St. Louis: Elsevier.

Delgado, C., & Mitchell, M. M. (2016). A survey of current valued academic leadership qualities in nursing. *Nursing Education Perspectives*, 37(1), 10. https://doi.org/10.5480/14-1496.

Dickinson, J., Fowler, A., & Griffiths, T. -L. (2022). Pracademics? Exploring transitions and professional identities in higher education. *Studies in Higher Education*, 47(2), 290–304. https://doi.org/10.1080/03075079.2020.1744123.

Dolan, H., Amidon, B. J., & Gephart, S. M. (2021). Evidentiary and theoretical foundations for virtual simulation in nursing education. *Journal of Professional Nursing: Official Journal of the American Association of Colleges of Nursing*, 37(5), 810–815. https://doi.org/10.1016/j.profnurs.2021.06.001.

Donaghy, P., Gillies, C., & McCann, N. (2023). Using a digital escape room to engage first year pre-registration nursing students in evidence-based practice learning: a case study. *Journal of Learning Development in Higher Education* [Preprint], 27. https://doi.org/10.47408/jldhe.vi27.1003.

Dowling, T., Metzger, M., & Kools, S. (2021). Cultivating inclusive learning environments that foster nursing education program resiliency during the Covid-19 pandemic. *Journal of Professional Nursing*, 37(5), 942–947. https://doi.org/10.1016/j.profnurs.2021.07.010.

Dursun Ergezen, F., Akcan, A., & Kol, E. (2022). Nursing students' expectations, satisfaction, and perceptions regarding clinical learning environment: a cross-sectional, profile study from Turkey. *Nurse Education in Practice*, 61, 103333. https://doi.org/10.1016/j.nepr.2022.103333.

Emrani, M., Khoshnood, Z., Farokhzadian, J., & Sadeghi, M. (2024). The effect of service-based learning on health education competencies of students in community health nursing internships. *BMC Nursing*, 23, 138. https://doi.org/10.1186/s12912-024-01799-y.

Felton, A., & Wright, N. (2017). Simulation in mental health nurse education: the development, implementation and evaluation of an educational innovation. *Nurse Education in Practice*, 26, 46–52. https://doi.org/10.1016/j.nepr.2017.06.005.

Fischer, S. A. (2016). Transformational leadership in nursing: a concept analysis. *Journal of Advanced Nursing*, 72(11), 2644–2653. https://doi.org/10.1111/jan.13049.

Flott, E., Ball, S., Hanks, J., Minnich, M., Kirkpatrick, A., Rusch, L., Koziol, D., Laughlin, A., & Williams, J. (2022). Fostering collaborative learning and leadership through near-peer mentorship among undergraduate nursing students. *Nursing Forum*, 57(5), 750–755. https://doi.org/10.1111/nuf.12755.

Foronda, C. L., Fernandez-Burgos, M., Nadeau, C., Kelley, C. N., & Henry, M. N. (2020). Virtual simulation in nursing education: a systematic review spanning 1996 to 2018. *Simulation in Healthcare: Journal of the Society for Simulation in Healthcare*, 15(1), 46–54. https://doi.org/10.1097/SIH.0000000000000411.

Greenleaf, R. K. (2002). *Servant Leadership: A Journey into the Nature of Legitimate Power and Greatness*. Paulist Press.

Greenway, M., & Acai, A. (2024). Academic leadership in nursing: a concept analysis. *Nurse Education Today*, 141, 106338. https://doi.org/10.1016/j.nedt.2024.106338.

Grossman, S., & Valiga, T. M. (2021). *The New Leadership Challenge: Creating the Future of Nursing* (6th ed.). Philadelphia: F.A. Davis.

Halstead, J. A. (2020). Fostering innovation in nursing education: the role of accreditation. *Teaching and Learning in Nursing*, 15(1), A4–A5. https://doi.org/10.1016/j.teln.2019.10.003.

Halton, J., Ireland, C., & Vaughan, B. (2024). The transition of clinical nurses to nurse educator roles - a scoping review. *Nurse Education in Practice*, 78, 104022. https://doi.org/10.1016/j.nepr.2024.104022.

Hays, J., & Reinders, H. (2018). Critical learnership: a new perspective on learning. *International Journal of Learning, Teaching and Educational Research*, 17(1), 1–25. https://doi.org/10.26803/ijlter.17.1.1.

Heydari, M. R., Taghva, F., Amini, M., & Delavari, S. (2019). Using Kirkpatrick's model to measure the effect of a new teaching and learning methods workshop for health care staff. *BMC Research Notes*, 12(1), 388. https://doi.org/10.1186/s13104-019-4421-y.

Hill, B. (2024). The importance of belongingness and friendships within the nursing community. *British Journal of Nursing*, 33(6), 310–310. https://doi.org/10.12968/bjon.2024.33.6.310.

Huber, D. L. (ed.) (2018). *Leadership and Nursing Care Management* (6th ed.). St. Louis: Elsevier.

Huston, C. J., & Marquis, B. L. (2024). *Leadership Roles and Management Functions in Nursing: Theory and Application* (11th ed.). Philadelphia: Wolters Kluwer.

Jackson, D. (2008). Servant leadership in nursing: a framework for developing sustainable research capacity in nursing. *Collegian*, 15(1), 27–33. https://doi.org/10.1016/j.colegn.2007.10.001.

Kang, S., Ho, T. T. T., & Nguyen, T. A. P. (2018). Capacity development in an undergraduate nursing program in Vietnam. *Frontiers in Public Health*, 6, 146. https://doi.org/10.3389/fpubh.2018.00146.

Kim, H. -O., Lee, I., & Lee, B. -S. (2022). Nursing leaders' perceptions of the state of nursing leadership and the need for nursing leadership education reform: a qualitative content analysis from South Korea. *Journal of Nursing Management*, 30(7), 2216–2226. https://doi.org/10.1111/jonm.13596.

Lee, M., Shin, S., Lee, M., & Hong, E. (2024). Educational outcomes of digital serious games in nursing education: a systematic review and meta-analysis of randomized controlled trials. *BMC Medical Education*, 24(1), 1458. https://doi.org/10.1186/s12909-024-06464-1.

Mills, A., Ryden, J., & Knight, A. (2020). Juggling to find balance: hearing the voices of undergraduate student nurses. *British Journal of Nursing*, 29(15), 897–903. https://doi.org/10.12968/bjon.2020.29.15.897.

Mrayyan, M. T., & Al-Rjoub, S. (2024). Does nursing leaders' humility leadership associate with nursing team members' psychological safety? A cross-sectional online survey. *Journal of Advanced Nursing*, 80(9), 3666–3678. https://doi.org/10.1111/jan.16117.

Mulholland, K., Nichol, D., & Gillespie, A. (2023). "It feels like you're going back to the beginning...": addressing imposter feelings in early career academics through the creation of communities of practice. *Journal of Further and Higher Education*, 47(1), 89–104. https://doi.org/10.1080/0309877X.2022.2095896.

Neville, K., Conway, K., Maglione, J., Connolly, K. A., Foley, M., & Re, S. (2021). Understanding servant leadership in nursing: a concept analysis. *International Journal for Human Caring*, 25(1), 22–29. https://doi.org/10.20467/HumanCaring-D-20-00022.

Neville-Norton, M., & Cantwell, S. (2019). Curriculum mapping in nursing education: a case study for collaborative curriculum design and program quality assurance. *Teaching and Learning in Nursing*, 14(2), 88–93. https://doi.org/10.1016/j.teln.2018.12.001.

Northouse, P. G. (2021). *Leadership: Theory and Practice* (9th ed.). Thousand Oaks: SAGE Publishing.

Nursing and Midwifery Council (2018a). *Standards of proficiency for registered nurses.* https://www.nmc.org.uk/standards/standards-for-nurses/standards-of-proficiency-for-registered-nurses/ Accessed: (11 March 2025).

Nursing and Midwifery Council (2018b). *Standards of proficiency for registered nursing associates.* https://www.nmc.org.uk/standards/standards-for-nursing-associates/standards-of-proficiency-for-nursing-associates/ Accessed: (11 March 2025).

Nursing and Midwifery Council (2021). *Royal Pharmaceutical Society's competency framework for all prescribers.* https://www.nmc.org.uk/standards/standards-for-post-registration/standards-for-prescribers/royal-pharmaceutical-societys-competency-framework-for-all-prescribers/ Accessed: (11 March 2025).

Nursing and Midwifery Council (2022a). *Standards of proficiency for community nursing specialist practice qualifications (SPQ).* https://www.nmc.org.uk/standards/standards-for-post-registration/standards-of-proficiency-for--community-nursing-specialist-practice-qualifications/ Accessed: (11 March 2025).

Nursing and Midwifery Council (2022b). *Standards of proficiency for specialist community public health nurses (SCPHN).* https://www.nmc.org.uk/standards/standards-for-post-registration/standards-of-proficiency-for-specialist-community-public-health-nurses2/ Accessed: (11 March 2025).

Nursing and Midwifery Council (2025a). *Quality assurance of education.* https://www.nmc.org.uk/education/quality-assurance-of-education/ Accessed: (9 March 2025).

Nursing and Midwifery Council (2025b). *Standards.* https://www.nmc.org.uk/standards/ Accessed: (11 March 2025).

Scheffer, M. M. J., Lasater, K., Atherton, I. M., & Kyle, R. G. (2019). Student nurses' attitudes to social justice and poverty: an international comparison. *Nurse Education Today*, 80, 59–66. https://doi.org/10.1016/j.nedt.2019.06.007.

Semple, L., & Currie, G. (2022). "It opened up a whole new world": An innovative interprofessional learning activity for students caring for children and families. *International Journal of Educational Research Open*, 3, 100106. https://doi.org/10.1016/j.ijedro.2021.100106.

Sezer, H., & Şahin, H. (2021). Faculty development program for coaching in nursing education: a curriculum development process study. *Nurse Education in Practice*, 55, 103165. https://doi.org/10.1016/j.nepr.2021.103165.

Sherman, R. O. (2019). The case for servant leadership. *Nurse Leader*, 17(2), 86–87. https://doi.org/10.1016/j.mnl.2018.12.001.

Spears, L. (1996). Reflections on Robert K. Greenleaf and servant-leadership. *Leadership & Organization Development Journal*, 17(7), 33–35. https://doi.org/10.1108/01437739610148367.

Svinicki, M. D., & McKeachie, W. J. (2014). *McKeachie's Teaching Tips: Strategies, Research, and Theory for College and University Teachers* (14th ed.). Belmont: Wadsworth.

Tavares, N. (2022). The use and impact of game-based learning on the learning experience and knowledge retention of nursing undergraduate students: a systematic literature review. *Nurse Education Today*, 117, 105484. https://doi.org/10.1016/j.nedt.2022.105484.

The Quality Assurance Agency for Higher Education (2025). *Quality assurance for the Nursing and Midwifery Council.* https://www.qaa.ac.uk/nmc Accessed: (9 March 2025).

Todt, K., & Covington, S. (2023). Servant-leadership in nursing education. *International Journal of Servant-Leadership*, 17, 317–337. https://doi.org/10.33972/ijsl.384.

Tropello, P. D., & DeFazio, J. (2014). Servant leadership in nursing administration and academia shaping future generations of nurses and interdisciplinary team providers to transform healthcare delivery. *Nurse Leader*, 12(6), 59–66. https://doi.org/10.1016/j.mnl.2014.09.010.

Tuckman, B. (1965). Developmental sequence in small groups. *Psychological Bulletin*, 63(6), 384–399. https://web.mit.edu/curhan/www/docs/Articles/15341_Readings/Group_Dynamics/Tuckman_1965_Developmental_sequence_in_small_groups.pdf?utm_source=chatgpt.com.

Wilkinson, C. (2020). Imposter syndrome and the accidental academic: an autoethnographic account. *International Journal for Academic Development*, 25(4), 363–374. https://doi.org/10.1080/1360144X.2020.1762087.

Yoder-Wise, P. S., & Sportsman, S. (eds.) (2023). *Leading and Managing in Nursing* (8th ed.). St. Louis: Elsevier.

CHAPTER 4

Ethical and Cultural Competence

Luis Teixeira

Florence Nightingale Faculty of Nursing, Midwifery and Palliative Care, Department of Adult Nursing, King's College London, UK

AIM

To explore the integration of ethical and cultural competence within nursing education and practice, equipping readers with the theoretical foundations, practical strategies, and reflective insights necessary to support inclusive, values-based, and culturally responsive care.

LEARNING OUTCOMES

By the end of this chapter, readers will be able to:

1. Define ethical and cultural competence and explain their significance in contemporary nursing education and clinical practice.

2. Evaluate key ethical theories and cultural competence models relevant to nurse education and professional conduct.

3. Identify challenges and barriers to embedding ethical and cultural competence in curricula, and describe strategies to overcome them.

4. Reflect on how lived experience, mentorship, and institutional support contribute to the development of ethically and culturally competent practitioners.

CHAPTER INTRODUCTION

In a world increasingly marked by cultural diversity, social complexity, and technological advancement, the ethical and cultural dimensions of nursing practice have never been more critical. Nurses today are expected not only to deliver safe and effective clinical care but also to navigate the moral intricacies of healthcare systems and engage sensitively with patients from varied cultural, social, and linguistic backgrounds. As such, fostering ethical and cultural competence in nursing education is no longer a peripheral concern; it is central to shaping nurses who are reflective, inclusive, and professionally accountable in an ever-evolving healthcare landscape.

This chapter explores how nursing education can be a transformative space for cultivating ethical awareness and cultural responsiveness. Ethical competence involves more than knowing codes or principles; it requires critical thinking, moral courage, and the ability to balance professional values with contextual realities. Similarly, cultural competence is not a fixed achievement but a dynamic process, encompassing self-awareness, humility, and a commitment to equitable and person-centred care. Together, these competencies are foundational to delivering healthcare that respects human dignity, promotes social justice, and responds effectively to diverse patient needs.

Throughout this chapter, the integration of ethics and culture within nursing curricula is examined, alongside an exploration of experiential and reflective learning strategies; structural and pedagogical challenges encountered by educators are also addressed. A particular

Transformative Nursing Education, First Edition. Edited by Aby Mitchell and Barry Hill.

emphasis is placed on the promotion of equality and diversity within nursing education, with recognition that ethical and culturally competent practice is shaped within the educational environment. The role of technology in ethics education, the significance of ongoing faculty development, and the persistent tension between theoretical knowledge and practical application are also critically considered.

By bringing together evidence, critical reflection, and pedagogical strategies, this chapter provides a comprehensive exploration of how ethical and cultural competence can be meaningfully embedded within transformative nursing education. It invites educators, students, and practitioners alike to view these competencies not as additional content, but as integral to the mission of nursing and to the future of socially responsive healthcare.

INTEGRATING ETHICS INTO NURSING EDUCATION

Ethical competence is a cornerstone of professional nursing practice, shaping decision-making, patient care, and interprofessional collaboration. Nurses frequently encounter ethical dilemmas, from respecting patient autonomy and confidentiality to addressing end-of-life decisions and ensuring equitable resource allocation (Grace, 2022). Without a robust ethical foundation, nurses may struggle to navigate these challenges, potentially compromising patient care and professional integrity. For this reason, ethics must be comprehensively embedded in nursing education (Teixeira, 2025).

Ethical nursing practice is often framed through principlism, a widely recognised ethical framework that emphasises autonomy, beneficence, non-maleficence, and justice as core principles in healthcare decision-making (Beauchamp & Childress, 2019). These principles provide a framework for decision-making, allowing nurses to balance patient rights, professional responsibilities, and institutional constraints. However, ethical reasoning in nursing extends beyond the application of predefined principles; it requires critical thinking, situational awareness, and the ability to make informed judgments in complex, real-world scenarios (Johnstone, 2019). Given the increasingly multifaceted nature of healthcare, nursing education must ensure that students and practitioners develop the ethical competence necessary to uphold professional values in a rapidly evolving clinical environment.

THEORETICAL FOUNDATIONS OF ETHICS IN NURSING EDUCATION

A well-rounded ethics curriculum in nursing education must introduce students to foundational ethical theories, enabling them to approach dilemmas with a nuanced and critical perspective. Deontology, as articulated by Immanuel Kant, emphasises duty-based decision-making, where actions are guided by moral obligations rather than their outcomes (Kant et al., 2012). In contrast, utilitarianism, developed by John Stuart Mill, prioritises the greatest good for the greatest number, requiring individuals to consider the broader consequences of their actions (Mill, 1863).

Beyond these traditional frameworks, Aristotelian virtue ethics shifts the focus to moral character, advocating for professional virtues such as honesty, integrity, and compassion (Hursthouse, 1999). Meanwhile, the ethics of care, introduced by Carol Gilligan, highlights relational and context-dependent decision-making, emphasising empathy, interconnectedness, and patient-centred responsiveness (Gilligan, 2003). Each of these theories provides valuable insights for nursing practice, allowing students and practitioners to critically assess ethical dilemmas from multiple perspectives and develop well-reasoned approaches to complex situations. See Table 4.1 for a comparison of key ethical theories relevant to nursing education.

Table 4.1 Overview of Ethical Theories in Nursing Education

Ethical theory	Key focus	Application in nursing education
Deontology	Duty and rules	Emphasises professional obligations and ethical codes
Utilitarianism	Outcomes and consequences	Encourages considering patient benefit and harm on a broader scale
Virtue Ethics	Moral character and virtues	Promotes the development of traits like compassion, honesty, and courage
Ethics of Care	Relationships and context	Highlights empathy, care, and interpersonal engagement with patients
Principlism (Bioethics)	Four principles: autonomy, beneficence, non-maleficence, justice	Commonly used framework in clinical reasoning and ethics curriculum

In addition to these theories, bioethics has emerged as a contemporary framework addressing ethical issues at the intersection of health sciences, technology, and society. Rooted in healthcare practice, bioethics applies ethical reasoning to clinical dilemmas, patient rights, and medical advancements. One of its key approaches, principlism, emphasises four core principles—autonomy, beneficence, non-maleficence, and justice—as a structured yet flexible guide for ethical decision making in healthcare (Beauchamp & Childress, 2019). While principlism provides a structured and widely accepted foundation for ethical reasoning (Herring, 2022), it is primarily rooted in Western bioethics, which tends to prioritise individual autonomy and rights-based ethics. However, ethical decision-making in nursing is inherently contextual, influenced by cultural values, social norms, and healthcare systems that may emphasise collectivism, relational ethics, or duty-based moral reasoning. By integrating both classical ethical theories and contemporary bioethical frameworks, nursing education can better promote the development of a nuanced and adaptable ethical foundation—one that supports practitioners in addressing the evolving challenges of contemporary practice.

CHALLENGES IN NURSING ETHICS EDUCATION

Despite its significance, integrating ethics into nursing education presents several challenges. One of the primary difficulties is the subjectivity and cultural variability of ethical dilemmas. Unlike clinical procedures that adhere to standardised, evidence-based guidelines, ethical decision-making is often influenced by individual beliefs, cultural norms, and societal values. A decision that is ethically justifiable in one cultural or institutional context may be perceived differently in another, necessitating an educational approach that promotes open dialogue and critical reflection rather than rigid moral absolutism.

Another persistent challenge is moral distress, which arises when nurses recognise the ethically appropriate action but feel powerless to act due to institutional barriers, hierarchical structures, or legal constraints (Jameton, 2013; Salari et al., 2022). This is particularly relevant for nursing students in clinical placements, where they may witness ethical breaches—such as inadequate pain management or disregard for patient preferences—yet hesitate to challenge authority figures. Without proper guidance and support, students may develop a sense of ethical resignation, leading to moral disengagement and diminished advocacy in their future practices. Addressing this issue requires a nursing curriculum that emphasises patient advocacy, key ethical theories and approaches, and coaching opportunities while in supervised clinical practice, so students are equipped to navigate ethical challenges with confidence and professional integrity.

METHODS FOR INTEGRATING ETHICS INTO NURSING CURRICULA

To foster ethical competence, nursing curricula should integrate theory, experiential learning, and reflective practice in a way that mirrors the complexities of real-world practice environments. Case-based learning has been widely recognised as an effective approach, allowing students to analyse ethical dilemmas drawn from actual clinical cases and develop reasoned responses to ethically ambiguous situations (Teixeira, 2020; Miron & Bricknell, 2024). This method not only reinforces theoretical knowledge but also enhances moral reasoning and ethical decision-making skills.

Similarly, simulation-based education has gained prominence as a valuable tool in ethics education. Role-playing exercises, virtual patient interactions, and high-fidelity simulations provide students with hands-on experiences in ethical decision-making, allowing them to practice responding to challenging scenarios in a controlled and safe environment for learning and growth (Mitchell, 2024). These simulations have been shown to enhance ethical sensitivity, strengthen professional judgment, and improve communication skills, all of which are crucial for ethical nursing practice.

Beyond structure coursework, reflective practice is a key strategy for integrating ethics into nursing education. Encouraging students to engage in self-reflection—whether through journaling, debriefing sessions, or guided ethical discussions—allows them to critically assess their own values, biases, and decision-making processes (Hansen et al., 2024). Indeed, reflection fosters ethical awareness and self-regulation, enabling nursing students and practitioners to incorporate ethical principles in a meaningful and consistent way.

THE ROLE OF PROFESSIONAL STANDARDS AND GUIDELINES

In the United Kingdom, the integration of ethics into nursing education is also guided by regulatory frameworks set by the Nursing and Midwifery Council (NMC). Central to this is *The Code: Professional standards of practice and behaviour for nurses, midwives and nursing associates* (Nursing and Midwifery Council (NMC), 2018), which outlines core values such as respect, integrity, accountability, and commitment to person-centred care. These principles provide a clear ethical foundation for both students and practitioners, informing educational content and professional expectations. Furthermore, the *Standards for pre-registration nursing programmes* (NMC, 2023a) and the *Standards of proficiency for registered nurses* (NMC, 2024) demand that ethical competence is embedded across the entire educational and professional development journey. These standards require nursing students to develop skills in ethical reasoning, reflective practice, and advocacy, preparing them to manage complex, value-laden decisions in diverse clinical contexts.

Rather than viewing ethics as an isolated subject, these frameworks promote its integration across theoretical and practical learning. Students are expected to demonstrate ethical understanding in real-life placements, uphold public trust, and respond to moral challenges with professional judgment. Moreover, by aligning nursing education with broader legal and policy frameworks, regulatory bodies such as the NMC ensure that ethical practice is grounded in current societal standards and human rights principles.

LEARNING AND LIFE: THE INTERCONNECTION

Ethical and cultural competence in nursing is not acquired solely through academic education; it is shaped through lived experiences, personal reflection, and ongoing engagement with diverse individuals and communities. This subchapter explores how the development of these competencies extends beyond classroom boundaries and into the broader context of students' lives and professional development. By examining the influence of personal values, cultural backgrounds,

clinical placements, and interprofessional collaboration, this section highlights the dynamic interplay between learning and life. It also considers the importance of reflective practice and the role of mentorship in shaping ethically aware and culturally responsive nurses. Understanding this interconnection is essential to preparing practitioners who can adapt to real-world complexity with empathy, critical insight, and professional integrity.

ACTIVITY BOX

Title: *Teaching Ethical and Cultural Competence Through Practice-Based*

Design a short reflective teaching activity that could be used with students during placement or skills sessions to develop ethical and cultural competence.

You might:

- Use a real or fictional placement scenario that raises an ethical or cultural issue (e.g. consent and language barriers, culturally sensitive end-of-life care).

- Include prompts for student reflection that encourage values clarification and link to NMC Code principles.
- Identify the role of the practice assessor or academic assessor in supporting reflection and professional growth.
- Consider how to adapt the activity for different learner levels or diverse student groups.

This task encourages you to apply your understanding of ethics and culture to your own teaching practice, while promoting inclusive, value-based learning in clinical education.

THE ROLE OF ETHICS AND CULTURE BEYOND THE CLASSROOM

Nursing ethics education does not conclude at graduation; it marks the beginning of a lifelong journey of ethical growth and learning. Ethical competency in nursing is widely considered a meta-competence, underpinning all areas of professional practice (Hemberg & Hemberg, 2020). Nurses continually encounter new ethical dilemmas as healthcare evolves, from emerging technologies to complex care systems, requiring them to regularly update and reflect on their ethical knowledge. Professional standards across the world state the 'obligation of lifelong learning'

(International Council of Nurses (ICN), 2021, p. 13) as essential to ethical practice, emphasising the ongoing nurse's responsibility to maintain competence. This means nurses must engage in continuing professional development, mentorship, and self-reflection throughout their careers to uphold ethical standards. Indeed, ethical competence develops progressively through repeated application and integration of ethical sensitivity, knowledge, reflection, and action in clinical practice; moreover, students describe their ethical development as 'being on a journey towards ethical competence' (Hansen et al., 2024) forged by real-life experiences and guided reflection.

Such facts reinforce that ethical competency is not a static skill obtained in the classroom but a lifelong learning process, enriched by each individual and/or collective interaction with service users, carers, professionals, and decisions made.

Every nursing student and practitioner brings a set of personal values and cultural influences that inevitably shape their ethical perspective. Ethical decision-making is not done in a vacuum of universal principles alone; rather, it is filtered through one's own cultural lens and value system. Studies have shown that nurses from different cultural or national backgrounds may emphasise different ethical concerns or approaches when faced with dilemmas, reflecting their diverse cultural norms and social contexts (Chen et al., 2025). It is also important to note that, while core professional values are shared, the expression of those values in patient care was significantly influenced by each country's cultural and religious context (Lesińska-Sawicka & Kızılırmak, 2024). In an era of globalised healthcare, nurses often work in multicultural teams and care for diverse patient populations, so they must be aware of how culture impacts ethical judgments. Cultural background can affect views on issues like autonomy, family involvement, end-of-life care, or truth-telling, sometimes leading to differing yet professionally valid decisions that are culturally conditioned. Recognising this interplay, nursing education encourages students to engage in self-awareness and dialogue about their own values and biases. By understanding how personal values and culture shape ethics, nurses can strive for cultural humility and make more balanced, inclusive ethical decisions that respect patients' diverse backgrounds (Royal College of Nursing (RCN), 2024). This alignment of ethics and culture beyond the classroom lays the groundwork for truly person-centred, culturally sensitive care.

EXPERIENTIAL LEARNING IN ETHICAL AND CULTURAL COMPETENCE

Experiential learning opportunities, notably clinical placements and service learning, are pivotal in translating ethical and cultural theory into competent practice. In clinical placements, nursing students step beyond the structured classroom setting and confront real-world scenarios that test and refine their ethical reasoning. During these rotations, students routinely face ethical problems that require them to apply classroom knowledge and, importantly, to develop new ethical skills on the spot (Hansen et al., 2024). In fact, such hands-on experiences have been shown to accelerate ethical growth; indeed, students' ethical competence is forged in practice as they navigate genuine patient care situations, often grappling with ambiguous or grey areas that classroom case studies cannot fully emulate.

Service-learning adds a complementary dimension by engaging students with underserved or culturally diverse communities. Unlike clinical training focused on skill acquisition, service-learning encourages social justice, empathy, and advocacy (Dombrowsky et al., 2019). Indeed, students involved in service-learning develop stronger cultural awareness and a more holistic understanding of care, cultivating habits of listening, inclusion, and respect for difference. By merging active practice with reflection, these experiential learning modalities ensure that ethical and cultural competence are not just academic concepts but lived, internalised capabilities.

Ethical decisions in healthcare are rarely made in isolation. Interprofessional education (IPE), where nursing students collaborate with peers from other relevant fields/subjects, prepares them for the team-based nature of clinical ethics; it develops mutual understanding and respectful negotiation of different professional values (Zenani et al., 2023). Simulation-based IPE, in particular, enhances ethical sensitivity by placing students in realistic scenarios that demand collaboration (Mönkkönen et al., 2021). These exercises build confidence and highlight how interprofessional dialogue supports morally sound, person-centred decision-making.

Figure 4.1 illustrates the integration of key processes required to develop ethical and cultural competence in nursing education. At the centre is the shared core of ethical

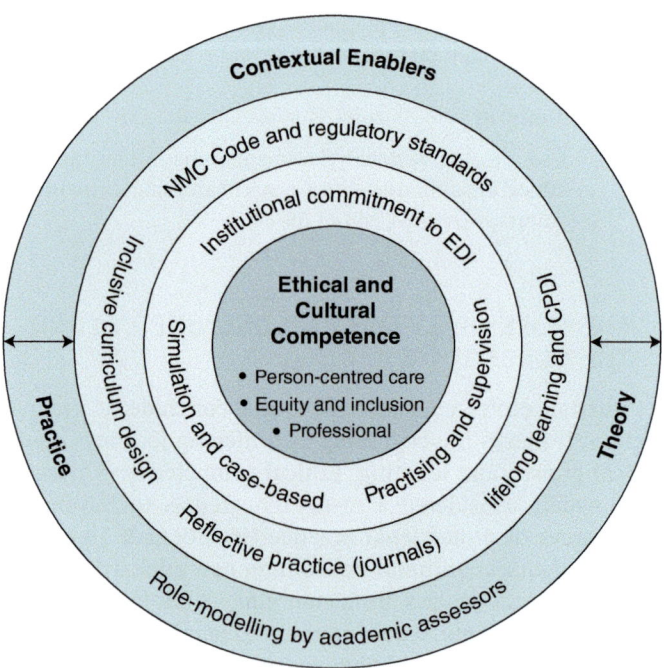

FIGURE 4.1 The ECCE model: ethical and cultural competence in education

and cultural competence, underpinned by person-centred care, equity and inclusion, and professional judgement. These core competencies are developed through a range of pedagogical processes represented in the middle ring, including reflective practice, simulation and case-based learning, inclusive curriculum design, academic and practice assessor support, and lifelong learning. These processes are supported and influenced by broader contextual enablers shown in the outer ring: the NMC Code and regulatory standards, institutional commitment to equity, diversity, and inclusion (EDI), and the alignment of clinical and academic settings.

The model positions ethical and cultural competence as dynamic and relational rather than fixed achievements. The arrows connecting theory and practice highlight the continuous, bidirectional process by which competence is cultivated through classroom learning and lived experience. It also reinforces that ethical and cultural competence must be deliberately fostered through the design of both curriculum content and the wider learning environment. The ECCE Model offers nurse educators a practical and visual way to scaffold teaching, supervision, and assessment strategies that prepare students for ethical and inclusive practice in real-world settings.

REFLECTIONS ON PERSONAL AND PROFESSIONAL GROWTH

Reflection is not just a pedagogical tool in nursing education; it is an essential process through which ethical awareness is deepened, and professional values are internalised. By engaging in structured reflection, nursing students and practitioners learn to pause and examine how their thoughts, feelings and actions align with ethical principles. This introspective process strengthens moral reasoning by encouraging individuals to consider the motivations behind their decisions and the potential impact on others, including patients and colleagues (Font Jiménez et al., 2023). Importantly, reflection bridges the gap between theory and practice. Classroom discussions on autonomy or justice gain new meaning when students reflect on how they navigated those principles during a difficult encounter. As Hansen et al. (2024) note, this kind of self-examination fosters deeper ethical insight and helps learners prepare for future dilemmas with greater clarity and confidence. When cultivated as a habit, reflective practice contributes to a lifelong process of ethical growth, promoting thoughtful, compassionate nursing across one's career.

Just as reflection shapes ethical understanding internally, mentors and role models reinforce it externally by demonstrating how ethical and culturally responsive nursing is lived in practice. Observing a senior nurse advocate for a patient, communicate across cultural boundaries, or speak up against injustice offers students a tangible example of professionalism in action (Hemberg & Hemberg, 2020). These role models provide more than technical guidance; they help shape identity. Through their behaviour, they model integrity, inclusion, and ethical courage—values that students are likely to emulate. When such mentorship is intentional and culturally competent, it empowers students not only to develop their own ethical voice but also to carry forward the profession's moral commitments with confidence and integrity (Tage et al., 2025).

PROMOTING EQUALITY AND DIVERSITY IN NURSING EDUCATION

Promoting equality and diversity is fundamental to transforming nursing education and equipping future professionals to deliver culturally competent, ethical care. As the nursing workforce increasingly reflects a wider range of identities and experiences, education must evolve to address disparities, integrate inclusive pedagogy, and create learning environments where all students and practitioners thrive.

UNDERSTANDING DIVERSITY IN NURSING

The demographic landscape of healthcare is changing rapidly. In the UK and internationally, multicultural populations demand care from equally diverse nursing teams. Yet the profession still struggles with underrepresentation across ethnicity, gender, socioeconomic background, and disability. For instance, approximately 25% of NHS staff come from ethnic minority backgrounds, and approximately 10% of nurses registered in the UK are men (Chastney et al., 2024; National Health Service (NHS) Digital, 2025; NMC, 2023b). Although these and other disparities have narrowed slightly in recent years, the figures still highlight the ongoing need to widen access and improve representation in nursing education.

A diverse nursing workforce enhances the quality of care by improving communication, cultural understanding, and patient trust. Patients often report better experiences when treated by professionals who share or understand their cultural background (Luhanga et al., 2023). However, disparities persist in student access, faculty representation, and clinical learning opportunities. Students from minority backgrounds may face subtle form of bias or exclusion during placements, affecting their learning and sense of belonging (Singh Grewal et al., 2024). Similarly, the lack of diverse faculty limits students' exposure to a broad range of perspectives and role models. Addressing these disparities in nursing education—from admissions and curriculum design to faculty hiring—is crucial for creating a workforce prepared to meet diverse health needs. Recommendations from experts include actively recruiting more faculty from minority groups and widening access for underrepresented students (Nolan et al., 2021). By acknowledging and closing these gaps, nursing as a profession can move toward greater inclusivity and social justice in healthcare.

INCORPORATING EQUALITY, DIVERSITY, AND INCLUSION IN NURSING CURRICULA

Inclusive education begins with curricula that reflect the realities of a multicultural world. Nursing programmes are increasingly embedding equality, diversity, and inclusion (EDI) as foundational principles, not optional content. This includes integrating topics such as health inequalities, systemic racism, cultural safety, and social determinants of health across modules.

Effective strategies for embedding EDI in nursing education include the use of culturally diverse case studies, inclusive language and images in teaching materials, and simulation scenarios that reflect a range of patient identities and contexts. For example, faculty might implement simulation exercises featuring patients from different ethnicities, religions, or LGBTQ+ identities to foster students' ability to provide culturally appropriate care. Culturally responsive simulation has been highlighted as an effective means to improve nurses' preparation for working with a broad range of patient populations (Markey et al., 2021). Likewise, case studies and unfolding clinical scenarios can be deliberately chosen to cover health issues in various communities. These techniques help students move beyond a one-size-fits-all model of care and develop skills to assess and respond to individual patient needs. See Table 4.2 for strategies that support embedding cultural competence in nursing education.

Culturally responsive teaching is equally vital, being recognised as skill for nurse educators since it creates a learning atmosphere where all students can thrive (Leibold et al., 2022). This involves educators being aware of their own cultural biases and adapting their teaching to students' diverse learning needs and backgrounds. Specific techniques include using inclusive language, acknowledging different communication styles, and validating the experiences of students from all cultures. Overall, embedding EDI in the curriculum means not only teaching about diversity, but teaching in a way that respects and leverages diversity among students.

Furthermore, increasing faculty diversity enhances inclusivity in both content and delivery. A more representative teaching body provides students with varied role models and perspectives while enriching classroom discussions. Faculty development programmes focused on inclusive teaching have been shown to improve student engagement and support the retention of underrepresented learners (Nolan et al., 2021).

Table 4.2   Strategies for Embedding Cultural Competence in Nursing Education

Strategy	Description	Intended outcome
Diverse Case Studies	Inclusion of patients from varied cultural backgrounds	Enhances awareness and contextualises clinical decision-making
Inclusive Simulation Scenarios	Role-play with LGBTQ+, ethnic minority, or faith-specific patient profiles	Builds empathy and cultural assessment skills
Reflective Practice Assignments	Journals and debriefs focused on cultural identity and bias	Promotes cultural humility and self-awareness
Community Engagement Projects	Involvement with local cultural groups or service users	Fosters practical understanding and community responsiveness
Culturally Responsive Teaching	Adapting teaching style to reflect and respect student diversity	Encourages equity, safety, and belonging within learning environments

INNOVATION BOX

Title: *Culturally Responsive Simulation for Ethical Practice*

A growing innovation in nurse education is the use of *culturally responsive simulation* to teach both ethical reasoning and cultural humility. Unlike traditional simulation, these scenarios are specifically designed to include patients from diverse backgrounds and to explore value-laden situations such as refusal of care, spiritual needs at the end of life, or communication barriers in consent.

By embedding cultural and ethical complexity into simulation, educators support students to critically apply principles from ethical theories, regulatory guidance (such as the NMC Code), and reflective practice. Evidence shows that these simulations help learners develop confidence, challenge assumptions, and practise inclusive communication in a safe learning space (Markey et al., 2021; Mitchell, 2024).

This approach ensures simulation is not just technical skills-based but also promotes deep learning around respect, dignity, and professional judgement—especially when debriefing is facilitated with sensitivity and openness.

ADDRESSING IMPLICIT BIAS AND STRUCTURAL INEQUALITY

While curriculum changes are important, individual and institutional biases must also be confronted to achieve true equity in nursing education. Implicit biases—unconscious attitudes or stereotypes that can influence behaviour—are common among healthcare providers, including nurses (Nolan et al., 2021). If unaddressed, these biases can affect how nursing students are taught, evaluated, and mentored, as well as how future nurses will care for patients. Bias training initiatives, particularly those that promote cultural humility, are increasingly integrated into nursing education to support self-awareness and equity-oriented practice (Smallheer et al., 2022).

However, standalone training is not enough. Long-term change depends on continuous engagement and structural reform. This includes reviewing admissions processes for fairness, diversifying course materials, and fostering environments where difficult conversations about race, privilege, and inequity are encouraged. As some have noted, nursing education has often adopted a colour-blind stance that fails to acknowledge systemic barriers (Burnett et al., 2020). Breaking this silence is essential to advancing meaningful inclusion. For instance, an admissions committee might adopt holistic review to appreciate applicants' diverse experiences beyond grades alone, thus reducing structural barriers for those from disadvantaged backgrounds. In the classroom, educators can deliberately counter stereotypes - for example, highlighting contributions of nurses from various ethnicities and genders in course contents. Indeed, increasing the visibility of minority nurses in front-line and leadership roles helps break down stereotypical images of who a nurse is (Dobson, 2022).

Nurse educators play a key role in modelling equity and challenging stereotypes. By presenting a more complete history of nursing, featuring contributions from diverse figures, and confronting stereotypes in teaching materials, educators help shape a more inclusive professional identity. They also support inclusive practice by affirming the voices of underrepresented students and advocating for equity within academic structures. This suggests that empowering students to take part in equity work—like forming nursing student diversity committees or anti-racism action groups—can complement formal curriculum efforts (Nolan et al., 2021). Ultimately, addressing implicit bias and structural inequality in nursing education requires a dual approach: personal transformation and institutional reform.

CREATING AN INCLUSIVE LEARNING ENVIRONMENT

Beyond curriculum and faculty development, fostering a truly inclusive environment means ensuring that every student feels respected, safe, and supported. Research shows that students from minority backgrounds often experience feelings of isolation or report microaggressions during placements or in the classroom (Singh Grewal et al., 2024). These experiences negatively impact retention, confidence, and academic success; creating a genuinely inclusive learning environment is as important as curricular content—students learn best when they feel safe and supported.

Support systems for students from underrepresented backgrounds are a key pillar of an inclusive nursing programme. Mentorship and peer support can significantly improve students' sense of belonging and capability. Many nursing schools have developed mentorship programmes pairing minority students with faculty or senior student mentors who share similar backgrounds or experiences; some institutions have established affinity groups or network to build community and reduce isolation (Dowling et al., 2021). Such initiatives signal to students that their institution is invested in their success.

Policies that address discrimination—both within the institution and in clinical settings—are critical. Discrimination does occur in clinical training settings; surveys of NHS staff in England found that ethnic minority healthcare workers reported higher levels of bullying and racism from colleagues and even patients (Chastney et al., 2024). Clear reporting mechanisms, training for placement supervisors/assessors, and visible zero-tolerance policies on racism and harassment reinforce a culture of respect (RCN, 2024). Collaboration with clinical/practice learning partners is essential to ensure inclusive practices continue off-campus. Finally, inclusive education is a collective responsibility. Creating space for dialogue, acknowledging diverse holidays and traditions, and fostering peer-led inclusion initiatives all contribute to a culture where diversity is celebrated. Such efforts not only enhance student experience but also prepare future nurses to be advocates for equity and justice in practice.

ADDRESSING CHALLENGES IN DEVELOPMENT, DELIVERY, AND EDUCATION

Developing ethical and cultural competence in nursing education requires overcoming significant challenges in curriculum design, faculty development, and the translation of theory into practice. Despite widespread agreement on the importance of ethical awareness and cultural sensitivity in nursing, nursing programmes may struggle to uniformly integrate these competencies. This subchapter explores key barriers to developing ethical and cultural competence, the importance of faculty preparedness and institutional support, and strategies to bridge the gap between theoretical instruction and practical implementation.

BARRIERS TO ETHICAL AND CULTURAL COMPETENCY DEVELOPMENT

One major challenge is the inconsistent approach to ethics education across nursing programmes. Indeed, there is no universal standard for what ethical content is taught or how it is delivered, leading to considerable variability in nursing curricula (Copeland, 2022; Groothuizen, 2024). In practice, this lack of standardisation means some students may graduate with robust training in ethical decision-making while others have only minimal exposure, hampering consistent ethical competence in the profession.

Similarly, integrating cultural competence into traditionally structured curricula has faced resistance. Historically, many nursing programmes treated cultural competence as an optional or supplemental topic rather than core content. Educators in a European multi-country study perceived cultural competence content as 'an addition to, and not an essential component of, their modules' (Antón-Solanas et al., 2021, p. 17), listing multiple barriers to integration. Common obstacles include overloaded curricula that leave little room for additional content, as well as discomfort or uncertainty in addressing topics like race, gender, or religion in class. Moreover, faculty have observed that some students (and even colleagues) display close-mindedness or rigidity of thought when confronting culturally sensitive issues, reflecting prejudices that mirror wider societal biases. These attitudes can lead to pushback against or superficial engagement with cultural competence training. Indeed, efforts to introduce cultural competence and racial awareness are complex by nature and often perceived as challenging for nurse educators, sometimes leading educators to feel uncomfortable or vulnerable when teaching these topics (Arveklev & Tengelin, 2024). Such resistance highlights the need to reframe cultural competence as fundamental to nursing practice rather than an extraneous add-on.

FACULTY PREPAREDNESS AND INSTITUTIONAL SUPPORT

Overcoming the above barriers requires well-prepared faculty and strong institutional commitment. Faculty play a pivotal role in modelling ethical and culturally competent behaviour, yet many feel underprepared to teach this content. Continuous faculty development in ethics and cultural competence is therefore essential. As noted, a lack of formal training in ethics among nursing educators can be a common issue (Copeland, 2022), and many may also lack training in pedagogical strategies for cultural competence (Antón-Solanas et al., 2021).

Without adequate preparation, even well-intentioned educators may find it challenging to facilitate difficult discussions on ethical dilemmas or cultural disparities. Educational institutions and nursing schools must invest in professional development programmes that equip educators with up-to-date knowledge and teaching skills in these domains. For example, Rahimi et al. (2023) demonstrated that a targeted training programme significantly improved nursing faculty's cultural competence, moving participants from basic competency to culturally proficient levels. Indeed, these authors highlighted the significance of the issue and suggested that ongoing education initiatives aimed at enhancing nurse educators' cultural competence should be given priority. Similar efforts can be made for ethics education, such as workshops on clinical ethics case facilitation or mentorship by nurse ethicists, to build faculty confidence in teaching ethics.

Institutional support is equally critical. Embedding ethical and cultural competence in the curriculum requires more than individual faculty effort; it demands an organisational commitment. Nursing programmes need to explicitly include these competencies as learning outcomes and allocate sufficient time and resources for them. This might mean revising curricula to create dedicated courses on integrating relevant content across courses in a scaffolded manner. Institutional leaders and accrediting bodies set the tone: when cultural safety and ethics are prioritised in accreditation standards and programme reviews, schools are more likely to devote attention to them. International and national frameworks reinforce this mandate. The European Commission has charged higher education institutions with a responsibility to promote social, civil, and transcultural competences and foster values like inclusion and non-discrimination (Antón-Solanas et al., 2021). In the UK, the Nursing and Midwifery Council's standards (NMC, 2018; NMC, 2024) expect registered nurses to practice with respect for diversity and professionalism, which in turn implies that education providers must ensure these areas are taught. However, translating such high-level expectations into concrete curriculum elements can be challenging. A study of nursing lecturers in Europe highlighted the need for clearer guidelines and support: faculty note a lack of support to formally train faculty members in cultural teaching and insufficient effort by authorities to integrate transcultural nursing into curricula (Antón-Solanas et al., 2021). Addressing this requires leadership from institutions—for instance, appointing curriculum champions or committees to oversee ethics and diversity education, providing faculty release time to attend training, and rewarding teaching innovations in these areas. When institutions visibly back these competencies (through policies, funding, and recognition), it empowers educators to persist in what can sometimes be difficult educational conversations.

BALANCING THEORY AND PRACTICAL IMPLEMENTATION

Perhaps one of the most persistent challenges is translating ethical and cultural theory into clinical practice. While students may learn ethical principles or cultural frameworks in the classroom, they often struggle to apply them within the dynamic and complex settings of healthcare. This theory–practice gap is well-documented across nursing education globally and is particularly evident in areas such as informed consent, communication across cultures, and advocacy in ethically ambiguous situations (Saifan et al., 2021). Furthermore, discrepancies between academic ideals and clinical realities can lead to moral distress or confusion among students, especially when ethical values discussed in class are not modelled in practice. Bridging this gap requires stronger collaboration between academic and clinical staff. Joint teaching, clinical case reflections, and the presence of ethical and culturally aware mentors in placement settings can help students contextualise and apply their learning more effectively (Saifan et al., 2021).

Simulation-based learning and structured reflection activities also offer promising avenues. They allow students to rehearse ethical decision-making and cultural interactions in safe environments before encountering them in real-world scenarios (Honkavuo, 2021). Moreover, involving clinical partners who share institutional commitments to equity and ethical practice helps reinforce consistency between theory and practice.

At a broader level, nursing education must also work to align itself with healthcare systems that operationalise inclusive, ethical care. If new graduates enter environments where ethical standards or inclusive values are deprioritised, it risks undermining the very competencies they have acquired. Embedding ethical and cultural principles across academic, clinical, and institutional contexts is thus key to sustaining impact.

ENHANCING CULTURAL COMPETENCE

Cultural competence has become an essential pillar of transformative nursing education amid increasingly diverse patient populations. Developing this competence is necessary for addressing health disparities and improving healthcare quality for underserved groups. Therefore, nursing educators are tasked with not only teaching cultural knowledge but also fostering the empathy and adaptability needed for practice in multicultural settings.

DEFINING CULTURAL COMPETENCE IN NURSING

In nursing, cultural competence is commonly defined as a combination of knowledge, skills, and attitudes that are applied in intercultural care contexts. It refers to nurses' ability to understand and respond effectively to patients' cultural beliefs, health practices, and communication styles in order to provide respectful, person-centred care (Červený et al., 2022; Reeve & Lavery, 2023). Moreover, delivering care that is culturally congruent with patients' values should be considered as a human right rather than as a privilege.

Culturally competent care is effective when it is congruent with the patient's own values and life context (Gradellini et al., 2021). For instance, a competent nurse will acknowledge how culture influences a patient's health perceptions and decision-making, thereby building trust and improving outcomes. Importantly, cultural competence is not a static trait one either has or lacks, but a continuous learning process. It requires cultivating attitudes of openness, respect, and curiosity so that nurses continually learn from each new patient encounter. As Campinha-Bacote's model emphasises, cultural competence is an ongoing process involving five constructs—cultural awareness, cultural knowledge, cultural skills, cultural encounters, and cultural desire (Campinha-Bacote, 2002)—meaning that true competence extends beyond factual knowledge to include a genuine willingness to engage with and learn from people of other cultures.

Contemporary discourse in nursing education advocates moving beyond cultural competence toward cultural humility (Lekas et al., 2020). While cultural competence implies an ability that can be fully mastered, cultural humility is a lifelong commitment to self-evaluation and growth. Indeed, checklist-style competence training can inadvertently lead to stereotyping or 'othering' of patients. In contrast, cultural humility emphasises an approach of ongoing self-reflection, recognising one's biases and knowledge limits, and treating each patient as the expert on their own cultural identity. This approach also aligns with an intersectional understanding of culture, acknowledging that individuals embody multiple social identities that intersect to shape their health experience.

CULTURAL COMPETENCE TRAINING STRATEGIES

Nurse educators have been employing a range of innovative strategies to enhance students' cultural competence. Experiential learning techniques are particularly effective, as they allow students to practice cultural skills in realistic contexts. For example, simulation-based training with patients from diverse backgrounds has been shown to improve and develop nursing students' cultural competence (Qin & Chaimongkol, 2021; Mitchell, 2023; Reis Da Silva & Mitchell, 2024). In simulated patient encounters, students navigate language barriers, interpret cultural cues, and practice respectful communication in a safe learning environment. Such simulations, especially when combined with case studies and facilitated debriefings, build students' confidence and empathy in cross-cultural interactions. Another powerful method is the use of storytelling and reflective narratives (Mitchell, 2024). By hearing patients' or peers' stories from different cultural perspectives, students gain insight into how culture impacts health beliefs and patient experiences. Indeed, these personal stories make abstract concepts tangible, allowing students to develop greater empathy and self-awareness.

Beyond classroom simulations, immersion experiences play an important role in cultural competence training. Local community engagement is one approach: by partnering with neighbourhood organisations, cultural centres, or immigrant support groups, students interact directly with people from diverse backgrounds and learn about their customs and healthcare needs in context (Garcia, 2023). Such community-based initiatives not only enhance cultural knowledge but also foster social responsibility, as students learn to meet people where they are and tailor care to address real-world health disparities. Likewise, international exchange programmes and study abroad experiences provide deep cultural immersion (Louis et al., 2025)—indeed, students who participate in theory-guided global immersion programmes show measurable gains in cultural awareness and a transformative appreciation of diversity.

MEASURING CULTURAL COMPETENCY OUTCOMES

Assessing outcomes in cultural competence education is both necessary and challenging. Various tools and frameworks have been developed to evaluate nursing students' cultural competence, but no single method captures this multidimensional construct perfectly (Červený et al., 2022). Self-report instruments and surveys have been used to gauge students' cultural knowledge, awareness, and confidence. For instance, the *Inventory for Assessing the Process of Cultural Competence* (IAPCC) (Campinha-Bacote, 2002) and its student version (IAPCC-SV) (Fitzgerald et al., 2009) are widely used scales that measure the five key constructs of cultural competence in learners. Newer assessment tools continue to emerge; a recent example is the *BENEFITS-CCCSAT* instrument, a 26-item tool covering domains such as respect for cultural diversity, culturally sensitive communication, and perceived challenges in providing culturally competent care (Yava et al., 2023).

Although the instruments mentioned above provide structured ways to track students' progress, measuring cultural learning beyond theoretical knowledge remains challenging. Self-assessments can be limited by social desirability bias or students' lack of insight into their own biases. Moreover, increases in factual knowledge or declarative understanding do not always translate into changed attitudes or behaviours in practice. Because of this, nursing programmes are also turning to performance-based assessments. Objective Structured Clinical Examinations (OSCEs) with cultural scenarios allow faculty to observe how students apply cultural competence in a clinical interaction (Lee et al., 2020). Reflective journals and debriefings can likewise reveal growth in cultural humility and empathy that might not register on a quiz (Červený et al., 2022); a persistent challenge is the absence of universally accepted benchmarks for cultural competence in nursing education. Indeed, each student's journey is unique and ongoing, making it important to use multiple assessment methods and to emphasise qualitative feedback. Ultimately, evaluative strategies aim to ensure that students not only know about cultural differences but can effectively bridge cultural gaps and demonstrate cultural sensitivity in their care. By prioritising comprehensive assessment, nursing educators can better gauge and guide the development of true cultural competence that continues beyond the classroom.

TECHNOLOGY IN ETHICS EDUCATION

Technology has emerged as both a powerful facilitator and a complex subject in the teaching of ethics and cultural competence within nursing education. Digital innovations—from simulation-based learning and online modules to artificial intelligence (AI) and virtual reality (VR)—are transforming how students engage with ethical reasoning, professional values, and cross-cultural care. At the same time, the ethical implications of technology use in healthcare require critical engagement. This subchapter explores the dual role of technology: as a medium through which ethics is taught, and as a domain where new ethical challenges must be addressed.

THE ROLE OF TECHNOLOGY IN TEACHING ETHICS AND CULTURAL COMPETENCE

One of the most promising developments in ethics education is the integration of interactive case-based learning through digital-learning suites/applications, virtual simulations, and virtual placements (Miron & Bricknell, 2024; Tanaka & Tezuka, 2022; Hill & Mitchell, 2024). These approaches immerse students in realistic clinical cases, allowing them to grapple with ethical dilemmas in a low-risk setting. For instance, students may be presented with scenarios involving informed consent, end-of-life care, or cultural misunderstandings in patient communication. Virtual simulations have been shown to enhance students' ethical sensitivity, critical thinking, and moral confidence (Rasesemola & Molabe, 2025). Importantly, when simulations incorporate culturally diverse patient profiles, they support the development of cultural competence as well, helping students practice respectful communication, navigate unfamiliar health beliefs, and adapt to varied care expectations (Fung et al., 2023).

Beyond virtual learning contexts, AI and machine learning offer novel approaches to ethics education. Indeed, AI-driven systems can present adaptive learning pathways where students are guided through decision trees and receive feedback on clinical reasoning and professional values (Teixeira et al., 2024). These intelligent systems challenge learners to justify their decisions while exposing them to the complexity of ethical trade-offs. However, AI is not just a pedagogical tool; it is increasingly a feature of modern healthcare, raising ethical questions that must be addressed in the classroom (Kwak et al., 2022). As AI is already influencing diagnostic pathways, resource allocation, and patient monitoring, nursing students must be taught to critically evaluate AI recommendations, understand algorithmic bias, and uphold human-centred care values in the face of automated input (El Arab et al., 2025). The convergence of AI and ethics education thus reflects a broader shift: nurses must now be fluent in both clinical and digital ethics.

E-LEARNING AND ONLINE MODULES FOR ETHICS EDUCATION

The rise of e-learning and online platforms has expanded the accessibility of ethics education. Learning management systems and asynchronous modules provide students with opportunities to engage in ethical discussions, complete self-paced case analyses, and participate in virtual seminars. Online formats are especially beneficial in reaching geographically dispersed students and offering consistent instruction across diverse educational settings (Tavani et al., 2024). Features such as embedded videos, interactive quizzes, and branching scenarios can stimulate reflection and deepen understanding.

Nevertheless, online ethics education also presents pedagogical and equity-related challenges. One risk is that complex ethical discourse may be oversimplified in modular formats, potentially reducing ethics to a checklist of principles rather than a lived, relational practice. The absence of real-time dialogue can limit opportunities for learners to challenge each other's perspectives, explore ambiguity, and process emotional responses. Furthermore, students from lower-resourced settings may lack stable internet access or digital literacy, reinforcing disparities in learning opportunities (Molato & Sehularo, 2022). Educators must be mindful of these dynamics when designing and delivering online ethics content, incorporating synchronous elements, discussion forums, and accessible formats to foster deeper engagement.

To address some of these limitations, educational institutions are increasingly turning to VR and augmented reality (AR) technologies to enhance experiential learning. These tools simulate complex care environments where students must apply ethical reasoning in context—for example, deciding how to allocate scarce resources in a critical care scenario, or managing a cross-cultural interaction during a home visit. Research has shown that VR-based training can improve students' emotional engagement, empathy, and recall of ethical principles (Sombilon et al., 2024). In particular, VR has been effective in helping students practice ethical leadership, teamwork, and conflict

resolution—skills that are difficult to teach through traditional methods alone. However, the integration of VR and AR must be intentional and ethically grounded. Scenarios must be inclusive, avoiding stereotypes and considering accessibility for students with disabilities. Informed consent, emotional debriefing, and psychological safety protocols are essential, especially when scenarios simulate distressing or ethically charged events (Sombilon et al., 2024). The design of VR experiences must reflect diversity in patient profiles, cultures, and clinical situations to avoid inadvertently reinforcing narrow views of health and care.

ETHICAL CONSIDERATIONS IN TECHNOLOGY USE

As technology becomes embedded in nursing practice, it becomes a subject of ethical inquiry. One of the most pressing concerns is data privacy and confidentiality. Electronic health records (EHRs), mobile health apps, and cloud-based storage systems require nurses to manage patient information in ways that comply with legal and professional standards. Breaches of confidentiality, whether through careless data handling, phishing attacks, or unauthorised access, can have serious consequences for patient trust and safety. Ethics education must therefore include modules on digital professionalism, information governance, and data protection regulations (Ibrahim et al., 2024). Case-based learning can help students explore scenarios such as a nurse overhearing a colleague discussing patient information in a public space or deciding how much information to document in an HER that could be accessed by multiple team members. These exercises reinforce the principle that ethical behaviour in digital settings is as critical as in face-to-face care and that nurses must be vigilant stewards of patient information in all formats.

The rise of telehealth has also introduced new ethical complexities. While remote consultations improve access for patients in rural or underserved areas, they can also introduce inequities (Solimini et al., 2021). In fact, not all patients have equal access to devices, internet, or digital literacy, creating a risk of digital exclusion. Additionally, telehealth raises questions about privacy, consent, and relational care. Thus, nurse educators must prepare students to apply ethical principles and frameworks in these modalities. This includes understanding the limitations of virtual care, setting clear professional boundaries, and advocating for equitable access. The ability to build rapport, assess patient well-being, and address emotional cues over digital platforms also requires new communication competencies, which can be developed through telehealth simulation and guided reflection (Sawin et al., 2024).

Finally, AI-assisted clinical decision-making poses some of the most profound ethical questions for the future of nursing. While AI has the potential to enhance diagnostic accuracy and reduce human error, it also introduces risks of depersonalisation, overreliance, and embedded bias (Teixeira, 2024). For instance, algorithms trained on non-representative data may produce recommendations that disadvantage certain patient groups, perpetuating health disparities rather than addressing them. Therefore, nurses must be taught to critically assess AI-generated recommendations, advocate for patient-centred care, and uphold their professional judgment in the face of automation. Nursing ethics education should emphasise that accountability for clinical decisions remains with the human provider, even when those decisions are informed by machine input. Moreover, students should understand the social and institutional dimensions of AI ethics, such as who designs these systems, whose values are embedded in them, and how transparency is maintained (El Arab et al., 2025).

Debates around AI and other technologies also open opportunities to examine broader ethical values: trust, relational care, equity, and human dignity. Ethics education can support students in developing a critical digital literacy that goes beyond technical proficiency to encompass reflective, values-driven practice. Encouraging interprofessional dialogue and case-based analysis helps nursing students see how ethical reasoning applies across technology, policy, and patient interaction. By engaging with these technologies not only as users but as ethical agents, future and current nurses will be better prepared to navigate the digital landscapes of healthcare. This requires, though, a shift in focus: from viewing technology as a neutral tool to understanding it as a space where ethical and cultural competence must be actively practised and continually re-examined.

TAKE-HOME POINTS

- Ethical and cultural competence are essential components of nursing education that support safe, person-centred, and equitable care.

- These competencies must be taught through immersive, reflective, and inclusive strategies that bridge theory and practice.

- Faculty preparedness, institutional commitment, and curriculum integration are key to embedding these values and supporting lifelong ethical development.

CPD REFLECTIVE QUESTIONS

1. How does my own cultural background influence the way I respond to ethical dilemmas in clinical practice?

2. In what ways can I support students or colleagues to develop ethical sensitivity and cultural humility in everyday learning environments?

3. What strategies could I adopt in my teaching or practice to ensure that equity, inclusion, and respect are modelled and maintained consistently?

REFERENCES

Antón-Solanas, I. et al. (2021). Nursing lecturers' perception and experience of teaching cultural competence: a European qualitative study. *International Journal of Environmental Research and Public Health*, 18(3), 1357.

Arveklev, S. H., & Tengelin, E. (2024). Learning to teach at a norm-critical clinical learning centre: a phenomenographic study. *Nurse Education Today*, 139, 106250.

Beauchamp, T. L., & Childress, J. F. (2019). *Principles of Biomedical Ethics* (8th ed.). New York: Oxford University Press.

Burnett, A. et al. (2020). Dismantling racism in education: in 2020, the year of the nurse & midwife, "it's time." *Nurse Education Today*, 93, 104532.

Campinha-Bacote, J. (2002). The process of cultural competence in the delivery of healthcare services: a model of care. *Journal of Transcultural Nursing*, 13(3), 181–184.

Červený, M. et al. (2022). Methods of increasing cultural competence in nurses working in clinical practice: a scoping review of literature 2011-2021. *Frontiers in Psychology*, 13, 936181.

Chastney, J. et al. (2024). "To tell you the truth I'm tired": a qualitative exploration of the experiences of ethnically diverse NHS staff. *BMJ Open*, 14(1), e070510.

Chen, X. et al. (2025). Development and psychometric properties of the nursing ethical decision-making ability scale. *BMC Medical Ethics*, 26(1), 35–11.

Copeland, D. (2022). Liberal arts and ethics education in nursing: a national survey. *Journal of Professional Nursing*, 42, 73–88.

Dobson, L. (2022). 9 Strategies for increasing diversity and inclusivity in nursing education. *Canadian Nurse*. https://www.canadian-nurse.com/blogs/cn-content/2022/05/30/9-strategies-for-increasing-diversity-and-inclusiv#:~:text=education%20www.canadian,2019.

Dombrowsky, T. et al. (2019). Service-learning and clinical nursing education: a Delphi inquiry. *The Journal of Nursing Education*, 58(7), 381–391.

Dowling, T. et al. (2021). Cultivating inclusive learning environments that foster nursing education program resiliency during the Covid-19 pandemic. *Journal of Professional Nursing*, 37(5), 942–947.

El Arab, R. A. et al. (2025). The role of AI in nursing education and practice: umbrella review. *Journal of Medical Internet Research*, 27, e69881.

Fitzgerald, E. M. et al. (2009). Psychometric testing of the inventory for assessing the process of cultural competence among healthcare professionals - student version (IAPCC-SV©). *Journal of Theory Construction & Testing*, 13(2), 64–68.

Font Jiménez, I. et al. (2023). Reflective based learning for nursing ethical competency during clinical practices. *Nursing Ethics*, 30(4), 598–613.

Fung, J. T. C. et al. (2023). Virtual simulation and problem-based learning enhance perceived clinical and cultural competence of nursing students in Asia: a randomized controlled cross-over study. *Nurse Education Today*, 123, 105721.

Garcia, R. (2023). Community-based cultural connections: a cornerstone of culturally congruent care in nursing education. *Cultural Connections Issue*. https://www.acenursing.org/bridges/community-based-cultural-connections-a-cornerstone-of-culturally-congruent-care-in-nursing-education#:~:text=By%20participating%20in%20community,of%20the%20individuals%20they%20serve

Gilligan, C. (2003). *In a Different Voice: Psychological Theory and Women's Development*. 38th print. Cambridge, Massachusetts: Harvard University Press.

Grace, P. J. (2022). *Nursing Ethics and Professional Responsibility in Advanced Practice*. (4th ed.). Burlington, MA: Jones & Bartlett Learning.

Gradellini, C. et al. (2021). Cultural competence and cultural sensitivity education in university nursing courses. A scoping review. *Frontiers in Psychology*, 12, 682920.

Grewal, C. S., Khan, M. B., Panesar, J. K. K., Asher, S., & Mehan, N. (2024). Exploring BAME student experiences in healthcare courses in the United Kingdom: a systematic review. *Journal of Advances in Medical Education and Professionalism*, 12(1):8–17. https://doi.org/10.30476/JAMP.2023.98882.1825.

Groothuizen, J. E. (2024). Axiological reflection for nursing ethics education: the missing link in understanding value conflicts. *Nursing Ethics*, 32(4), 1230–1239.

Hansen, S. et al. (2024). Nurturing ethical insight: exploring nursing students' journey to ethical competence. *BMC Nursing*, 23(1), 568.

Hemberg, J., & Hemberg, H. (2020). Ethical competence in a profession: healthcare professionals' views. *Nursing Open*, 7(4), 1249–1259.

Herring, J. (2022). *Medical Law and Ethics* (9th ed.). Oxford University Press.

Hill, B., & Mitchell, A. (2024). Virtual placements in nursing education. *British Journal of Nursing (Mark Allen Publishing)*, 33 (12), 536–537.

Honkavuo, L. (2021). Ethics simulation in nursing education: nursing students' experiences. *Nursing Ethics*, 28 (7–8), 1269–1281.

Hursthouse, R. (1999). *On Virtue Ethics*. Oxford: Oxford University Press.

Ibrahim, A. M. et al. (2024). Balancing confidentiality and care coordination: challenges in patient privacy. *BMC Nursing*, 23(1), 564.

International Council of Nurses (ICN) (2021). *The ICN code of ethics for nurses*. https://www.icn.ch/sites/default/files/2023-06/ICN_Code-of-Ethics_EN_Web.pdf

Jameton, A. (2013). A reflection on moral distress in nursing together with a current application of the concept. *Journal of Bioethical Inquiry*, 10(3), 297–308.

Johnstone, M.-J. (2019). *Bioethics: A Nursing Perspective* (7th ed.). Chatswood, NSW: Elsevier.

Kant, I. et al. (2012). *Groundwork of the Metaphysics of Morals*. Revised edition / translation revised by Jens Timmermann. Cambridge: Cambridge University Press.

Kwak, Y. et al. (2022). Influence of AI ethics awareness, attitude, anxiety, and self-efficacy on nursing students' behavioral intentions. *BMC Nursing*, 21(1), 1–267.

Lee, Y.-H. et al. (2020). Objective structural clinical examination for evaluating learning efficacy of cultural competence cultivation programme for nurses. *BMC Nursing*, 19(1), 1–114.

Leibold, N. et al. (2022). Culturally responsive teaching in nursing education: a faculty development project. *Creative Nursing*, 28(3), 154–160.

Lekas, H.-M. et al. (2020). Rethinking cultural competence: shifting to cultural humility. *Health Services Insights*, 13, 1178632920970580.

Lesińska-Sawicka, M., & Kızılırmak, A. (2024). Ethical values held by nursing students. Comparative study in two country. *BMC Nursing*, 23(1), 521–528.

Louis, K. S. et al. (2025). Nursing students' enhanced cultural competence after study abroad: a mixed-methods study. *The Journal of Nursing Education*, 64(3), 185–191.

Luhanga, F. et al. (2023). "Let's call a spade a spade. My barrier is being a Black student": challenges for black undergraduate nursing students in a western Canadian province. *Canadian Journal of Nursing Research*, 55(4), 457–471.

Markey, K. et al. (2021). Cultural competence development: the importance of incorporating culturally responsive simulation in nurse education. *Nurse Education in Practice*, 52, 103021.

Mill, J. S. (1863). *Utilitarianism, by John Stuart Mill*. England: Parker, Son and Bourn, 1863.

Miron, M., & Bricknell, M. (2024). Innovation in education: the military medical ethics 'playing cards' and smartphone application. *BMJ Military Health*, 170(1), 47–50.

Mitchell, A. (2023). Simulated patients. *British Journal of Nursing (Mark Allen Publishing)*, 32(22), 1070.

Mitchell, A. (2024). Creating lived experience simulations. *British Journal of Nursing (Mark Allen Publishing)*, 33(11), 522–523.

Molato, B. J., & Sehularo, L. A. (2022). Recommendations for online learning challenges in nursing education during the COVID-19 pandemic. *Curationis (Pretoria)*, 45(1), e1–e6.

Mönkkönen, K. et al. (2021). Interprofessional understanding of ethical dilemmas: learning experiences of simulation learning in social welfare and health care education. *Journal of Social Work Values and Ethics*, 18(2), 16–28.

National Health Service (NHS) Digital (2025). *NHS workforce statistics – December 2024*. https://digital.nhs.uk/data-and-information/publications/statistical/nhs-workforce-statistics/december-2024

Nolan, T. S. et al. (2021). Cultural humility: retraining and retooling nurses to provide equitable cancer care. *Clinical Journal of Oncology Nursing*, 25(5), 3–9.

Nursing and Midwifery Council (NMC) (2018). *The code: professional standards of practice and behaviour for nurses, midwives and nursing associates*. https://www.nmc.org.uk/globalassets/sitedocuments/nmc-publications/nmc-code.pdf

Nursing and Midwifery Council (NMC) (2023a). *Standards for education and training, part 3: standards for pre-registration nursing programmes*. https://www.nmc.org.uk/globalassets/sitedocuments/standards/2024/standards-for-pre-registration-nursing-programmes.pdf

Nursing and Midwifery Council (NMC) (2023b). *The NMC register: 1 April 2022–31 March 2023*. https://www.nmc.org.uk/globalassets/sitedocuments/data-reports/may-2023/0110a-annual-data-report-full-uk-web.pdf

Nursing and Midwifery Council (NMC) (2024). *Standards of proficiency for nurses*. https://www.nmc.org.uk/globalassets/sitedocuments/standards/2024/standards-of-proficiency-for-nurses.pdf

Qin, Y., & Chaimongkol, N. (2021). Simulation with standardized patients designed as interventions to develop nursing students' cultural competence: a systematic review. *Journal of Transcultural Nursing*, 32(6), 778–789.

Rahimi, M. et al. (2023). A virtual training program for improving cultural competence among academic nurse educators. *BMC Medical Education*, 23(1), 445–445.

Rasesemola, R. M., & Molabe, M. P. T. (2025). Enhancing student nurses' ethical skills via simulation-based learning: barriers and opportunities. *BMC Nursing*, 24(1), 147–149.

Reeve, L., & Lavery, J. (2023). Navigating cultural competence in district nursing. *British Journal of Community Nursing*, 28(7), 338–343.

Reis Da Silva, T. H., & Mitchell, A. (2024). Simulation in nursing: the importance of involving service users. *British Journal of Nursing (Mark Allen Publishing)*, 33(5), 262–265.

Royal College of Nursing (RCN) (2024). *Our equity, diversity and inclusion strategy*. https://www.rcn.org.uk/Professional-Development/publications/equity-diversity-and-inclusion-strategy-uk-pub-011-613

Saifan, A. et al. (2021). Solutions to bridge the theory-practice gap in nursing education in the UAE: a qualitative study. *BMC Medical Education*, 21(1), 1–490.

Salari, N. et al. (2022). The severity of moral distress in nurses: a systematic review and meta-analysis. *Philosophy, Ethics, and Humanities in Medicine: PEHM*, 17(1), 1–13.

Sawin, E. M. et al. (2024). Use of telehealth simulation to teach the enhanced primary care RN role through community/public health-focused simulations. *Public Health Nursing*, 41(6), 1588–1599.

Smallheer, B., et al. (2022). A scoping review of the priority of diversity, inclusion, and equity in health care simulation. *Clinical Simulation in Nursing*, 71, 41–64.

Solimini, R. et al. (2021). Ethical and legal challenges of telemedicine in the era of the covid-19 pandemic. *Medicina (Kaunas, Lithuania)*, 57(12), 1314.

Sombilon, E. V. et al. (2024). Ethical considerations when designing and implementing immersive realities in nursing education. *Curēus (Palo Alto, CA)*, 16(7), e64333.

Tage, P. K. S. et al. (2025). Nursing students' experiences with improving cultural competence through education and practices in rural Indonesia: a qualitative study. *Frontiers of Nursing*, 12(1), 37–45.

Tanaka, M., & Tezuka, S. (2022). A scoping review of alternative methods of delivering ethics education in nursing. *Nursing Open*, 9(6), 2572–2585.

Tavani, F. M. et al. (2024). The effects of e-learning using educational multimedia on the ethical decision-making and professionalism of nursing students during the COVID-19 pandemic: a quasi-experimental study. *BMC Medical Education*, 24(1), 1232–1239.

Teixeira, L. (2020). Seeing is believing. *New Vistas*, 6(2), 3–7.

Teixeira, L. (2024). AI integration in nursing practice: striking a balance between technology and the human touch. *British Journal of Nursing (Mark Allen Publishing)*, 33(15), 738–739.

Teixeira, L. (2025). 10 simple rules: addressing ethical issues in nursing education (awaiting publication in BJN? May 2025).

Teixeira, L. et al. (2024). Virtual reality with artificial intelligence-led scenarios in nursing education: a project evaluation. *British Journal of Nursing (Mark Allen Publishing)*, 33(17), 812–820.

Yava, A. et al. (2023). Developing the better and effective nursing education for improving transcultural nursing skills cultural competence and cultural sensitivity assessment tool (BENEFITS-CCCSAT). *BMC Nursing*, 22(1), 1–331.

Zenani, N. E. et al. (2023). The contribution of interprofessional education in developing competent undergraduate nursing students: integrative literature review. *BMC Nursing*, 22(1), 315.

CHAPTER 5

Innovation and Practical Application in Nursing Education

Sadie Diamond-Fox

School of Healthcare and Nursing Sciences, Faculty of Health and Wellbeing, Northumbria University, UK

AIM

To examine the role of technological innovation and digital pedagogy in transforming nursing education, with a focus on flexible learning, competency-based frameworks, interprofessional collaboration, and sustainability.

LEARNING OUTCOMES

By the end of this chapter, readers will be able to:

1. Analyse the benefits and limitations of digital and mobile learning tools in nursing education, including their impact on knowledge retention, student engagement, and accessibility.

2. Evaluate the use of simulation, virtual patients, and AI-assisted tools in developing clinical reasoning and decision-making skills.

3. Explore the application of competency-based education (CBE) models supported by digital portfolios and adaptive learning platforms.

4. Critically appraise the ethical, cultural, and sustainability considerations of implementing educational technologies in a global health context.

CHAPTER INTRODUCTION

Nursing education is undergoing a profound transformation, driven by rapid advancements in technology, evolving healthcare demands, and the need for more flexible and accessible learning models. Traditional pedagogical approaches, while foundational, must adapt to accommodate diverse learner needs, foster interprofessional collaboration, and integrate innovative teaching strategies that enhance both technical proficiency and critical thinking. This chapter explores how educators can utilise digital learning resources, immersive technologies, and competency-based frameworks to revolutionise nursing education. By doing so, educators can ensure graduates are not only clinically competent but also reflective, adaptive, and ethically grounded healthcare professionals.

Additionally, the chapter examines the efficacy of digital interventions, assessing how technologies such as artificial intelligence (AI), virtual reality (VR), and simulation-based learning enhance knowledge retention and skill acquisition. A structured framework for technology-driven feedback and curriculum design will be presented, emphasising sustainability, cultural competence, and ethical considerations.

FLEXIBLE AND ACCESSIBLE LEARNING RESOURCES

Nursing education must continually evolve to meet the dynamic and complex needs of healthcare. The traditional model of rigid, classroom-based learning is no longer sufficient to prepare nurses for the realities of modern practice. The increasing diversity of learners, the expansion of digital healthcare, and the growing emphasis on lifelong learning necessitate flexible and accessible educational strategies. Flexibility in nursing education enables students to engage with learning materials in a way that suits their professional, personal, and geographical circumstances, ultimately supporting a more adaptable and competent nursing workforce.

Flexibility is particularly crucial as nursing education moves towards competency-based education (CBE), where students progress based on demonstrated knowledge and skills rather than time spent in a classroom (Frank et al., 2010). Table 5.1 highlights the differences between traditional education models and CBE. The CBE approach aligns with global efforts to enhance learning autonomy, encourage reflective practice, and improve workforce readiness. By providing multiple pathways for learning, educators can tailor experiences to individual needs, fostering greater engagement, retention, and application of knowledge in clinical practice (Jeffries, 2020).

ADDRESSING THE DIVERSE NEEDS OF LEARNERS

One of the primary drivers of flexible learning in nursing education is the diversity of students entering the profession. Many nursing students are mature learners, career changers, or working professionals balancing their studies with employment and family responsibilities. A one-size-fits-all approach to education can create barriers for these individuals, limiting access to learning and professional development. By incorporating blended learning models, asynchronous content delivery, and self-paced learning, educators can offer greater flexibility while maintaining high standards of education (McCutcheon et al., 2015).

For example, distance learning and online programmes allow students to engage with theoretical content remotely, reducing the need for frequent travel and making education more accessible to those in rural or underserved areas. This is particularly relevant given the increasing

shortage of healthcare professionals in remote regions, where technology-enabled learning could help bridge workforce gaps (World Health Organization (WHO), 2021). Similarly, part-time and modular study options enable learners to tailor their education to their individual circumstances, preventing financial or time constraints from becoming obstacles to professional advancement.

Moreover, studies suggest that flexible learning supports student well-being, work-life balance, and academic success. In a study by O'Doherty et al. (2018), nursing students reported that online learning allowed them to better manage personal responsibilities while maintaining academic performance. This adaptability is vital for supporting the retention and progression of students who might otherwise struggle to complete their education due to life commitments.

BLENDED LEARNING AND HYBRID MODELS

Blended learning, which integrates face-to-face and online education, has become a widely accepted approach in nursing education. This model allows students to access digital lectures, virtual simulations, and interactive discussions online, while still benefiting from in-person

clinical placements and hands-on training. The flexibility of blended learning ensures that students receive the best of both worlds—autonomy in theoretical learning and experiential opportunities in clinical settings (Rowe et al., 2012).

Table 5.1 Comparison of Traditional vs. Competency-Based Education (CBE)

	Traditional education	Competency-based education (CBE)
Learning Approach	Time-based (fixed duration)	Outcome-based (skill mastery)
Assessment	Standardised exams	Skill demonstrations and continuous feedback
Progression	Based on time spent in courses	Based on demonstrated competence
Student Pace	Uniform for all learners	Individualised learning paths
Technology Integration	Limited digital tools	AI, VR, adaptive learning

Hybrid learning further extends this concept by incorporating immersive technologies such as VR, augmented reality (AR), and AI to create realistic training environments. These experiential learning tools bridge the gap between theory and practice while allowing students to engage with content flexibly at their own pace.

A review by Padilha et al. (2019) found that VR-based simulations in nursing education significantly enhanced clinical decision-making, critical thinking, and engagement compared to traditional learning methods. Immersive learning technologies also provide opportunities to simulate rare, complex, or high-risk scenarios, ensuring that students are exposed to critical cases they may not encounter frequently in practice (Verkuyl et al., 2019).

Furthermore, the integration of mobile learning (m-learning) offers additional flexibility, enabling students to access content anytime, anywhere via smartphones and tablets. This aligns with constructivist learning theories, which suggest that learners benefit most when they can engage with material in meaningful, context-relevant ways (Kolb, 1984). Research by Guze (2015) found that m-learning enhances student engagement, retention, and self-directed learning, particularly among adult learners.

ACTIVITY BOX

Title: *Designing a Digital Learning Strategy for Your Nursing Module*

Select a module you currently teach or plan to teach. Reflect on how technology-enhanced learning can be integrated into it.

Step 1: Map the current teaching format and identify where flexibility could be introduced (e.g. asynchronous discussion boards, mobile access to content).

Step 2: Choose one or more digital strategies (e.g. microlearning, AI-driven adaptive learning, virtual patients) to embed.

Step 3: Consider the needs of diverse learners in your cohort—how would your strategy improve engagement, inclusion, and accessibility?

Step 4: Share and peer-review each other's digital learning strategy in a collaborative Padlet or online discussion forum.

Reflective Prompt: What are the anticipated barriers to implementing your strategy, and how might you address them?

SUPPORTING LIFELONG LEARNING AND PROFESSIONAL DEVELOPMENT

The fast-paced nature of healthcare means that nurses must continually update their knowledge and skills to keep up with emerging best practices, new technologies, and evolving patient needs. Flexible learning pathways support lifelong learning and professional development, ensuring that nurses remain competent throughout their careers (Frenk et al., 2010). Short courses, microlearning modules, and mobile-friendly learning platforms offer accessible ways for nurses to update their knowledge without committing to long-term, full-time study. Microlearning, which involves breaking content into small, easily digestible units, has been shown to enhance knowledge retention and engagement (Hug, 2010). For instance, nurses using mobile-based microlearning modules report greater satisfaction with learning due to its on-the-go accessibility and real-time application in practice (Schmidt-Kraepelin et al., 2019).

Additionally, open educational resources (OERs), such as freely available research articles, digital textbooks, and online courses, provide cost-effective learning opportunities that are particularly valuable for nurses working in low-resource settings (Hew & Cheung, 2014). The WHO (2021) has advocated for the global expansion of OERs as a means of promoting equitable access to nursing education. Lifelong learning is further supported by professional e-portfolios and digital badging systems, which allow nurses to track their learning and demonstrate competencies over time. These evidence-based documentation systems not only support career progression but also align with CBE models, ensuring that nurses remain accountable for their professional development.

CHALLENGES AND CONSIDERATIONS

While flexible learning offers numerous benefits, there are also challenges that must be addressed to ensure its effectiveness and accessibility (Table 5.2). Flexible learning is not simply a convenience but a necessity in modern nursing education. By embracing diverse learning formats, digital tools, and hybrid models, educators can ensure

Table 5.2 Challenges and Considerations to Promote Effectiveness and Accessibility

Challenges	Considerations for educators
Digital Divide and Access Disparities	• Some students may lack reliable internet access or technological resources, creating inequities in learning opportunities
	• Institutions must invest in inclusive digital strategies, such as providing loaned devices or subsidising broadband access for disadvantaged learners (Czerniewicz et al., 2020)
Maintaining Engagement in Online Learning	• While digital learning offers flexibility, it also presents risks of isolation and disengagement (Means et al., 2013)
	• Hybrid models with synchronous interactions, virtual study groups, and digital mentorship can help mitigate this issue (Salmon, 2014)
Faculty Development and Support	• Educators must be trained in digital pedagogy to effectively implement flexible learning models (Torrisi-Steele & Drew, 2013)
	• Institutions should offer ongoing faculty development to enhance digital literacy and teaching effectiveness

that nursing students are equipped with the knowledge and skills they need—wherever and whenever they need them. The integration of blended learning, immersive simulations, and mobile learning supports diverse learner needs, enhances professional development, and ultimately strengthens patient care outcomes. However, addressing accessibility barriers, maintaining student engagement, and supporting educators is essential for realising the full potential of flexible learning.

As nursing education continues to evolve, flexibility must remain at the heart of curriculum design, ensuring that learning is not only accessible but also adaptable, inclusive, and sustainable.

DIGITAL AND MOBILE LEARNING INNOVATIONS

The rapid advancement of digital technologies has transformed nursing education, offering greater flexibility, accessibility, and engagement for learners. Digital and mobile learning innovations provide interactive, personalised, and scalable solutions that support both formal education and lifelong learning in nursing. By leveraging digital tools such as mobile learning (m-learning), microlearning, AI, and OERs, nursing education can become more inclusive, responsive, and effective.

Mobile learning (m-learning) refers to educational content delivered via mobile devices, allowing learners to access materials anytime, anywhere (Gikas & Grant, 2013). The use of smartphones, tablets, and cloud-based applications in nursing education enables students to engage with learning materials while balancing clinical placements, work commitments, and personal responsibilities. A study by George et al. (2014) found that nursing students who used mobile-based learning platforms demonstrated improved knowledge retention and critical thinking skills compared to those using traditional methods. Mobile apps such as Medscape, UpToDate, and BMJ Best Practice provide real-time access to clinical guidelines, supporting evidence-based practice (EBP) and enhancing students' ability to apply theoretical knowledge in practical settings.

M-learning aligns with constructivist and self-directed learning theories, empowering students to take control of their education by engaging with content on-demand and in real-world contexts (Kolb, 1984). In addition, gamified mobile learning applications, such as Kahoot! and Osmosis, enhance motivation and engagement, reinforcing learning through quizzes and interactive challenges (Schmidt-Kraepelin et al., 2019). Despite its advantages, m-learning also presents challenges, including device compatibility issues, internet access disparities, and potential distractions from non-educational content (Czerniewicz et al., 2020). Educators must therefore implement structured mobile learning strategies, ensuring content is aligned with curriculum objectives and includes interactive components to maintain engagement.

MICROLEARNING AND JUST-IN-TIME LEARNING

Microlearning involves delivering content in small, focused units, typically in video, infographic, or interactive quiz format. This approach is particularly beneficial for busy healthcare professionals, as it allows learning to occur in short, manageable sessions that fit into clinical schedules (Hug, 2010). Research has shown that microlearning improves retention rates by up to 20% compared to traditional lecture-based approaches, due to its alignment with cognitive load theory, which suggests that learners absorb information more effectively in small chunks (Mayer & Moreno, 2010).

Examples of microlearning in nursing education include:

- Short instructional videos demonstrating clinical skills (e.g. wound care, catheterisation).

- Case-based learning scenarios that present a patient case followed by guided decision-making exercises.

- Podcast-style learning for evidence-based practice updates, allowing nurses to learn while commuting or exercising.

Microlearning also supports just-in-time learning (JITL), where students access information precisely when they need it—such as reviewing procedure guidelines before performing a clinical task (Guze, 2015). This method enhances knowledge application, reduces errors, and improves confidence in clinical settings.

OPEN EDUCATIONAL RESOURCES (OERS) AND DIGITAL EQUITY

OERs are freely accessible, high-quality educational materials that promote knowledge-sharing and reduce financial barriers in nursing education (Hew & Cheung, 2014).

Examples of OERs include:

- Massive Open Online Courses (MOOCs) from platforms such as Coursera, FutureLearn, and OpenWHO.

- Free digital textbooks and clinical practice guidelines from organisations like the WHO and NHS Digital.

- Collaborative Wikis and online repositories for evidence-based nursing practice.

OERs democratise education by providing access to high-quality resources regardless of geographical location or institutional affiliation. However, challenges such as content reliability, lack of standardisation, and digital literacy gaps must be addressed to maximise their impact (Hew & Cheung, 2014).

ARTIFICIAL INTELLIGENCE (AI) AND PERSONALISED LEARNING

AI is revolutionising education by offering personalised, data-driven, and adaptive learning experiences. In nursing education, AI-driven tools provide individualised learning pathways, automate administrative processes, and enhance clinical decision-making training. AI can analyse student performance, predict learning needs, and provide real-time feedback, enabling a more efficient and student-centred approach to education (Huang et al., 2020).

AI applications in nursing education include adaptive learning systems, virtual patient simulations, AI-driven assessments, and intelligent tutoring systems (ITS). These technologies enhance engagement, improve retention, and support CBE by ensuring that students receive tailored content suited to their progress and needs (Dede, 2020). However, ethical concerns regarding data privacy, algorithmic bias, and the role of AI in human decision-making must be addressed to ensure its responsible implementation (Topol, 2019).

AI-driven adaptive learning platforms use machine learning algorithms to adjust content delivery based on student engagement and performance. These platforms personalise education by:

- Identifying knowledge gaps and delivering targeted remediation content.

- Adjusting difficulty levels based on a learner's progress.

- Providing real-time feedback to enhance self-directed learning.

An example of AI-driven learning is Socratic by Google, which helps students by analysing queries and guiding them towards relevant resources. Similarly, platforms such as Smart Sparrow and Carnegie Studies suggest that AI-enabled adaptive learning systems can provide personalised learning paths, adjusting content and pacing to individual learners' needs (Roll & Wylie, 2016).Research suggests that adaptive learning enhances engagement, reduces cognitive overload, and improves competency acquisition (Aleven et al., 2016). For nursing students, this means more efficient skill development, reduced failure rates, and enhanced clinical reasoning (Chen et al., 2021).

AI-DRIVEN VIRTUAL PATIENTS AND SIMULATION TRAINING

Virtual patients (VPs) powered by AI simulate realistic clinical interactions, enabling nursing students to practise clinical decision-making in a risk-free environment. AI-powered simulations can dynamically adapt patient responses based on student input, providing a more interactive and responsive learning experience compared to traditional case-based learning.

Examples of AI-driven virtual patient systems include:

- SimMan 3G (Laerdal): Uses AI to simulate human physiological responses in high-fidelity simulations.

- Body Interact: An interactive AI-driven clinical simulation that provides real-time patient interactions.

- GIGXR's HoloPatient: Uses AI and AR to create lifelike virtual patients in mixed-reality learning environments.

A systematic review by Verkuyl et al. (2019) found that AI-enhanced simulation training improves clinical judgement, situational awareness, and patient safety outcomes. Unlike traditional simulation, AI-driven VPs learn from student decisions, evolving scenarios in real-time to better reflect the unpredictability of clinical practice.

AI is increasingly integrated into clinical decision support systems (CDSS), helping nurses and healthcare providers make more accurate diagnoses and treatment decisions. In education, AI-driven CDSS allows students to practise evidence-based clinical reasoning through real-world case studies (Topol, 2019). For example, IBM Watson Health provides AI-assisted diagnostics by analysing patient data and offering evidence-based recommendations. By training with such systems, nursing students can develop stronger critical thinking skills, data interpretation abilities, and diagnostic reasoning. Additionally, AI-enhanced electronic health records (EHR) simulations enable students to engage in clinical documentation exercises, improving their familiarity with patient management systems used in hospitals.

AI-DRIVEN FORMATIVE AND SUMMATIVE ASSESSMENTS

AI is also transforming student assessment by providing automated grading, instant feedback, and predictive analytics to identify students at risk of failing. AI-driven natural language processing (NLP) systems can analyse written responses and assess competency levels, communication skills, and reasoning processes.

Examples include:

- AI-powered essay scoring systems, such as Gradescope, which may be used to evaluate nursing students' clinical reflections.

- AI chatbots, like Jill Watson at Georgia Tech, which provide instant feedback on discussion forums.

- Virtual Objective Structured Clinical Examinations, where AI evaluates student interactions with virtual patients.

A study by Zawacki-Richter et al. (2019) found that AI-assisted assessment improves student performance by offering immediate, detailed feedback, reducing grading bias, and identifying learning trends.

ETHICAL CONSIDERATIONS AND CHALLENGES OF AI IN NURSING EDUCATION

While AI presents transformative opportunities for nursing education, its implementation raises several ethical, pedagogical, and practical challenges. Ensuring that AI is used responsibly, equitably, and transparently is essential to maintaining academic integrity, student autonomy, and professional accountability.

AI systems rely on algorithms trained on existing datasets, which can introduce biases that impact student learning experiences. If an AI-driven learning tool is developed using data that does not represent diverse student populations, it may disproportionately benefit some groups while disadvantaging others (Obermeyer et al., 2019). Algorithmic bias may result in AI assessments favouring students from specific demographic backgrounds, potentially reinforcing disparities in academic performance. Furthermore, AI-generated learning pathways might misinterpret individual needs, leading to unintended discrimination in adaptive learning environments. Nursing educators must regularly audit AI systems to ensure they are trained on diverse, inclusive, and representative datasets. To mitigate bias, AI-driven education must be continuously refined with input from diverse student populations, educators, and ethicists to ensure fairness and accuracy.

AI in education relies on large-scale data collection, raising concerns about student privacy, informed consent, and data security (Huang et al., 2020). AI-driven platforms track student progress, assess learning behaviours, and analyse performance metrics to deliver personalised educational experiences. However, improper data handling can result in breaches of confidentiality, unauthorised data access, or misuse of student information. There are a number of key privacy considerations to consider which are outlined in Table 5.3. Educational institutions should establish clear AI data governance policies, ensuring that student rights, confidentiality, and digital ethics are prioritised.

Table 5.3 Considerations for AI Data Governance

Considerations	Details
Who owns the data?	Institutions must clarify whether students retain control over their educational data or if it belongs to third-party AI providers
How is student data protected?	Institutions must ensure compliance with General Data Protection Regulation (GDPR) and ethical AI principles, ensuring secure data encryption and anonymisation
Informed consent and transparency	Students should be fully aware of how their data is used, with the option to opt out of AI-driven data analysis

THE ROLE OF EDUCATORS IN AI-DRIVEN NURSING EDUCATION

A common concern is whether AI will replace traditional educators, reducing the human element in nursing education. While AI can enhance learning by automating assessments, providing real-time feedback, and offering personalised study plans, it cannot replace the critical thinking, mentorship, and emotional intelligence that educators bring to nursing education (Luckin et al., 2016). AI-driven learning must be faculty-guided, ensuring that AI serves as a supplementary tool rather than an autonomous instructor. Nursing educators must be trained in AI literacy, understanding how to interpret AI-generated insights and effectively integrate technology into teaching. AI should be used to enhance, not replace, traditional teaching methods, ensuring that nursing students still receive human-centred mentorship and ethical guidance. Educators play a vital role in shaping AI implementation, ensuring that technology supports rather than diminishes the quality of nursing education.

Implementing AI-driven learning systems requires significant investment in digital infrastructure, faculty training, and ongoing software updates. Institutions with limited resources may struggle to afford high-quality AI tools, leading to disparities in access to AI-enhanced education (Zawacki-Richter et al., 2019). High costs of AI-powered platforms can create a digital divide, where wealthier institutions have access to superior educational technology while others are left behind. Limited digital literacy among faculty and students may hinder AI adoption, requiring comprehensive training programs. Furthermore, unequal access to internet connectivity and digital devices may prevent students in low-resource settings from benefiting fully from AI-enhanced education. To ensure equitable AI integration, institutions must invest in faculty development, provide financial support for AI adoption, and address digital accessibility issues to ensure that all students benefit equally from AI-driven learning.

ETHICAL RESPONSIBILITY IN AI-ASSISTED CLINICAL DECISION-MAKING

As AI is increasingly used to train nursing students in clinical decision-making, concerns arise about over-reliance on AI recommendations. Nursing students must learn to critically evaluate AI-generated clinical suggestions rather than blindly following machine-driven decisions. AI should be used to support, not replace, human judgement in patient care scenarios. Students must be trained in clinical reasoning skills alongside AI-based diagnostics to ensure they understand the limitations and potential errors in AI-generated recommendations. AI algorithms in clinical education must be transparent, with clear explanations of how decisions are made to prevent black-box decision-making. Educators must reinforce ethical nursing principles, patient safety, and human oversight to prevent AI dependency in clinical practice.

The integration of AI into nursing education presents unparalleled opportunities but also significant ethical and practical challenges. Addressing concerns related to algorithmic bias, data privacy, educator roles, financial accessibility, and AI-driven decision-making is essential to ensure that AI serves as a tool for enhancing nursing education rather than replacing human judgement.

As AI continues to evolve, nursing education must prioritise ethical AI governance, faculty training, and digital equity to harness its full potential responsibly. By maintaining a balance between technological innovation and human oversight, AI can transform nursing education into a more efficient, personalised, and ethically sound learning environment.

INTERPROFESSIONAL AND COLLABORATIVE LEARNING THROUGH TECHNOLOGY

Collaboration is a fundamental skill in nursing, requiring effective teamwork, communication, and shared decision-making among healthcare professionals. Interprofessional education (IPE), which brings together students from different healthcare disciplines, enhances collaborative competence and patient-centred care (Barr et al., 2014). Digital technologies play a pivotal role in facilitating interprofessional and collaborative learning through virtual platforms, simulation-based training, and real-time communication tools.

Virtual case-based learning (VCBL) involves interactive, team-based problem-solving scenarios that simulate real-world healthcare challenges. These platforms allow nursing students to collaborate with medical, pharmacy, physiotherapy, and social work students in virtual patient case discussions.

By integrating discussion forums, collaborative case studies, and interactive decision-making tools, VCBL ensures that students learn how to communicate effectively and resolve conflicts in multidisciplinary teams before entering clinical practice (Reeves et al., 2016).

SIMULATION-BASED TEAM TRAINING

Simulation is widely recognised as an effective method for enhancing teamwork, leadership, and crisis management skills in nursing (Jeffries, 2020). Digital simulation platforms, including VR, AR, and AI-driven virtual patients, provide realistic scenarios where interprofessional teams can practise communication, delegation, and emergency response strategies. High-fidelity simulation labs allow students to engage in real-time, scenario-based teamwork exercises. In addition, VR-based interprofessional simulations recreate emergency situations, such as cardiac arrests, where nurses, doctors, and paramedics must work together under pressure. AI-powered debriefing tools provide real-time feedback on team performance, communication, and leadership. A systematic review by Verkuyl et al. (2019) found that interprofessional simulation training significantly improves patient safety outcomes by enhancing coordination and reducing medical errors.

COLLABORATIVE DIGITAL PLATFORMS FOR COMMUNICATION AND PEER LEARNING

In addition to structured learning, technology facilitates informal collaboration and peer learning through cloud-based communication tools. Platforms such as Microsoft Teams, Slack, and Padlet enable students and faculty to engage in discussions, share resources, and provide real-time feedback. Studies suggest that social learning through digital platforms improves engagement and knowledge retention by allowing students to actively interact, ask questions, and reflect on their learning (Salmon, 2014). However, successful implementation requires training on digital literacy, guidance on professional online communication, and strategies to maintain student engagement in virtual discussions (Torrisi-Steele & Drew, 2013). Digital and mobile learning innovations, combined with interprofessional and collaborative learning strategies, enhance flexibility, engagement, and knowledge application in nursing education. Technologies such as mobile learning, AI-driven adaptive platforms, simulation-based training, and virtual case-based learning are transforming the way nurses learn and collaborate. However, ensuring equitable access, addressing digital literacy gaps, and fostering meaningful student engagement remain critical considerations for future advancements.

ASSESSING THE EFFICACY OF DIGITAL INTERVENTIONS

As digital learning becomes increasingly integrated into nursing education, it is essential to assess its effectiveness, impact on student learning outcomes, and overall contribution to competency development. Evaluation ensures that digital tools such as e-learning platforms, simulation-based training, and AI-driven tutoring enhance nursing education rather than merely replacing traditional teaching methods. To determine the efficacy of digital learning, educators must focus on measuring learning outcomes, engagement, knowledge retention, and competency development through evidence-based approaches.

The effectiveness of digital learning in nursing education can be evaluated through multiple dimensions, including learning outcomes, student engagement, knowledge retention, and competency development. Each of these factors plays a crucial role in determining whether digital interventions enhance nursing education and contribute to high-quality, evidence-based practice.

One of the primary indicators of effectiveness is learning outcomes, which assess whether students meet the intended educational objectives. Learning outcomes can be evaluated through a combination of formative and summative assessments, including quizzes, written reflections, clinical case studies, and objective structured clinical examinations (OSCEs). Digital learning platforms often incorporate automated assessment tools that provide real-time feedback, enabling students to track their progress and address knowledge gaps. Studies have shown that well-designed e-learning modules and simulation-based training significantly enhance knowledge acquisition, clinical reasoning, and problem-solving skills, making them as effective—if not more so—than traditional teaching methods.

Another critical factor in evaluating digital learning is student engagement and motivation, as active participation correlates with better retention, deeper understanding, and improved academic performance. Digital learning platforms utilise various engagement strategies, including gamification, interactive case studies, and collaborative online discussions. Features such as scenario-based quizzes, virtual patient cases, and adaptive learning pathways help maintain student interest and motivation. However, some research suggests that purely online learning can lead to reduced engagement if students lack opportunities for social interaction and faculty support (Means et al., 2013). Hybrid learning models that combine digital learning with face-to-face interaction have been found to be more effective in sustaining engagement (Rowe et al., 2012).

Knowledge retention is another important measure of digital learning effectiveness, as it determines whether students can recall and apply what they have learned over time. Research suggests that microlearning and spaced repetition techniques improve long-term retention by reducing cognitive overload and reinforcing key concepts at optimal intervals (Mayer & Moreno, 2010). Simulation-based learning has also been shown to enhance retention, as students gain hands-on experience in realistic scenarios, making learning more experiential and memorable. Furthermore, multimodal learning, which incorporates a mix of video, text, interactive elements, and practical applications, enhances cognitive processing and recall, leading to stronger knowledge retention in nursing students (Padilha et al., 2019).

Finally, competency development is a fundamental goal of nursing education, and digital learning plays a significant role in helping students achieve the necessary clinical and professional competencies. CBE focuses on ensuring that students demonstrate proficiency in clinical skills, critical thinking, and decision-making rather than simply completing coursework. Digital learning tools support competency development through AI-driven adaptive learning, which adjusts difficulty levels based on student progress, and virtual patient simulations, which enable students to practise real-world clinical decision-making in a risk-free environment. Additionally, digital assessments, e-portfolios, and clinical skill tracking systems allow educators to monitor student progress and provide targeted feedback to ensure skill mastery. A meta-analysis found that simulation-based digital learning significantly improves clinical competency, making it an effective tool for bridging the gap between theory and practice.

Evaluating digital learning in nursing education requires a comprehensive approach that considers learning outcomes, engagement, retention, and competency development (Table 5.4). Research indicates that blended learning, interactive simulations, and AI-driven adaptive platforms provide significant advantages over traditional methods, particularly when designed with evidence-based principles in mind. However, to maximise effectiveness, digital learning must be pedagogically sound, engaging, and tailored to student needs, ensuring that it enhances both knowledge acquisition and practical skill development.

Evidence-based Approaches to Evaluating Digital Learning

Evaluating digital learning requires evidence-based methodologies that align with pedagogical best practices. Research on e-learning, simulation-based training, and AI-driven tutoring provides valuable insights into how digital interventions contribute to nursing education. By examining these approaches, educators can determine the most effective strategies for integrating digital tools into nursing curricula.

E-learning and online platforms have been extensively studied in nursing education, with research highlighting their impact on student satisfaction, knowledge retention, and skill development. Studies indicate that

Table 5.4 Metrics for Measuring Digital Learning Success

	Measurement method	Example
Learning Outcomes	Exam scores, clinical assessments	Knowledge retention studies
Engagement	Student participation rates	LMS analytics, discussion forums
Knowledge Retention	Pre/post-test comparisons	Longitudinal studies
Competency Development	Virtual OSCEs, skill tracking	VR-based skill simulations

blended learning approaches, which combine online instruction with face-to-face learning, tend to produce higher student satisfaction and improved clinical knowledge (McCutcheon et al., 2015). Self-paced e-learning modules offer flexibility and accessibility, allowing students to learn at their own convenience. However, one of the challenges of purely online learning is the requirement for strong learner self-motivation and discipline. Collaborative e-learning tools, such as discussion forums and virtual teamwork projects, help mitigate this issue by fostering peer-to-peer learning and critical thinking. Systematic reviews suggest that e-learning is as effective as, if not superior to, traditional lectures when well-designed and interactive (Means et al., 2013).

Simulation-based training has become a cornerstone of digital nursing education, providing a risk-free environment where students can develop clinical reasoning, teamwork, and procedural skills. High-fidelity simulations that utilise VR, AR, and AI allow nursing students to practise complex procedures and emergency scenarios in a controlled setting. Research has shown that simulation-based learning enhances confidence, clinical judgement, and decision-making skills (Jeffries, 2020). VR-based simulations, in particular, have been found to increase skill transfer to real-world clinical practice, ensuring that students are better prepared for hands-on patient care (Padilha et al., 2019). Additionally, structured debriefing and reflective practice within simulation training further enhance learning outcomes by encouraging students to analyse their experiences and improve future performance (Verkuyl et al., 2019).

AI-driven tutoring and adaptive learning technologies are emerging as powerful tools in nursing education, enabling personalised learning pathways that adapt to individual student progress. AI-powered tutoring systems adjust content difficulty in real time, ensuring that students receive instruction tailored to their needs (Aleven et al., 2016). AI-driven analytics also help educators identify struggling students early, allowing for timely intervention and personalised support.

Conversational AI chatbots have been introduced in some nursing programmes to provide instant feedback, reinforce knowledge, and enhance student engagement. By leveraging AI, nursing education can become more efficient, responsive, and data-driven, improving learning outcomes while maintaining a student-centred approach. Overall, research supports the effectiveness of e-learning, simulation-based training, and AI-driven tutoring in nursing education. These digital interventions enhance knowledge acquisition, competency development, and student engagement, making them valuable additions to traditional teaching methods. However, their success depends on careful instructional design, faculty training, and student support to ensure that digital learning remains both effective and equitable. Future research should focus on long-term impacts, standardisation of digital assessments, and integration of AI-driven personalisation in nursing curricula.

FRAMEWORKS FOR TECHNOLOGY AND FEEDBACK IN NURSING EDUCATION

The integration of technology into nursing education necessitates structured frameworks that support effective teaching, assessment, and student development. Feedback is a crucial element in nursing education, guiding learners in critical thinking, clinical reasoning, and skill acquisition. Technological advancements have transformed feedback mechanisms, enabling real-time, personalised, and data-driven evaluations that enhance student learning experiences.

One key framework used in nursing education is the Technology-Enhanced Feedback Model (TEFM), which integrates learning analytics, AI, and digital assessment tools to provide timely, meaningful, and adaptive feedback. AI-driven learning platforms can analyse student performance trends, offering personalised study recommendations and automated feedback on assignments and clinical competencies. This approach allows educators to move beyond traditional grading systems and provide students with targeted insights into their strengths and areas for improvement (Aleven et al., 2016).

Another widely used model is the Feedback Spiral in Digital Learning, which emphasises a continuous feedback loop where students receive immediate, actionable feedback from simulation-based training, virtual case studies, and peer interactions. High-fidelity simulations with VR and AR allow nursing students to receive automated feedback on clinical decision-making, enhancing their situational awareness and competence in real-world scenarios (Verkuyl et al., 2019).

Technology also facilitates peer-to-peer and collaborative feedback, particularly through discussion forums, e-portfolios, and digital assessment dashboards. These tools enable students to reflect on their learning, track progress, and engage in formative feedback exchanges with instructors and peers. The incorporation of automated and human-mediated feedback mechanisms ensures that students develop competency-based skills in an interactive and student-centred learning environment.

In summary, frameworks for technology and feedback in nursing education must be structured, evidence-based, and student-focused. Digital technologies offer scalable, personalised, and continuous assessment opportunities, ultimately enhancing learning outcomes, engagement, and professional development in nursing education.

INNOVATION BOX

Title: *The Digital Competency Loop: A Feedback-Driven Approach to AI in Nursing Education*

This innovative approach builds on the concept of adaptive learning by embedding AI-driven feedback directly into competency tracking systems. The *Digital Competency Loop* involves four continuous stages:

1. **Engage** (the student interacts with AI-driven simulations or platforms)
2. **Analyse** (performance data is gathered and reviewed by the system)
3. **Respond** (personalised feedback and remediation content is provided)
4. **Demonstrate** (the student re-engages to demonstrate improved competence)

What makes this approach distinctive is its continuous, low-stakes, formative design, where failure is treated as a springboard for personalised learning, rather than a summative endpoint. By making feedback an active agent in the learning process, the loop improves performance while supporting confidence and retention.

DIGITAL FEEDBACK IN INTERPROFESSIONAL EDUCATION

Interprofessional education (IPE) is essential in nursing, as it prepares students to collaborate with professionals from other healthcare disciplines. Digital technology has transformed how feedback is delivered in IPE, making assessments more collaborative, data-driven, and immediate. Digital feedback mechanisms enhance communication, teamwork, and decision-making skills, ensuring that nursing students are well-equipped to function in interdisciplinary healthcare teams.

One approach to digital feedback in IPE is collaborative digital assessments, where students receive feedback from multiple disciplines rather than solely from nursing educators. Cloud-based platforms and electronic portfolios enable joint feedback from doctors, physiotherapists, pharmacists, and other healthcare professionals, providing students with diverse perspectives on their clinical reasoning and teamwork skills. Research has shown that multi-source digital feedback helps students develop a broader understanding of interprofessional roles, enhancing their ability to work effectively in patient-centred care teams (Reeves et al., 2016).

Virtual simulation-based teamwork assessments are another innovative way to evaluate interdisciplinary performance. In these digital simulations, students from different healthcare backgrounds collaborate in high-fidelity, AI-powered virtual scenarios, such as managing a deteriorating patient or responding to an emergency. AI and analytics tools track student interactions, evaluating communication, leadership, and role clarity within the team. Immediate, data-driven feedback provides insights into team dynamics, response efficiency, and clinical decision-making, allowing students to refine their approach to interprofessional teamwork (Verkuyl et al., 2019).

An example of AI-assisted feedback in a multidisciplinary nursing education program is the use of automated feedback systems in virtual patient simulations. AI-driven platforms, such as Body Interact and SimX, analyse student interactions with virtual patients and provide real-time feedback on clinical reasoning, communication, and interprofessional collaboration. This AI-generated feedback helps students identify strengths and areas for improvement, promoting a culture of reflective practice and continuous learning in interprofessional education.

By integrating digital feedback tools into IPE, nursing education can foster stronger interprofessional relationships, enhance patient safety, and prepare students for the complexities of modern healthcare teamwork.

CURRICULUM DESIGN AND CONTEMPORARY EDUCATION

The landscape of nursing education is evolving rapidly, with curriculum design shifting towards CBE. This transformation responds to the growing need for outcome-driven learning, where students are assessed based on their ability to demonstrate mastery of skills and knowledge rather than the traditional model of time-based progression. CBE ensures that nursing graduates are clinically competent, critically reflective, and prepared for real-world healthcare challenges. The integration of digital tools and technologies into competency assessments is central to this shift, enabling a more personalised, flexible, and efficient approach to nursing education.

To support the effective integration of digital tools in nursing education, a structured model can help educators visualise the connections between pedagogical design, technological enablers, and expected outcomes. Figure 5.1 presents the Diamond-Fox Model of Integrated Digital Education. Figure 5.1 illustrates how digital technologies are not standalone tools, but interconnected components of a broader educational system that promotes competency, ethical awareness, accessibility, and sustainability. The model is designed to support curriculum teams in aligning technology-enhanced teaching strategies with learner needs, professional standards, and global health priorities.

This diagram presents the Diamond-Fox Model of Integrated Digital Education, a visual framework structured around four interconnected principles essential to designing and delivering effective digital nurse education. At its centre lies *Integrated Digital Education*, which is supported and shaped by four equally important domains:

1. **Accessibility** – ensuring learners can engage with education regardless of location, background, or available resources

2. **Flexibility** – enabling multiple modes of learning, such as asynchronous content, mobile access, and varied pacing

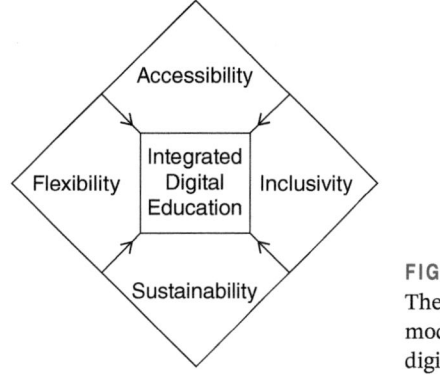

FIGURE 5.1
The diamond-fox model of integrated digital education

3. **Sustainability** – promoting eco-conscious delivery methods and long-term viability of educational models

4. **Inclusivity** – embedding equity, cultural sensitivity, and diverse learner representation in all aspects of digital delivery

Each principle is connected through iterative feedback loops, reflecting the model's emphasis on interconnectedness and adaptability. Rather than treating digital tools or teaching methods in isolation, this model positions them within a broader values-led, student-centred system. The Diamond-Fox Model can be used during curriculum design, programme validation, and team planning to ensure that innovation is always underpinned by principles of fairness, access, and pedagogical purpose.

THE SHIFT TO COMPETENCY-BASED EDUCATION (CBE)

Traditional nursing education models often rely on fixed curricula, set instructional hours, and standardised examinations. However, this time-bound approach does not necessarily ensure that students have mastered clinical skills, decision-making, and professional competencies. In contrast, CBE prioritises learning outcomes, ensuring that students progress only when they demonstrate proficiency in key competencies rather than merely completing required coursework (Frank et al., 2010). This model aligns with the realities of clinical practice, where nursing professionals must apply critical thinking, leadership, and problem-solving skills in unpredictable healthcare environments.

CBE fosters individualised learning pathways, allowing students to progress at their own pace. Some learners may excel in certain areas and require more support in others, and CBE ensures that students receive targeted instruction and remediation where necessary. Furthermore, CBE places a strong emphasis on reflective practice and continuous self-assessment, helping students develop lifelong learning habits essential for professional growth in a rapidly evolving healthcare landscape.

INTEGRATION OF DIGITAL TOOLS IN COMPETENCY ASSESSMENT

The integration of digital tools in competency assessment has significantly enhanced the efficiency, objectivity, and scalability of CBE in nursing education. Digital platforms allow for real-time tracking of student progress, personalised feedback, and adaptive assessments, ensuring that learners receive targeted support and development opportunities.

One key innovation in CBE is the use of AI-driven learning analytics, which track student performance across various assessments and clinical simulations. These analytics help educators identify competency gaps, enabling tailored learning plans for individual students. AI-powered feedback systems provide automated insights, ensuring that students receive immediate, data-driven evaluations of their strengths and areas for improvement (Aleven et al., 2016).

Additionally, virtual simulation tools and high-fidelity mannequins provide interactive, experiential learning experiences, allowing students to demonstrate clinical competencies in realistic healthcare scenarios. Digital simulations help assess critical thinking, patient safety, and emergency response skills, ensuring that students meet established clinical performance standards before entering real-world practice (Padilha et al., 2019).

E-portfolios and digital competency tracking systems have also revolutionised how nursing students document their learning journeys. These platforms enable students to compile evidence of skills acquisition, reflections, and peer/faculty feedback, creating a comprehensive record of professional development. Such tools not only support formative and summative assessment but also help nursing graduates showcase their competencies to employers.

In conclusion, CBE represents a fundamental shift in nursing education, prioritising mastery over seat time and ensuring that students are fully prepared for clinical practice. The integration of digital tools in competency assessment enhances the effectiveness of this model, enabling personalised learning, real-time feedback, and data-driven decision-making. As healthcare continues to evolve, nursing curricula must embrace CBE principles and leverage digital innovations to create future-ready, competent nursing professionals.

SUSTAINABILITY IN DIGITAL LEARNING AND NURSING EDUCATION

Sustainability is becoming a key priority in nursing education, particularly as digital learning continues to transform how knowledge is delivered and assessed. Integrating sustainable practices into digital learning not only reduces environmental impact but also enhances accessibility, equity, and global health outcomes. By leveraging cloud-based solutions, e-learning platforms, and digital-first curriculum models, nursing education can contribute to both climate sustainability and the achievement of Sustainable Development Goals (SDGs).

MINIMISING THE CARBON FOOTPRINT OF DIGITAL EDUCATION

A crucial aspect of sustainability in digital learning is minimising the carbon footprint of educational technologies. Traditional on-premise learning solutions, such as physical computer labs, servers, and printed educational materials, require significant energy and resource consumption. By contrast, cloud-based learning platforms offer a more sustainable alternative. Cloud computing reduces hardware dependency, optimises server efficiency, and enables remote access, decreasing the need for travel and paper-based learning materials (Tim & Rana, 2022).

Cloud-based Learning Management Systems (LMS), such as Moodle, Blackboard, and Canvas, store educational resources digitally, allowing students to access course materials anytime, anywhere. This shift reduces reliance on textbook printing, physical classroom space, and energy-intensive infrastructure. Additionally, virtual simulation tools, such as VR-based clinical training, eliminate the need for single-use simulation materials, promoting an eco-friendlier approach to competency-based learning.

However, the shift to digital learning must be balanced with sustainable data management practices, as data centres contribute to global energy consumption. Institutions should prioritise green cloud services that use renewable energy sources and energy-efficient data processing to reduce the carbon footprint of digital education (Masanet et al., 2020).

E-LEARNING FOR GLOBAL HEALTH EQUITY

Sustainability in digital learning extends beyond environmental considerations to social and educational equity. E-learning has the potential to bridge educational gaps in underserved areas, ensuring that nursing students in low-resource settings have access to high-quality education regardless of geographical barriers (WHO, 2021).

Digital learning eliminates traditional cost and access barriers, allowing students from developing countries, rural areas, and conflict zones to participate in nursing education through open-access courses, mobile learning applications, and low-bandwidth e-learning platforms. Massive Open Online Courses (MOOCs), offered by institutions such as

Coursera, edX, and FutureLearn, provide free or low-cost nursing education to global learners, fostering health equity and capacity-building. Additionally, digital platforms facilitate international collaborations, allowing students and educators to engage in global case discussions, cross-border research, and tele-mentoring. These initiatives support the World Health Organization's (WHO) Global Strategic Directions for Nursing and Midwifery, which emphasise scalable, technology-driven nursing education to strengthen the global healthcare workforce (WHO, 2021).

PROMOTING SUSTAINABLE DEVELOPMENT GOALS (SDGS) THROUGH NURSING EDUCATION

The United Nations (2015) SDGs provide a framework for integrating sustainability, health equity, and lifelong learning into nursing education. Digital learning plays a crucial role in supporting these goals by making education more accessible, environmentally sustainable, and globally inclusive. By leveraging e-learning technologies, cloud-based resources, and digital-first curriculum models, nursing education can contribute to multiple SDGs while preparing healthcare professionals for a rapidly changing world.

One of the most directly relevant SDGs to nursing education is SDG 3: Good Health and Well-being. By expanding access to high-quality, digital nursing education, institutions can produce better-trained healthcare professionals, ultimately leading to improved patient outcomes. Digital learning allows nursing students to gain critical skills and knowledge regardless of their geographic location, ensuring that healthcare workers in rural, underserved, or developing regions receive the same high-quality training as those in more resource-rich environments.

Another essential goal is SDG 4: Quality Education, which emphasises inclusive and equitable learning opportunities. Digital education platforms help bridge educational gaps by providing open-access courses, mobile learning applications, and online resources to students who may not have access to traditional classroom-based education. This is particularly beneficial for nurses in remote areas, conflict zones, or economically disadvantaged regions, where physical access to training institutions is limited. By reducing these barriers, e-learning fosters a more diverse and globally connected nursing workforce.

Sustainability in nursing education also aligns with SDG 12: Responsible Consumption and Production. The shift to digital learning significantly reduces reliance on printed materials, travel emissions, and resource-intensive classroom settings. By adopting cloud-based solutions, virtual simulations, and paperless assessments, institutions can minimise waste and lower the environmental footprint of nursing education. This transition supports the broader goal of sustainable healthcare practices, where reducing unnecessary resource consumption is crucial to environmental responsibility.

Additionally, digital learning supports SDG 13: Climate Action by promoting low-emission, eco-friendly educational solutions. Traditional, in-person learning models require physical infrastructure, commuting, and high energy consumption, all of which contribute to carbon emissions. By transitioning to cloud-based, digital-first learning solutions, nursing education can significantly lower its environmental impact. Virtual learning platforms, teleconferencing for lectures, and AI-driven adaptive learning help institutions operate more sustainably while ensuring that nursing students receive comprehensive and high-quality training.

To further align with these sustainability goals, educational institutions should embed climate and sustainability education into nursing curricula. Topics such as climate-resilient healthcare, environmental health, and disaster preparedness should be integrated into nursing training to ensure that future healthcare professionals understand and address the links between health, climate change, and social equity (Watts et al., 2020). By educating nurses on sustainable healthcare practices, eco-friendly patient care, and climate adaptation strategies, the nursing profession can play a pivotal role in global sustainability efforts.

Incorporating the SDG framework into nursing education is not just about reducing environmental impact—it is about creating a healthcare workforce that is equipped to tackle global challenges. Digital learning serves as a powerful enabler of these goals, fostering a sustainable, inclusive, and forward-thinking approach to nursing education.

FUTURE DIRECTIONS

Emerging technologies will continue to reshape nursing education, offering new opportunities for interactive, personalised, and scalable learning. AI will play a key role in automating assessments, providing real-time feedback, and supporting personalised learning pathways. VR and AR will enhance simulation-based training, allowing students to practise high-risk clinical scenarios in safe, controlled environments. Blockchain technology has the potential to revolutionise credentialing and competency tracking, ensuring that nursing qualifications are secure, verifiable, and transferable across institutions. Additionally, gamification strategies, such as game-based learning and competitive challenges, will further enhance student engagement and motivation.

As the field evolves, nursing educators must take a proactive role in integrating these innovations while maintaining ethical, equitable, and sustainable learning practices. This requires a commitment to faculty development, digital literacy, and evidence-based pedagogy, ensuring that technological advancements align with student needs and healthcare priorities. Institutions should also prioritise sustainability in digital learning, reducing the environmental impact of nursing education while promoting global accessibility and lifelong learning opportunities.

Looking ahead, the future of nursing education lies in its ability to adapt to emerging technologies, prioritise competency-based learning, and uphold ethical and sustainable educational principles. Educators must embrace innovation and digital transformation to equip the next generation of nurses with the skills, critical thinking, and resilience required for modern healthcare practice.

TAKE-HOME POINTS

1. Technology-enhanced learning, when designed with evidence-based pedagogy, can improve engagement, competency acquisition, and access in nursing education.

2. AI-driven feedback, simulation-based learning, and mobile learning strategies support flexible, personalised pathways aligned to competency-based frameworks.

3. Ethical, cultural, and sustainability considerations must be embedded in the planning and delivery of digital nursing education to ensure equitable, inclusive practice.

CPD REFLECTIVE QUESTIONS

1. How do I currently integrate technology into my teaching, and are these methods aligned with evidence-based learning strategies?

2. In what ways can I ensure that digital learning resources are accessible and inclusive for all students, regardless of background or location?

3. How might I address ethical and data governance concerns when using AI or analytics in the assessment and feedback of nursing students?

REFERENCES

Aleven, V., Roll, I., McLaren, B. M., & Koedinger, K. R. (2016). Help helps, but only so much: research on help seeking with intelligent tutoring systems. *International Journal of Artificial Intelligence in Education*, 26(1), 205–223.

Barr, H., Koppel, I., Reeves, S., Hammick, M., & Freeth, D. (2014). *Effective Interprofessional Education: Argument, Assumption and Evidence.* John Wiley & Sons.

Chen, X., Xie, H., Hwang, G. J., & Chen, W. (2021). A multi-perspective study on artificial intelligence in education: grants, conferences, journals, software tools, institutions, and researchers. *Computers & Education: Artificial Intelligence*, 2, 100012.

Czerniewicz, L., Agherdien, N., Badenhorst, J., Belluigi, D., Chambers, T., Chili, M., De Villiers, M., Felix, A., Gachago, D., Gokhale, C., Ivala, E., Kramm, N., Madiba, M., Mistri, G., Mgqwashu, E., Pallitt, N., Prinsloo, P., Solomon, K., Strydom, S., Swanepoel, M., Waghid, F., & Wissing, G. (2020). A wake-up call: equity, inequality and COVID-19 emergency remote teaching and learning. *Postdigital Science and Education*, 2(3), 946–967.

Dede, C. (2020). *The 60-Year Curriculum: New Models for Lifelong Learning in the Digital Economy.* Routledge.

Frank, J. R., Snell, L. S. & Cate, O. T. (2010). Competency-based medical education: theory to practice. *Medical Teacher*, 32(8), 638–645.

Frenk, J., Chen, L., Bhutta, Z. A., Cohen, J., Crisp, N., Evans, T., Fineberg, H., Garcia, P., Ke, Y., Kelley, P., Kistnasamy, B., Meleis, A., Naylor, D., Pablos-Mendez, A., Reddy, S., Scrimshaw, S., Sepúlveda, J., Serwadda, D., & Zurayk, H. (2010). Health professionals for a new century: transforming education to strengthen health systems in an interdependent world. *The Lancet*, 376(9756), pp. 1923–1958. https://doi.org/10.1016/S0140-6736(10)61854-5.

George, P. P., Papachristou, N., Belisario, J. M., Wang, W., Wark, P. A., & Cotic, Z. (2014). Online eLearning for undergraduates in health professions: a systematic review of the impact on knowledge, skills, attitudes and satisfaction. *Journal of Global Health*, 9(1), 010406.

Gikas, J., & Grant, M. M. (2013). Mobile computing devices in higher education: student perspectives on learning with cellphones, smartphones & social media. *The Internet and Higher Education*, 19, 18–26.

Guze, P. A. (2015). Using technology to meet the challenges of medical education. *Transactions of the American Clinical and Climatological Association*, 126, 260.

Hew, K. F., & Cheung, W. S. (2014). Students' and instructors' use of massive open online courses (MOOCs): motivations and challenges. *Educational Research Review*, 12, 45–58.

Huang, R., Spector, J. M., & Yang, J. (2020). *Educational Technology: A Primer for the 21st Century*. Springer.

Hug, T. (2010). Mobile learning as "microlearning": conceptual considerations. *International Journal of Mobile and Blended Learning*, 2(4), pp. 47–57.

Jeffries, P. R. (2020). *The NLN Jeffries Simulation Theory*. Wolters Kluwer.

Kolb, D. A. (1984). *Experiential Learning: Experience as the Source of Learning and Development*. Prentice-Hall.

Luckin, R., Holmes, W., Griffiths, M., & Forcier, L. B. (2016). *Intelligence Unleashed: An Argument for AI in Education*. Pearson Education.

Masanet, E., Shehabi, A., Lei, N., Smith, S., & Koomey, J. (2020). Recalibrating global data center energy-use estimates. *Science*, 367(6481), 984–986.

Mayer, R. E., & Moreno, R. (2010). Techniques that reduce extraneous cognitive load and manage intrinsic cognitive load during multimedia learning. *Cognitive Load Theory*, 131–152.

McCutcheon, K., Lohan, M., Traynor, M., & Martin, D. (2015). A systematic review evaluating the impact of online or blended learning vs. face-to-face learning of clinical skills in undergraduate nursing education. *Journal of Advanced Nursing*, 71(2), 255–270.

Means, B., Toyama, Y., Murphy, R., Bakia, M., & Jones, K. (2013). The effectiveness of online and blended learning: a meta-analysis of the empirical literature. *Teachers College Record*, 115(3), 1–47.

Obermeyer, Z., Powers, B., Vogeli, C., & Mullainathan, S. (2019). Dissecting racial bias in an algorithm used to manage the health of populations. *Science*, 366(6464), 447–453.

O'Doherty, D., Dromey, M., Lougheed, J., Hannigan, A., Last, J. & McGrath, D. (2018). Barriers and solutions to online learning in medical education – an integrative review. *BMC Medical Education*, 18(1), 130. https://doi.org/10.1186/s12909-018-1240-0.

Padilha, J. M., Machado, P. P., Ribeiro, A., Ramos, J., & Costa, P. (2019). Clinical virtual simulation in nursing education: randomized controlled trial. *Journal of Medical Internet Research*, 21(3), e11529.

Reeves, S., Fletcher, S., Barr, H., Birch, I., Boet, S., Davies, N., McFadyen, A., Rivera, J., & Kitto, S. (2016). A BEME systematic review of the effects of interprofessional education: BEME guide no. 39. *Medical Teacher*, 38(7), 656–668.

Roll, I. & Wylie, R. (2016). Evolution and revolution in artificial intelligence in education. *International Journal of Artificial Intelligence in Education*, 26(2), pp. 582–599.

Rowe, M., Frantz, J., & Bozalek, V. (2012). The role of blended learning in the clinical education of healthcare students: a systematic review. *Medical Teacher*, 34(4), e216–e221.

Salmon, G. (2014). *E-tivities: The key to Active Online Learning*. Routledge.

Schmidt-Kraepelin, M., Thiebes, S., Tran, M., & Sunyaev, A. (2019). What's in the game? Developing a taxonomy of gamification concepts for health apps. *Proceedings of the 52nd Hawaii International Conference on System Sciences*.

Tim H. W., & Rana M. E. (2022). A review of cloud computing on sustainable development: contribution, exploration and potential challenges. *2022 International Conference on Data Analytics for Business and Industry (ICDABI)*. https://doi.org/10.1109/ICDABI56818.2022.10041482.

Topol, E. (2019). *Deep Medicine: How Artificial Intelligence Can Make Healthcare Human Again*. Basic Books.

Torrisi-Steele, G. and Drew, S., (2013). The literature landscape of blended learning in higher education: The need for better understanding of academic blended practice. *International Journal for Academic Development*, 18(4), pp. 371–383.

United Nations (2015). *Sustainable development goals: 17 goals to transform our world*. Online. https://www.un.org/en/exhibits/page/sdgs-17-goals-transform-world. Accessed: (9 December 2025).

Verkuyl, M., Lapum, J. L., Hughes, M., McCulloch, T., Liu, L., Mastrilli, P., & St-Amant, O. (2019). Virtual gaming simulation in nursing education: a mixed-methods study. *Clinical Simulation in Nursing*, 29, 9–14.

Watts, N., Amann, M., Arnell, N., Ayeb-Karlsson, S., Beagley, J., Belesova, K., Boykoff, M., Byass, P., Cai, W., Campbell-Lendrum, D., Capstick, S., Chambers, J., Coleman, S., Dalin, C., Daly, M., Dasandi, N., Dasgupta, S., Davies, M., Di Napoli, C., Dominguez-Salas, P., Drummond, P., Dubrow, R., Ebi, K. L., Eckelman, M., Ekins, P., Escobar, L. E., Georgeson, L., Golder, S., Grace, D., Graham, H., Haggar, P., Hamilton, I., Hartinger, S., Hess, J., Hsu, S. -C., Hughes, N., Jankin Mikhaylov, S., Jimenez, M. P., Kelman, I., Kennard, H., Kiesewetter, G., Kinney, P. L., Kjellstrom, T., Kniveton, D., Lampard, P., Lemke, B., Liu, Y., Liu, Z., Lott, M., Lowe, R., Martinez-Urtaza, J., Maslin, M., McAllister, L., McGushin, A., McMichael, C., Milner, J., Moradi-Lakeh, M., Morrissey, K., Munzert, S., Murray, K.A., Neville, T., Nilsson, M., Sewe, M. O., Oreszczyn, T., Otto, M., Owfi, F., Pearman, O., Pencheon, D., Quinn, R., Rabbaniha, M., Robinson, E., Rocklöv, J., Romanello, M., Semenza, J. C., Sherman, J., Shi, L., Springmann, M., Tabatabaei, M., Taylor, J., Triñanes, J., Shumake-Guillemot, J., Vu, B., Wilkinson, P., Winning, M., Gong, P., Montgomery, H., & Costello, A. (2020). The 2020 report of the Lancet Countdown on health and climate change: responding to converging crises. *The Lancet*, 397(10269), 129–170.

World Health Organization (WHO) (2021). *Global strategic directions for nursing and midwifery (2021–2025)*. https://www.who.int/publications/i/item/9789240033863. Accessed: (9 December 2025).

Zawacki-Richter, O., Marín, V.I., Bond, M., & Gouverneur, F. (2019). Systematic review of research on artificial intelligence applications in higher education – where are the educators? *International Journal of Educational Technology in Higher Education*, 16, Article 39. https://doi.org/10.1186/s41239-019-0171-0.

CHAPTER 6

Transformative Simulation

Aby Mitchell

Florence Nightingale Faculty for Nursing, Midwifery and Palliative Care, King's College London, UK

AIM

To explore the transformative role of simulation in nursing education, focusing on experiential learning, debriefing strategies, emotional intelligence, cultural competence, and simulation as a tool for system improvement, intervention, and inclusive practice.

LEARNING OUTCOMES

By the end of this chapter, readers will be able to:

1. Apply experiential learning theory, particularly Kolb's cycle, to the design and delivery of simulation in nursing education.

2. Evaluate structured debriefing frameworks and tools that enhance reflective practice and improve clinical judgment.

3. Analyse the role of simulation in developing emotional intelligence, cultural competence, and social skills for person-centred care.

4. Explore how simulation can support quality improvement, system change, and inclusive co-designed learning experiences in healthcare education.

CHAPTER INTRODUCTION

The practice of simulation dates back to ancient times when military forces used models and live exercises to refine battle strategies. In healthcare, simulation was first introduced in the 1960s to help surgeons master complex procedures. Over time, it has become an essential training method in medical and nursing education (Piedrahita-Mejía & Cardona-Cano, 2022). Simulation is defined as a technique that replicates real healthcare scenarios, providing a safe space for practice, assessment, and skill development without risk to patients (SSH).

Simulation has become a key component of healthcare education. Simulation has become a transformative tool in nursing education, significantly enhancing the way students develop and practice clinical skills (Lavoie & Clarke, 2017; Jeffries, 2021). To ensure students are well-prepared for clinical practice, nursing programs combine theoretical instruction with hands-on experience. A long-standing challenge for educators has been addressing the 'theory-practice gap', which highlights the difficulty in translating classroom learning into real-world application (Laursen, 2015). The *Institute of Medicine's* (2011) report, *The Future of Nursing*, underscores how integrating simulation with experiential learning provides a structured approach for developing essential clinical competencies (Institute of Medicine, 2011).

STANDARDS AND FRAMEWORKS GUIDING SIMULATION

Several organisations have established standards to ensure the quality and effectiveness of simulation in healthcare education:

- **Association for Simulated Practice in Healthcare (ASPiH):** ASPiH provides a comprehensive framework outlining the attributes required to design and deliver effective simulation-based education. These standards emphasise the importance of aligning simulation activities with learning outcomes, ensuring fidelity, and incorporating structured debriefing sessions.

- **Society in Europe for Simulation Applied to Medicine (SESAM):** SESAM's accreditation program recognises institutions that demonstrate high-quality simulation-based medical education, focusing on core values and educational principles that underpin simulation programmes.

- **Nursing and Midwifery Council (NMC):** The NMC supports the integration of simulated practice learning (SPL) in pre-registration nursing programs, allowing approved education institutions to deliver a proportion of practice learning through simulation. This approach enables students to develop competencies in a safe and structured setting.

DISTINGUISHING SKILLS SESSIONS FROM SIMULATION SESSIONS

Understanding the difference between skills sessions and simulation sessions is essential for curriculum planning:

- **Skills Sessions:** These focus on the acquisition and practice of specific technical skills, such as intravenous cannulation or wound dressing, often using task trainers or low-fidelity models.

- **Simulation Sessions:** These involve immersive scenarios that replicate complex clinical situations, requiring students to integrate technical skills with critical thinking, communication, and teamwork. High-fidelity mannequins or standardised patients are commonly used to enhance realism.

EXPERIENTIAL LEARNING IN NURSING

The effectiveness of simulation in education is rooted in various learning theories. Experiential learning emphasises the importance of hands-on experiences in skill acquisition (Falloon, 2019). Social learning theory suggests that observing and interacting with peers enhances clinical performance (Johnson, 2020). Additionally, cognitive load theory highlights that students can only absorb a limited amount of theoretical information at a time, and simulation helps manage this load while fostering decision-making skills in high-pressure environments (Szulewski et al., 2021).

Each element of the learning cycle needs to be incorporated into the educational experience for experiential learning to be the most efficient, and learners need to be mindful of and actively engaged in each element's activities (Kolb, 1984). Incorporating structured activities during the conceptual and experimental phases of experiential learning, along with real-world exposure and observation through reflection, helps learners become aware of every step of the learning process (Kolb, 1984).

Kolb's theory of experiential learning describes the process of data memorisation to critical thinking in which they deliberate and operate data to aid the decision-making process (Kolb, 1984). This theory is dependent not only on the inclusion of four central stages and all elements for learning Figure 6.1 but also on the learner's awareness of these elements. The awareness of all these elements and the strategic application of knowledge within these elements rely on metacognition, the conscious awareness of learning (Chmil et al., 2015). Metacognition is an essential component of clinical nursing judgment, or the ability to think in terms of the nursing process. Clinical judgement can only be assessed when there is evidence of behaviours allowing for the evaluation of the level of mastery in cognitive, psychomotor, and affective domains. These allow for evaluation by the instructor and self-evaluation from the learner (Table 6.1). For experiential learning to be most effective, each stage of the learning cycle must be integrated into the educational experience, with learners actively participating and remaining aware of each phase (Kolb, 1984). Structured activities during the conceptual and experimental stages, combined with real-world exposure and reflective observation, support learners in recognising and engaging with each step of the learning process (Kolb, 1984). See Figures 6.1 and 6.2 for example.

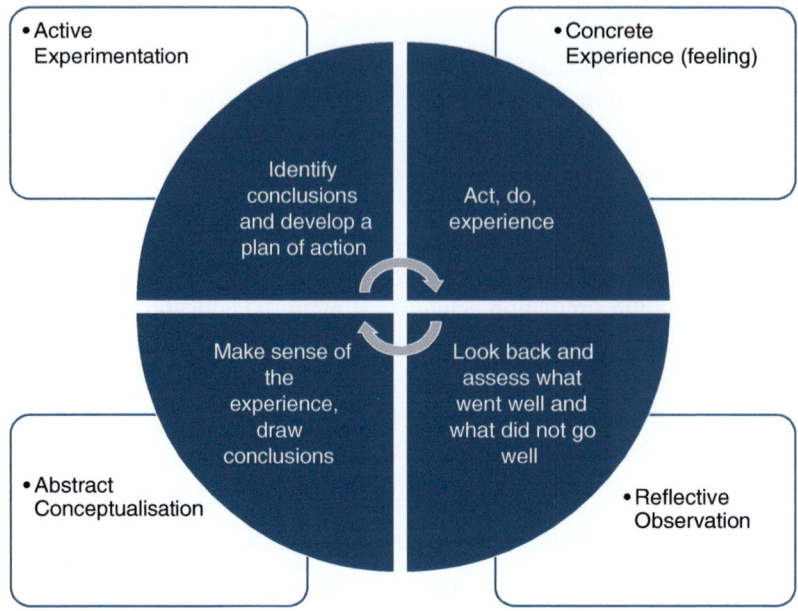

FIGURE 6.1   Designing simulations based on Kolb's experiential learning cycle (Table 6.1)

Table 6.1   Application of Kolb's Experiential Learning Cycle to Simulation Design

Stage	Purpose	Facilitator role	Learner role	Techniques/strategies
Concrete Experience	Provide a realistic and engaging simulation that forms the basis for learning	Facilitate the simulation without intervening, ensuring immersion	Actively participate in the scenario; engage fully in the experience	• Clear briefing and learning outcomes • Defined roles (learner, peers, instructor) • Peers observe and record using tools (SOAP notes, timekeeper, scribe)
Reflective Observation	Encourage learners to analyse what happened and how they responded	Guide a safe, open debriefing discussion	Reflect on performance and share perspectives with peers	• Immediate debrief after simulation • Reflective questioning (what went well, challenges, team dynamics) • Peer feedback • Link reflections to theory and practice
Abstract Conceptualisation	Help learners connect experiences to theoretical models and frameworks	Facilitate discussion linking practice to theory; share resources	Analyse experiences and synthesise ideas to form general principles	• Conceptual discussion (e.g. teamwork, communication models) • Case analysis of alternative approaches • Resource sharing (guidelines, literature, frameworks)
Active Experimentation	Apply new insights and test strategies in future practice	Support learners in applying new approaches; provide constructive feedback	Develop and trial new strategies in future simulations or practice	• Action planning (individual or team) • Role play alternative approaches • Performance checklists/rubrics • Self-assessment and peer/instructor feedback

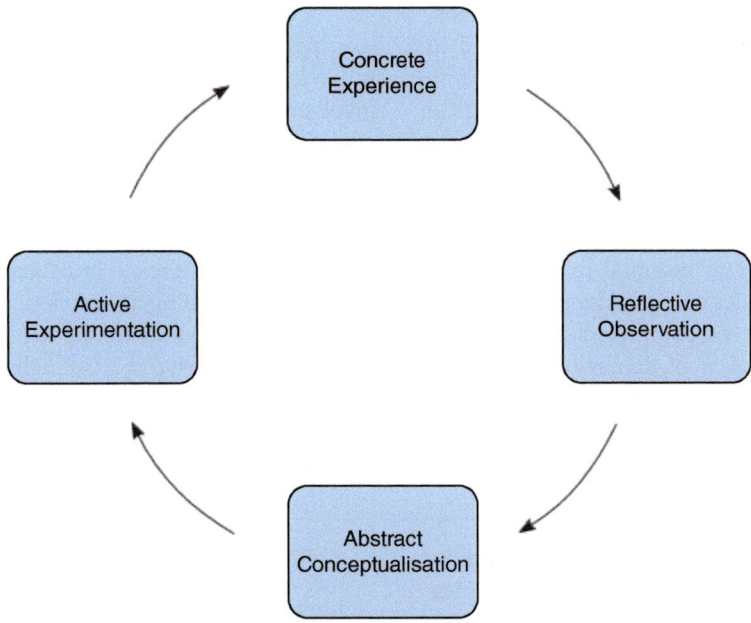

Concrete Experience: The participant encounters a concrete experience within the simulation. This might be a new experience of microaggression or a similar experience of microaggression that they have experienced in the past

Reflective Observation of the New Experience: The simulation was designed to evoke reflection in and on action using the Forum Theatre technique. The participant reflects on the new experience in the light of their existing knowledge. Areas of particular importance for the facilitator to highlight are any inconsistencies between experience and understanding and unconscious bias

Abstract Conceptualisation: Using Forum Theatre techniques participants are able to reflect in and on the action, giving rise to new ideas, or a modification of existing abstract concepts (the person has learned from their experience)

Active Experimentation: The newly created or modified concepts give rise to experimentation. The participant is able to apply their ideas and rehearse/practise new ways of responding to microaggressions

FIGURE 6.2 Application of the Kolb learning cycle to microaggression simulation

ASSESSMENT IN SIMULATION-BASED EDUCATION

Simulation can support both formative and summative assessment. Formative uses include observation, feedback, and reflection. Summative assessments can use structured tools such as Objective Structured Clinical Examinations (OSCEs), Direct Observation of Procedural Skills (DOPS), and checklists assessing technical and non-technical skills (e.g. communication, teamwork). Effective evaluation should align with learning outcomes, be transparent, and allow for learner feedback. Incorporating multiple perspectives (self, peer, facilitator) strengthens validity and supports professional growth.

Assessment in simulation-based education plays a critical role in ensuring that learners achieve desired competencies and can translate simulated experiences into clinical performance. High-quality assessment practices in simulation rely on well-defined objectives, valid and reliable tools, and trained evaluators to ensure consistent outcomes. Incorporating standardised patients, scenario fidelity, and evidence-based rubrics enhances the credibility of assessments and promotes learner engagement (Cook et al., 2011). Debriefing remains a cornerstone of simulation-based assessment, offering opportunities for critical analysis, emotional processing, and knowledge integration (Eppich & Cheng, 2015). Furthermore, assessing both technical proficiency and non-technical attributes, such as decision-making and situational awareness, reflects the complexity of real-world healthcare delivery (Gaba, 2004). As simulation becomes increasingly embedded in curricula, its assessment methodologies must evolve to reflect changes in educational standards, technological advancements, and interprofessional practice demands.

Learners move beyond conceptual knowledge to gain practical knowledge at the procedural and metacognitive levels. Developing higher-order thinking and active involvement can positively influence participant outcomes when using a simulation as a pedagogical tool.

PSYCHOLOGICAL SAFETY

Creating psychological safety is essential for maximising learning in simulation and debriefing sessions. This concept refers to an environment where individuals can engage, speak, and perform without fear of damaging their reputation, social standing, or career progression. For participants to feel secure, they must be confident that expressing themselves will not result in criticism or exclusion. Ensuring a supportive learning atmosphere involves structuring both the simulation and debriefing to foster openness. One effective way to establish this is through a pre-simulation briefing, where facilitators set expectations and reinforce the principles of a safe and respectful learning space.

SIMULATION MODALITIES AND FIDELITY

Simulation in nursing education can be categorised by fidelity, which refers to the realism or authenticity of the simulated experience. Low-fidelity simulations often involve task trainers and partial manikins for practising isolated skills (e.g., wound dressing or catheter insertion). Medium-fidelity simulations introduce more interactivity, such as programmable manikins with basic physiological responses. High-fidelity simulations offer highly realistic environments using advanced manikins, immersive clinical settings, and full scenarios with integrated team dynamics, allowing learners to engage in complex, multidisciplinary care delivery.

Simulation modalities also vary. These include:

- Manikin-based simulation (e.g., high-fidelity adult or paediatric manikins),

- Standardised patients or actors,

- Virtual simulations and VR/AR platforms, and

- Forum theatre or role-play-based simulations to enhance reflection and communication.

INTERPROFESSIONAL LEARNING THROUGH SIMULATION

Simulation provides an ideal platform for interprofessional education (IPE), where nursing students collaborate with learners from medicine, pharmacy, paramedicine, and allied health. It fosters understanding of professional roles, promotes mutual respect, and improves communication and teamwork. IPE simulation scenarios should be designed to reflect the complexity of real-world healthcare, including shared decision-making, clinical prioritisation, and responding to acute deterioration.

Structured IPE simulation enhances safety and collaborative practice by allowing students to rehearse team-based responses in a psychologically safe environment. These experiences are invaluable in helping learners develop confidence, clarify their professional identity, and appreciate the strengths and contributions of other disciplines. Embedding IPE within simulation supports the delivery of coordinated, person-centred care and reflects the realities of today's multidisciplinary healthcare systems.

DEBRIEFING

Debriefing remains the cornerstone of simulation-based education. Debriefing refers to the facilitated conversation about the simulation and experience and can occur during or after the event. Debriefing tools are used as a structured framework to evoke self and team reflection and as an opportunity to provide feedback and information to aid improvement. In contrast, feedback refers to specific information provided to the learners about their performance compared to a defined standard (Cheng et al., 2018).

Debriefing allows learning to reflect on specific aspects of the simulation from the concrete experience and events relating to what happened, the rationale for actions and inactions, and generate learnings from this experience to apply in future practice. Active experimentation with potential solutions leads to future experiences, and the experiential learning cycle starts again.

Debriefing has been shown to significantly improve the performance of teams and individuals when structured and effectively facilitated (Tannenbaum & Cerasoli, 2013). Debriding has been associated with improved knowledge, skills, and clinical behaviours when compared to no briefing or other teaching methodologies (Cheng et al., 2018). Post-event debriefing or within-event debriefing is deemed equally effective depending on the nature of the scenario, learner group, and learning outcomes for the session. Post-event debriefing tends to centre around reflection on action (Schön, 1983), educational strategies, guided/facilitated conversation, and personal experience, whilst in the event can promote deliberate practice, evoke reflection in action, performance critique, and real-time feedback to enhance performance. Debriefing of this nature includes a discussion with participants, not just providing feedback. Table 6.2 identifies the debrief modality and essential elements and techniques required.

DEBRIEFING TOOLS

Plus Delta

This approach uses a two-column format, with the 'plus' column highlighting effective behaviours or actions, while the 'delta' column identifies areas requiring improvement or adjustment. It provides a simple and structured method for guiding discussions, making it particularly useful for novice debriefers. Learners actively engage in the process by reflecting on the simulation experience, either in its entirety or specific aspects, and evaluating their own or the group's performance. The primary goal of this method is to encourage self-assessment, allowing participants to recognise strengths and identify opportunities for growth (Andrade, 2019).

'Debriefing with Good Judgement'

Reaction – Analysis – Summary

Rudolph et al. (2006) describe this model as a 3-phase conversational structure for debriefing, consisting of the phases: reaction, analysis, and summary.

Using this conversational structure, the first phase of the debriefing (reaction) focuses on the simulation participants exploring their responses, reactions, and the emotional impact of the simulation experience. In this phase, participants can 'blow off steam' before completing the remainder of the debriefing. The analysis focuses on what, why, and how actions evolved during the simulation. Allowing the facilitator and learners to identify gaps in knowledge and skills, understand the reason for the gaps, and work together on areas for development to close the gaps. The summary focuses on lessons learned, analysis, and takeaway points.

Diamond Debrief

Description – Analysis – Application

The diamond debrief is a similar three-phase model, which omits a specific reaction or defusing phase. The discursive structure of the model includes phases of

Table 6.2 The Science of Debriefing

Modality	Purpose	Essential elements	Techniques and strategies
Within-event (in-simulation/ concurrent/ micro-debriefing)	To provide immediate reflection and corrective feedback during the simulation, enhancing real-time performance	• Established ground rules • Psychological safety • Clearly defined learning objectives • Use of pauses and silence • Open-ended questions	• Rapid cycle deliberate practice (stop–action, error correction, rewind, and repeat) • Real-time directive feedback • Highlighting consequences of actions/omissions • Learner/team self-assessment • Circular questioning • Inquiry-based prompts
Post-event (terminal debriefing)	To enable structured reflection after the simulation, ensuring key learning objectives and critical events are discussed	• Established ground rules • Psychological safety • Clearly defined learning objectives • Use of pauses and silence • Open-ended questions	• Facilitator-led structured discussion (guided by debriefing models/phases) • Learner/team self-assessment and critique • Directive feedback • Circular questioning • Inquiry-based exploration • Guided self/team correction

description, analysis, and application. The diamond shape is designed to visually represent the idealised process of a debrief opening out to a facilitated discussion about the scenario before focusing on specific learning points. This model encourages a standardised approach to debriefing non-technical skills and can be used by more than one facilitator within the session (Jaye et al., 2015).

Gas Model

Gather – Analyse – Summarise

This three-phase model encourages a shared mental model amongst the team to gather information and provide a summary of the simulation events. The analysis phase focuses on learner-centred reflection. The facilitator provides prompt questions to promote rumination and reflective thought processes. The summary phase ensures that learning objectives have been revised and key teaching points are solidified (Salik & Paige, 2023).

Promoting Excellence and Reflective Learning in Simulation (Pearl)

Reaction – Description – Analysis – Summary

This is a four-phase blended debriefing framework designed to include appropriate integration of feedback, debriefing and/or guided reflection (Decker et al., 2021). The reactions phase sets the tone and context for the rest of the debriefing by establishing the learner's initial reactions, acknowledging emotions, and allowing time for processing. The description phase ensures that all learners and facilitators understand all the main elements of the scenario. This is an important phase to ensure everyone is working from the same diagnosis for the scenario and to avoid any confusion or misinterpretation. The analysis phase seeks to evoke learner self-assessment, identifying gaps in knowledge, areas for improvement, and positive behaviours through directive feedback and identifying further areas for exploration and discussion. In the final phase, the learner should share what they have learned and provide one or two take-home messages. The facilitator will provide a learner-centred summary to ensure all learning objectives have been assimilated (Cheng et al., 2016).

A number of debriefing adjuncts can be used to enhance the impact of the debriefing experience, including video-assisted debriefing, co-debriefing (whereby each facilitator focuses on a particular aspect), and employing a debriefing script (Table 6.3).

Table 6.3   Application of the PLUS Delta Debrief Tool

Debriefing tool	
Opening words and appreciation	Thank you for taking part in this simulation
PLUS	Please share some of the things that went well in this simulation
	What were the good things you and the team did?
	Ask the participants to comment on what aspects of the simulation were most rewarding
	How did they feel making decisions in the simulation?
	Consider aspects such as clinical reasoning, communication skills, team dynamics, and adherence to protocols
	What insights were gained from this experience? Relate these to the learning objectives and clinical practice
DELTA	What would you do differently next time?
	What would you change moving forward?
	How could the challenges be addressed?
	Discuss any aspects of the scenario where the participants felt concerned. What contributed to these feelings? Consider aspects such as clinical skills, decision-making abilities, team dynamics, communication, and time management. How could these be improved?
	Discuss any recurring strengths or areas for improvement what concrete steps could address these?
Summary	How would you summarise this experience?
	Ask the participants to identify what they learned from the session
	Explore ways to access the impact of the care given in the simulation and how these challenges may be addressed in the future
	Summarise the key takeaways from the learning experience

APPLICATION OF THE PLUS DELTA DEBRIEF TOOL

Poor debriefing in simulations can lead to missed learning opportunities, leaving learners unclear about their mistakes and how to improve. It may also reduce psychological safety, causing anxiety or defensiveness that hinders open reflection. Ultimately, this compromises skill development and the transfer of knowledge to real clinical practice, affecting patient safety. Table 6.4 identifies consequences of poor debriefing and possible solutions.

Table 6.4   Common Challenges in Simulation Debriefing with Associated Consequences and Practical Solutions

Limitation	Potential consequence	Possible solutions
Learners are not able or do not feel comfortable sharing emotions	• Emotions may hinder debrief effectiveness • Withholding emotions can reduce engagement	• Create a safe space to express emotions • Use open-ended questions • Allow silence and pauses • Acknowledge emotions as they arise
Learners are reluctant to share initial reactions (more vocal members dominate)	• Critical issues not fully explored • Quieter learners disengage	• Use open-ended questions • Embrace pauses to encourage contributions • Gently invite quieter participants to share
Learner does not feel listened to or cannot express key themes	• Learners feel disconnected and less engaged • Facilitator misses learner priorities	• Track key issues raised by learners • Address emerging issues during analysis • Summarise key themes before moving on
Misinterpretation of scenario or a lack of shared understanding	• Learners have inconsistent levels of understanding • Confusion or off-topic discussion	• Begin with a descriptive phase to clarify shared understanding • Validate perspectives across the group
Learner's perspective not shared with facilitator	• Confusion during analysis phase • Varying interpretations left unresolved	• After one learner shares, invite others to confirm mutual understanding
Positive behaviours not discussed	• Missed opportunities to reinforce strengths • Learning remains deficit-focused	• Intentionally discuss positive behaviours • Encourage learners to share what went well
Positive behaviours not reinforced by facilitator	• Missed opportunities to consolidate learning • Goals unmet	• Facilitator highlights positive behaviours • Provide guidance on areas for improvement
Debrief focuses only on one specific learning outcome	• Learners do not complete a full self-assessment	• Compile strengths and learning opportunities before focusing on one gap • Prompt learners to continue self-assessment after objective-specific discussion
Performance gaps not fully explored	• Superficial discussion with limited takeaways	• Use facilitation techniques tailored to time, nature of gap, and clarity of underlying rationale
Learner disagrees with facilitator's observation	• Learner becomes disengaged, defensive, or disruptive	• Base inquiry on clear, concrete observations • Use learner's own prior words to guide inquiry
Learner does not receive specific task feedback	• Learning needs not addressed • Learner disengages	• Provide task- and content-specific feedback
Insufficient time for learner-centred summary	• Learners do not articulate learning • Facilitator unable to consolidate objectives • Key take-home messages missed	• Allocate sufficient time for debrief • Facilitator shares take-home points after learners summarise

Source: Adapted from Cheng et al. (2016).

ACTIVITY BOX

Design a simulation-based learning activity on pressure ulcer prevention using Kolb's experiential learning cycle:

1. **Set learning outcomes**

   Define what students should achieve, such as

   a. recognising risk factors

   b. performing risk assessments

   c. implementing appropriate interventions

2. **Create a clinical scenario (Concrete Experience)**

   Develop a case involving a patient at risk of pressure ulcers. Choose a suitable modality such as a high-fidelity manikin, virtual simulation, or role play.

3. **Facilitate reflection (Reflective Observation)**

   After the scenario, guide a structured debrief where students reflect on their actions and emotions.

4. **Link to theory (Abstract Conceptualisation)**

   Encourage students to connect their experience with theoretical knowledge, clinical guidelines, or prior classroom content.

5. **Plan future action (Active Experimentation)**

   Support students to design an action plan or revised approach for future practice. Prompt individual reflection on how the activity has shaped their understanding and clinical decision making.

ROLES OF PRACTICE ASSESSORS AND SUPERVISORS

In the context of simulation, practice assessors and supervisors play pivotal roles in guiding and evaluating student learning:

- **Practice Supervisors:** These individuals support and supervise students during simulation activities, providing feedback and facilitating reflective discussions. They are responsible for creating a conducive learning environment that encourages student engagement and development.

- **Practice Assessors:** Practice assessors evaluate students' performance in simulation scenarios, ensuring that learning outcomes are met. They collaborate with academic staff to make informed decisions about students' progress and readiness for clinical practice.

SIMULATION GOVERNANCE, ETHICS AND CONSENT

Simulation activities must be underpinned by sound governance. This includes gaining informed consent for video capture, setting expectations for psychological safety, respecting confidentiality, and clear policies on data storage. Ethical issues can also arise when learners re-enact traumatic events, so trauma-informed approaches and facilitator awareness of learner wellbeing are essential. A local policy should outline roles, responsibilities, equipment safety, and procedures for escalation if learners experience distress during or after simulation.

FACULTY DEVELOPMENT AND EDUCATOR PREPAREDNESS

The quality of simulation-based education is critically dependent on the competence and confidence of the educators delivering it. Facilitators must possess not only clinical expertise but also the pedagogical skills to design effective scenarios, promote psychological safety, guide debriefings, and evaluate outcomes. However, many nursing educators transition into academic roles with limited formal training in simulation education, resulting in variable preparedness.

Structured faculty development programmes are essential for standardising quality and upskilling nurse educators in simulation pedagogy. This includes training in scenario writing, fidelity matching, technical equipment use, debriefing models, and learner assessment. Certification routes such as the *INACSL Healthcare Simulation Educator (CHSE)* credential and local simulation faculty pathways can support this.

Institutions should also promote reflective practice and peer support among simulation faculty to ensure ongoing development. Co-debriefing, team observation, and feedback mechanisms help educators evaluate and refine their own facilitation styles. Embedding simulation expertise into academic development strategies supports a culture of educator 'learnership', reinforcing that transformative simulation requires continuous growth for both learners and educators.

DEVELOPING EMOTIONAL, SOCIAL, AND CULTURAL INTELLIGENCE

Cultural competence is defined as a multidimensional concept, the capability of an individual to function effectively in situations characterised by cultural diversity. Metacognitive cultural intelligence (METACQ) is the level of cultural awareness demonstrated by an individual during cross-cultural interactions and includes planning, monitoring and revising mental models of cultural norms for groups of people (Galan-Lominchar et al., 2024). Cognitive cultural intelligence (COGCQ) refers to the understanding of norms, practices, and conventions across various cultures, gained through both educational and personal experiences. Behavioural cultural intelligence (BEHCQ) is the ability to demonstrate suitable verbal and nonverbal behaviours when interacting in culturally diverse settings (Galan-Lominchar et al., 2024).

Instructional design of simulations to develop cultural intelligence and include cultural competence and how cultural differences impact healthcare decisions should identify cultural considerations affecting the patient's perspective of treatment in the patient profile.

Learning objectives must ensure learners demonstrate a comprehensive understanding of cultural competence as a multidimensional concept in healthcare, recognising its significance in providing equitable and patient-centred care. Apply adaptive communication strategies to effectively engage with diverse patient populations and critically reflect on their interactions to enhance cultural awareness. Identification of cultural misunderstandings that may arise in healthcare settings, demonstrating an appreciation for the role of cross-cultural interactions in clinical decision-making and personalised patient care.

EXAMPLE OF A SIMULATION SCENARIO

Mrs. Liu, a 68-year-old Chinese immigrant with limited English proficiency who has been admitted for uncontrolled diabetes. Mrs. Liu's family insists on using herbal remedies alongside prescribed treatments, requiring students to navigate a patient-centred discussion that integrates cultural sensitivity, evidence-based practice, and shared decision-making. During the simulation learners must apply culturally appropriate communication strategies whilst respecting Mrs. Lui's cultural beliefs about traditional medicine and dietary practices. Through reflection and debriefing, students will explore the impact of cultural beliefs on health behaviours, develop adaptive communication skills, and practice delivering care that honours the patient's values while ensuring safety and efficacy in treatment.

EMOTIONAL INTELLIGENCE

Self-awareness is fundamental to psychological insight (Goleman, 1995). The framework for emotional intelligence contains five elements.

Self-awareness is the examination of how emotions affect behaviour using values to guide decision-making and self-assessment. Being aware of both mood and thought (Goleman et al., 2002). Emotional awareness requires recognition of emotions and acknowledging feelings, accepting feelings as they arise and reflecting on why the feeling is present and what can be learnt from this. Effective self-awareness improves empathy (Younas et al., 2019). Composed of affective, cognitive, attitude and ethical components to enable the learner to recognise, feel and understand the emotions of others (Rasheed, 2015; Younas et al., 2019). Simulation is an excellent forum to examine personal and group behaviours in high-intensity, complex or challenging situations. Within simulation, it is essential for learners to reflect on the usefulness of the response and the lessons to take away. Part of the debrief should be for learners to acknowledge the effects of their emotions on themselves and others. This is known as The Ripple Effect: Emotional contagion and influences on group behaviours (Barsade, 2002).

Embedding self-awareness in nursing simulations involves designing activities that encourage reflection and understanding of one's own strengths and weaknesses, biases, and emotional responses during simulated clinical scenarios. Provide the learners with tools that encourage students to analyse their actions, decision-making process, and emotional responses during the simulation. Ensure that the simulations mimic high-stress, ethically complex, or emotionally intense situations (e.g., end-of-life care, patient aggression, cultural misunderstandings). These moments naturally prompt introspection.

Example: if a patient's family becomes emotional, distressed or aggressive, learners can be asked to consider how this makes them feel and whether it affects their ability to remain professional. These reflective pause points can be facilitated by the educator or initiated by learners and are particularly effective when using forum theatre or other immersive simulation modalities that allow reflection in action.

Example: A simple approach is to build in short, structured pauses. For instance, facilitators might invite learners to take a brief 30-second pause and consider what emotions they are experiencing in that moment. The Gibbs reflective cycle can then be used alongside the debrief model to help unpack actions, thoughts and feelings in a structured way.

Example: Facilitators may also explore how emotions influenced decision making by asking questions such as what feelings shaped your actions and what assumptions were present at the time. Self-assessment tools can support this process, including situational emotional response scales or self-awareness measures such as the Emotional Regulation of Others and Self scale. These tools help capture the multidimensional aspects of self-awareness and identify areas for further development.

Utilise video recordings in simulation. Encourage learners to watch back their performance and self-reflect on behaviours. This method is valuable for greater insight into areas for personal development, triggers to emotional responses and changes in behaviours. Some simulation virtual reality platforms created modules whereby the learner can leave their avatar and watch the interaction again as an observer to critique their own performance.

Invite peer observers to give constructive feedback on body language, communication style, and emotional regulation. For example, how did the learner respond to the emotional tone of the simulated patient. What non-verbal cues did they pick up on? Role reversal is an excellent way to promote self-awareness. Encourage learners to play the role of patients, family members and other healthcare professionals to evoke deeper awareness. 360-degree feedback can be useful to improve performance and identify targeted areas for development, build relationships and improve team dynamics (Johnson, 2020).

Social competence in nursing includes communication, collaboration, conflict resolution, cultural sensitivity, and professionalism. Team-based simulations where learners can participate as part of the multi-disciplinary team enhance communication, delegation, and collaboration whilst the learner navigates their own scope of practice.

- Example Scenario: Rapid response to a deteriorating patient requiring teamwork and role clarity.

- Prompt: 'How did you ensure all voices were heard during the crisis'? What role did you assume during the event and how does this align with your scope of practice?

Simulations designed to encourage learners to manage conflicts, deal with difficult patients or coworkers, or navigate ethical dilemmas can strengthen confidence in assertive communication, empathy, and boundary setting. Creating these real-life scenarios in a psychologically safe environment (Mitchell et al., 2025).

- Example Scenario: A student nurse approaches a colleague to talk about a patient safety concern.

- Prompt: 'What approach did you take to express your concern respectfully'? How did you feel during this interaction? What would you do differently next time?

Create situations that demand cultural sensitivity, respect for diversity, and ethical decision-making to enhance learners respect for others' values and perspectives.

- Example Scenario: Caring for a non-English speaking patient who declines a treatment due to cultural beliefs.

- Prompt: 'How did you adapt your communication style to be culturally appropriate'? Was there anything you were not expecting in the conversation? How did you manage this?

SIMULATION FOR IMPROVEMENT, INTERVENTION, AND INVOLVEMENT

Simulation for improvement is concerned with using simulation to improve something which already exists to align with best practice principles, patient safety, and quality of care (Weldon et al., 2023). Simulation can be used to understand care processes to improve efficacy whilst maintaining patient safety, collaboration, and readiness for practice (Whitfill, 2018). Simulations for improvement could centre around a specific incident, a hypothetical challenging situation or a rehearsal for process, innovation, or navigating a change. Using simulation modalities to pause, review, and rewind is an excellent way to work on specific areas for development in teams or individuals.

Simulation for intervention can be used to change a situation or a way of doing things. This could be integrating novel workflows, protocols, and cognitive aids, with rapid changes to patient care and delivery (Dubé, 2020; Weldon et al., 2023). This approach can be used for sharing information at a large scale across multiple professional groups. An illustrative example of simulation serving as an intervention to modify workflows and protocols is detailed in the work by Dubé et al. (2020). In this study, systems-focused simulations were employed to proactively identify and address latent safety threats and inefficiencies within a newly established neurology clinic. The simulations facilitated the testing and refinement of new workflows, including the integration of novel roles and technologies, prior to the clinic's operational launch. This approach enabled the healthcare team to implement changes in a controlled environment, ensuring that adjustments were made before impacting actual patient care. The study underscores the value of simulation not only as a training tool but also as a strategic method for system redesign and quality improvement in healthcare settings (Weldon et al., 2023).

Simulation for Involvement emphasises inclusivity both in participation and co-design, ensuring that individuals and communities who may not otherwise be represented in healthcare education are actively included. This approach ensures that simulations reflect the diverse realities of patients navigating complex health systems. By involving simulated patients and service users, the patient voice is brought to the forefront, especially during relational moments of care. These participants provide real-time feedback on how scenarios feel from their perspective and offer recommendations to enhance clinical practice (Mitchell, 2023; Weldon et al., 2023). For example, Mitchell (2024) used co-designed simulations with people with learning disabilities in pre-registration nursing education to ensure their lived experiences shaped the learning process. Similarly, Weldon developed tools to engage future healthcare managers in redesigning care pathway processes through simulation, and Pillay et al. (2021) created a simulation rooted in equal, non-hierarchical collaboration between neonatal teams across units. Collectively, these examples demonstrate how simulation can serve as a platform for equity, patient partnership, and co-production in healthcare education and service redesign.

CONDUCTING GAP ANALYSIS IN SIMULATION

Simulation is a valuable tool for conducting gap analysis in healthcare education and clinical practice, as it enables the identification of discrepancies between current performance and desired standards in a controlled, replicable environment. By recreating real-world clinical scenarios, simulation allows educators and organisations to observe processes, uncover latent safety threats, and assess individual or team competencies against established benchmarks (Weinstock et al., 2015). This approach provides actionable insights into areas needing improvement, whether related to knowledge, technical skills, communication, or system processes. For example, a hospital may use in situ simulation to evaluate the effectiveness of its emergency response to paediatric cardiac arrest. The findings might reveal delays in initiating CPR or issues with equipment availability, prompting targeted interventions and system redesign. In this way, simulation-based gap analysis supports continuous quality improvement and patient safety initiatives by linking performance data to educational and organisational outcomes.

CO-DESIGN AND AUTHENTICITY IN SIMULATION

Co-design and authenticity are essential components in the development of high-quality simulation-based education, enhancing learner engagement and the relevance of the learning experience. Co-design involves collaborative development of simulation scenarios with input from clinicians, educators, patients, and learners themselves. This approach ensures that the simulation content reflects real-world challenges, clinical priorities, and contextual nuances (Mitchell, 2024). Authenticity, or fidelity, refers not only to the physical realism of the simulation but also to psychological and contextual fidelity, which influence how learners perceive and respond to the scenario (Dieckmann et al., 2007). Incorporating authentic clinical environments, realistic patient narratives, and interprofessional dynamics helps create immersive experiences that support deeper learning and transfer to clinical practice. For instance, involving patients in the co-design of simulations about delivering bad news can improve the emotional realism of the scenario and better prepare clinicians for sensitive communication. Co-designed simulations are more likely to reflect diverse perspectives, enhance inclusivity, and increase the perceived relevance of training among participants (Mitchell, 2024). Together, co-design and authenticity foster meaningful, learner-centred education that aligns with real clinical expectations and promotes professional growth. Table 6.5 provides a template for co-designing simulations.

Table 6.5 Co-design Simulation Template

Section	Description
1. **Simulation Title**	Clear, concise, and descriptive title for the scenario
2. **Purpose and Learning Objectives**	Define educational goals aligned with curriculum standards or competency frameworks (e.g. clinical skills, communication, teamwork)
3. **Contributors**	List co-designers (educators, clinicians, learners, patients) with their roles and contributions
4. **Scenario Overview**	Brief summary including setting, context, and rationale for the case
5. **Patient Profile**	Patient demographics, medical history, psychosocial elements, and patient input if applicable
6. **Setting and Resources**	Specify the simulated environment and required materials (e.g. equipment, standardised patients, staff)
7. **Pre-brief**	Orientation for learners, confidentiality agreements, psychological safety guidelines, and relevant background readings
8. **Simulation Format**	State delivery method (e.g. group work, with observers, online, in person)
9. **Scenario Flow**	Timeline of events, key decision points, and facilitator prompts. Include optional scenario branches (e.g. arrival of relative, MDT member)
10. **Assessment and Feedback**	Define assessment method (formative/summative), tools (e.g. checklists, rubrics), and feedback strategies (structured debrief, self-assessment)
11. **Debriefing Plan**	Describe debrief structure (e.g. PLUS-DELTA), focus areas (technical, emotional), and involvement of contributors
12. **Inclusivity and Cultural Considerations**	Explain how diversity, cultural safety, and equity are addressed. Include community or patient representative input
13. **Evaluation and Iteration**	Plan for collecting feedback and revising the scenario
14. **References and Supporting Materials**	Provide clinical guidelines, educational theory, patient narratives, and supplementary resources (slides, handouts, checklists)

USING SIMULATION TO INFLUENCE AND INFORM NURSING PRACTICE

Simulation plays a pivotal role in influencing and informing nursing practice by providing a safe, controlled environment where nurses can develop, test, and refine clinical skills, decision-making, and professional behaviours without risking patient safety. High-fidelity and in situ simulation allow nurses and multidisciplinary teams to engage in realistic, complex clinical scenarios, ranging from managing deteriorating patients to addressing ethical dilemmas—thereby enhancing clinical judgment, confidence, and teamwork (Cant & Cooper, 2017). Crucially, simulation is increasingly used to stress-test new policies, guidelines, environments, and technologies before implementation. For example, simulations can sense-check a clinical guideline or safety-check a redesigned clinical space before patient use, helping to identify latent threats and refine systems (Health Education England (HEE), 2020). Additionally, simulation supports the development of organisational safety culture by recreating serious harm incidents, enabling teams to learn from past errors, such as improper equipment use or unsafe restraint practices, and practice safe responses (Mitchell et al., 2023). This is particularly valuable in preparing staff for new models of care, including the use of technology to improve medication safety across prescribing, preparation, and administration. Simulation is also a key tool in broader national initiatives: collaborations with organisations such as the Health and Safety Investigations Board (HSIB) help explore complex areas of practice and embed safety recommendations. Through reflective debriefs, simulation helps students and professionals examine their roles, challenge assumptions, and consider systemic issues such as communication failures and organisational culture. This reflective, experiential learning fosters resilience and prepares nurses to respond effectively to the realities of clinical practice, contributing to safer, more adaptive healthcare systems.

CONTEMPORARY ISSUES IN HEALTHCARE SIMULATION

Contemporary issues in healthcare simulation increasingly revolve around the integration of emerging technologies such as virtual reality (VR), artificial intelligence (AI), and augmented reality (AR), which are transforming how healthcare professionals are trained and assessed. These innovations offer immersive, interactive environments that enhance realism and learner engagement, enabling the safe exploration of complex clinical scenarios (Pottle, 2019). VR allows learners to practise procedures repeatedly without risk to patients, while AI can provide adaptive feedback and personalised learning pathways, improving knowledge retention and clinical decision-making skills (Baylor, 2020).

AR, meanwhile, overlays digital information onto the physical environment, enhancing real-time learning during procedures or in-situ training (Akçayır & Akçayır, 2017). However, challenges such as cost, digital literacy disparities, and the need for robust evidence on educational impact remain significant. There is also ongoing debate around the ethical implications of AI-driven assessment and data use in simulation-based education (Topol, 2019). As simulation technology rapidly evolves, it is essential for educators and institutions to critically evaluate both the opportunities and limitations of these tools to ensure they support safe, equitable, and evidence-informed learning environments.

CASE STUDIES

Table 6.6 synthesises various examples from the literature on simulation case studies, highlighting key themes, methodologies, and outcomes across different settings. It brings together diverse approaches to simulation-based learning, illustrating how case studies have been used to explore challenges, innovations, and best practices. By consolidating these examples, the table offers a clear overview of the evidence base and supports a deeper understanding of simulation's impact in education and training.

INNOVATION BOX

Simulation Innovation: 'SafeStart VR' – A Voice-Controlled VR Simulation for Patient Safety Improvement

You are a junior nurse starting your morning shift on a busy medical ward. As you enter the virtual nurse's station, an AI-driven handover avatar (your colleague from the night shift) begins the shift report. The patient in question, *Mr. Adrian James*, was transferred overnight from A&E with abdominal pain and suspected infection.

The handover is loosely structured and contains subtle omissions (e.g., the nurse skips over medication history and allergy status due to time pressure). The patient's notes are available via the VR interface, including vital signs, early warning score (NEWS 5), and a flagged but unspoken penicillin allergy.

Your role is to:

- Verbally guide the simulation by asking appropriate questions during handover (e.g., 'Can you clarify his allergy status'?)

- Use voice commands to review digital charts and patient history

- Recognise risks in real time (e.g., incomplete antibiotic plan, penicillin being prescribed)

- Communicate concerns to the doctor avatar using SBAR and escalate when ignored

- Make safety-driven decisions (e.g., hold antibiotics, contact pharmacy)

AI Features

- Voice-activated branching dialogue: The scenario adapts in real time based on what you ask or miss

- Feedback engine: Offers immediate feedback on missed cues, communication gaps, and safety threats

- Digital twin analytics: Tracks and scores decision-making, assertiveness, and handover structure

- Reflective debrief: Post-simulation report with personalised insights and a comparison to best-practice guidelines

Post-simulation Tasks

- Participate in a facilitated debrief (in-person or virtual)

- Reflect on cognitive bias, missed cues, and communication gaps

- Draft an action plan for improving future handovers in your own clinical area

Table 6.6 Simulation Case Studies

Case example	Focus area	Simulation type	Participants	Key outcomes
Microaggression Simulation for Second-Year Nursing Students	Recognising and addressing microaggressions (race, age) in clinical settings	Real-world scenario simulation based on student feedback	Second-year nursing students	Improved awareness of microaggressions, experiential learning opportunity; highlighted the need for more structured training to address discrimination in healthcare practice Mitchell et al. (2025)
Virtual Reality with AI for Holistic Assessment	Holistic patient assessment using AI-led patient avatars	Two types: Menu-based and Voice-controlled AI VR simulations	Pre-registration adult nursing students ($n = 11$) from two UK universities	Identified advantages and challenges of both methods; voice-controlled felt more intuitive, menu-based gave more structure. Themes included technological literacy, learning transition, and VR as a learning tool. Helped with safe practice of complex assessments Teixeira et al. (2024)
Learning Disability and Autism Simulation with Baked Beans Theatre Company	Mandatory training in learning disabilities and autism care	High-fidelity simulation with actors/service users, facilitated debrief and peer-supported learning	Third-year nursing students across all fields	Improved communication and assessment skills highlighted the importance of inclusive, person-centred care and building patient trust. Reinforced safe and equitable healthcare delivery Mitchell and Leontino (2023)
Ligature Training Simulation for Mental Health Professionals	Managing ligature-related incidents in mental health settings	High-fidelity simulation in a realistic simulated environment over a two-day workshop	Mental health practitioners	Thematic analysis revealed three dominant themes: (1) Transformative experience – significant growth in knowledge and skill; (2) Transformed views – shifted attitudes towards the importance and impact of ligature training; (3) Patient-centred risk management and empowerment – greater awareness of involving patients in risk strategies. Demonstrated simulation's effectiveness in preparing staff for real-life ligature scenarios and enhancing patient safety. This research contributes significantly to best practice development in mental health training and underscores the role of immersive education in supporting professional growth and systemic improvement Mitchell et al. (2023)

CONCLUSION

Simulation plays a fundamental role in transformative nurse education, serving undergraduate students, registered practitioners, and the wider interdisciplinary team. It offers a safe and structured environment in which individuals and teams can develop, refine, and evaluate clinical skills, communication, decision-making, and teamwork. Beyond technical competence, simulation supports improvements in patient safety and the overall quality of care by enabling healthcare professionals to practise and reflect without risk to real patients.

The increasing demand for simulation is driven by multiple factors, including pressure on clinical placement capacity, the need to address areas for service improvement, and the imperative to foster cultural competence and awareness across diverse healthcare settings. High-quality simulations are underpinned by robust instructional design, authentic co-design with service users and stakeholders, and skilled facilitation during debriefing. These elements ensure that simulations are immersive, inclusive, and aligned with intended learning outcomes. As healthcare continues to evolve, simulation stands as a vital educational strategy for preparing a responsive, reflective, and patient-centred workforce.

TAKE-HOME POINTS

1. Effective simulation design aligns with experiential learning principles, supporting deeper understanding through active participation, reflection, theory application, and real-world testing.

2. Psychological safety, structured debriefing, and self-awareness are essential for maximising simulation's educational value and supporting learners' professional development.

3. Simulation is not only a teaching tool but a mechanism for improvement, innovation, and inclusive collaboration in education, service design, and policy development.

CPD REFLECTIVE QUESTIONS

1. How can I adapt my simulation teaching approach to better support learners' emotional and cultural intelligence?

2. Which debriefing model(s) do I currently use, and how do they align with the principles of structured reflective learning?

3. In what ways could I use simulation in my current setting to co-produce solutions with students, service users, or colleagues?

REFERENCES

Akçayır, M., & Akçayır, G. (2017). Advantages and challenges associated with augmented reality for education: a systematic review of the literature. *Educational Research Review*, 20, 1–11.

Andrade, H. L. (2019). A critical review of research on student self-assessment. *Frontiers in Education*, 4, 87. https://doi.org/10.3389/feduc.2019.00087.

Barsade, S. G. (2002). The ripple effect: emotional contagion and its influence on group behavior. *Administrative Science Quarterly*, 47(4), 644–675.

Baylor, A. L. (2020). Artificial intelligence and the future of teaching and learning. *EDUCAUSE Review*, 55(4).

Cant, R. P., & Cooper, S. J. (2017). Use of simulation-based learning in undergraduate nurse education: an umbrella systematic review. *Nurse Education Today*, 49, 63–71.

Cheng, A., Eppich, W., Grant, V., Sherbino, J., Zendejas, B., & Cook, D. A. (2018). Debriefing for technology-enhanced simulation: a systematic review and meta-analysis. In *Defining Excellence in Simulation Programs* (pp. 327–342).

Cheng, A., Grant, V., Robinson, T., Catena, H., Lachapelle, K., Kim, J., Adler, M., & Eppich, W. (2016). The promoting excellence and reflective learning in simulation (PEARLS) approach to health care debriefing: a faculty development guide. *Clinical Simulation in Nursing*, 12(10), 419–428. https://doi.org/10.1016/j.ecns.2016.05.002.

Chmil, J. V., Turk, M., Adamson, K., & Larew, C. (2015). Effects of an experiential learning simulation design on clinical nursing judgment development. *Nurse Educator*, 40(5), 228–232. https://doi.org/10.1097/NNE.0000000000000159.

Cook, D. A., Hatala, R., Brydges, R., Zendejas, B., Szostek, J. H., Wang, A. T., Erwin, P. J., & Hamstra, S. J. (2011). Technology-enhanced simulation for health professions education: a systematic review and meta-analysis. *Journal of the American Medical Association*, 306(9), 978–988.

Decker, S., Alinier, G., Crawford, S. B., Gordon, R. M., Jenkins, D., & Wilson, C. (2021). Healthcare simulation standards of best practice™: the debriefing process. *Clinical Simulation in Nursing*, 58, 27–32. https://doi.org/10.1016/j.ecns.2021.08.011.

Dieckmann, P., Gaba, D., & Rall, M. (2007). Deepening the theoretical foundations of patient simulation as social practice. *Simulation in Healthcare*, 2(3), 183–193.

Dubé, M., Kaba, A., Cronin, T., Barnes, S., Fuselli, T., & Grant, V. (2020). COVID-19 pandemic preparation: using simulation for systems-based learning to prepare the largest healthcare workforce and system in Canada. *Advances in Simulation*, 5, 22. https://doi.org/10.1186/s41077-020-00138-w.

Eppich, W., & Cheng, A. (2015). Promoting excellence and reflective learning in simulation (PEARLS): development and rationale for a blended approach to health care simulation debriefing. *Simulation in Healthcare*, 10(2), 106–115.

Falloon, G. (2019). Using simulations to teach young students science concepts: an experiential learning theoretical analysis. *Computers & Education*, 135, 138–159. https://doi.org/10.1016/j.compedu.2019.03.001.

Foronda, C., Fernandez-Burgos, M., Nadeau, C., Kelley, C. N., & Henry, M. N. (2020). Virtual simulation in nursing education: a systematic review spanning 1996 to 2018. *Simulation in Healthcare*, 15(1), 46–54.

Gaba, D. M. (2004). The future vision of simulation in health care. *Quality and Safety in Health Care*, 13(Suppl), i2–10.

Galan-Lominchar, M., Muñoz-San Roque, I., del Campo Cazallas, C., McAlpin, R., Fernández-Ayuso, D., & Ribeiro, A. S. F. (2024). Nursing students' internationalization: virtual exchange and clinical simulation impact cultural intelligence. *Nursing Outlook*, 72(2), 102137.

Goleman, D. (1995). *Emotional Intelligence: Why It Can Matter More Than IQ*. New York: Bantam Books.

Goleman, D., Boyatzis, R., & McKee, A. (2002). *Primal Leadership: Realizing the Power of Emotional Intelligence*. Boston: Harvard Business School Press.

HEE (2020). *Simulation-based education: enhancing patient safety and outcomes*.

Institute of Medicine (2011). *The Future of Nursing: Leading Change, Advancing Health*. Washington, DC: The National Academies Press.

Jaye, P., Thomas, L., & Reedy, G. (2015). 'The diamond': a structure for simulation debrief. *The Clinical Teacher*, 12(3), 171–175. https://doi.org/10.1111/tct.12300.

Jeffries, P. R. (2021). *The NLN Jeffries Simulation Theory* (2nd ed.). Philadelphia, PA: Wolters Kluwer.

Johnson, B. (2020). Observational experiential learning: theoretical support for observer roles in health care simulation. *Journal of Nursing Education*, 59(1), 7–14.

Kolb, D. A. (1984). *Experiential Learning: Experience as the Source of Learning and Development*. Englewood Cliffs, NJ: Prentice-Hall.

Laursen, S. L. (2015). Assessing undergraduate research in the sciences: the next generation. *CUR Quarterly*, 35(3), 9–14.

Lavoie, P., & Clarke, S. P. (2017). Simulation in nursing education. *Nursing*, 47(7), 18–20.

Mitchell, A. (2024). Creating lived experience simulations. *British Journal of Nursing*, 33(11), 522–523.

Mitchell, A., Bowyer, M., & Salmon, L. (2025). A simulated microaggression session for pre-registration nursing students. *British Journal of Nursing*, 34(7), 369–373.

Mitchell, A., Hill, B., & Murray, J. (2023). Exploring the lived experiences of mental health professionals: a phenomenological study on ligature training in a simulated environment. *Journal of Applied Learning & Teaching*, 6(Special Issue 1), 64–73.

Piedrahita-Mejía, J. C., & Cardona-Cano, R. (2022). The history of the simulation concept and its use in educational environments in the health sector. *Revista Cuidarte*, 19(4), 10–13. https://doi.org/10.21676/2389783X.4988.

Pillay, T., Clarke, L., Abbott, L., Surana, P., Shenvi, A., Deshpande, S., Cookson, J., Nash, M., Fawke, J., Rasiah, V., & Cusack, J. (2021). Optimising frontline learning and engagement between consultant-led neonatal teams in the West Midlands: a survey on the utility of an augmented simulation training technique. *Advances in Simulation*, 6, 29. https://doi.org/10.1186/s41077-021-00181-1.

Pottle, J. (2019). Virtual reality and the transformation of medical education. *Future Healthcare Journal*, 6(3), 181–185.

Rasheed, S. P. (2015). Self-awareness as a therapeutic tool for nurse/client relationship. *International Journal of Caring Sciences*, 8(1), 211–216.

Rudolph, J., Simon, R., Dufresne, R., & Raemer, D. (2006). There's no such thing as "nonjudgmental" debriefing: a theory and method for debriefing with good judgment. *Simulation in Healthcare*, 1(1), 49–55. https://doi.org/10.1097/01266021-200600110-00006.

Salik, I., & Paige, J. T. (2023). Debriefing the interprofessional team in medical simulation. In *StatPearls*. StatPearls Publishing. https://www.ncbi.nlm.nih.gov/books/NBK554526/.

Schön, D. A. (1983). *The Reflective Practitioner: How Professionals Think in Action*. New York: Basic Books.

Szulewski, A., Howes, D., Van Merriënboer, J. J. G., & Sweller, J. (2021). From theory to practice: the application of cognitive load theory to the practice of medicine. *Academic Medicine*, 96(1), 24–30. https://doi.org/10.1097/ACM.0000000000003524.

Tannenbaum, S. I., & Cerasoli, C. P. (2013). Do team and individual debriefs enhance performance? A meta-analysis. *Human Factors*, 55(1), 231–245. https://doi.org/10.1177/0018720812448394.

Teixeira, L., Mitchell, A., Martinez, N. C. & Salim, B. J. (2024). Virtual reality with artificial intelligence-led scenarios in nursing education: a project evaluation. *British Journal of Nursing*, 33(17), pp. 812–820. https://doi.org/10.12968/bjon.2024.0055.

Topol, E. (2019). *Deep Medicine: How Artificial Intelligence Can Make Healthcare Human Again*. Basic Books.

Weinstock, P., Kappus, L., Garden, A., & Burns, J. P. (2015). Simulation at the point of care: reduced-cost, in situ training via a mobile cart. *Pediatric Critical Care Medicine*, 16(3), 260–265.

Weldon, S. M., & colleagues. (2023). The seven simulation-based 'I's: a concept taxonomy review of transformative simulation in healthcare. *International Journal of Healthcare Simulation*, 1–13. https://doi.org/10.54531/tzfd6375.

Whitfill, T., Gawel, M., & Auerbach, M. (2018). A simulation-based quality improvement initiative improves pediatric readiness in community hospitals. *Pediatric Emergency Care*, 34(6), 431–435. https://doi.org/10.1097/PEC.0000000000001233.

Younas, A., Parveen, S., Sundus, A., & Inayat, S. (2019). Nurses' perspectives of self-awareness in nursing practice: a descriptive qualitative study. *Nursing & Health Sciences*, 22(2), 398–405. https://doi.org/10.1111/nhs.12671.

CHAPTER 7

Digital and Immersive Technologies in Nursing Education

Claire Ford[1] and Behnam Jafari Salim[2]

[1] *School of Healthcare and Nursing Sciences, Northumbria University, Newcastle upon Tyne, UK*
[2] *King's College London, London, UK*

AIM

To examine the role and impact of digital and immersive educational technologies, specifically virtual reality (VR), artificial intelligence (AI), augmented reality (AR), and 360-degree video, in transforming nursing education, with particular focus on pedagogy, practice-based learning, and curriculum integration.

LEARNING OUTCOMES

By the end of this chapter, readers will be able to:

1. Critically evaluate the pedagogical and practical applications of immersive technologies in pre- and post-registration nursing education.

2. Analyse the challenges and opportunities of integrating VR, AI, AR, and 360-degree video into online and hybrid learning environments.

3. Consider the influence of immersive technologies on nursing practice, clinical judgement, and student engagement.

4. Identify effective approaches for embedding immersive learning into nursing curricula through gamification and digital transformation frameworks.

CHAPTER INTRODUCTION

Nursing education is undergoing considerable transformation, shaped by the integration of advanced technologies such as virtual reality (VR), augmented reality (AR), mixed reality (MR), and artificial intelligence (AI). These approaches expand learning opportunities by strengthening experiential learning and supporting simulation-based education within both synchronous and asynchronous contexts.

Immersive technologies such as VR, AR, and MR enable students to engage in safe and controlled yet realistic clinical environments that develop critical thinking, clinical reasoning, decision-making, communication skills, and professional identity. The use of artificial intelligence in virtual learning environments offers the possibility of providing personalised, one-to-one, and standardised learning experiences at scale.

The Nursing and Midwifery Council (NMC) (2018) now permits the use of simulation-based learning for up to 600 of the required 2,300 practice learning hours. NHS England (2024) has reinforced this direction through national simulation and immersive technology frameworks, recognising their potential to address placement pressures and expand clinical capacity.

As nursing curricula respond to growing student numbers, placement challenges, and wider digital transformation within healthcare, immersive approaches offer meaningful enhancements to traditional teaching. Virtual teaching environments and AI-driven scenarios are being developed to expand capacity and personalise learning, particularly in pre-registration programmes.

Examples include the use of simulation for trauma or deterioration management, AI-led patient avatars for diagnostic reasoning, and structured virtual placements that map directly to clinical proficiencies and practice hours. These methods extend opportunities for clinical judgement, reduce placement variability, and support equitable access to complex learning experiences.

This chapter provides a critical overview of immersive technologies in nursing education, examining both their pedagogical foundations and practical applications. It highlights opportunities, limitations, and implementation challenges, and offers guidance for nurse educators seeking to embed immersive practices. Readers are encouraged to reflect on how immersive learning aligns with professional standards, student needs, and the future direction of digital healthcare.

SIMULATION IN NURSING EDUCATION: STANDARDS, ROLES, AND PEDAGOGICAL PRACTICES

Simulation has become a core element of nursing education, enabling students to engage in practice-based learning in controlled yet realistic environments. It provides opportunities to rehearse clinical skills, develop teamwork, and practise communication and decision-making without compromising patient safety. Simulation supports the development of clinical competence, builds confidence, and strengthens professional identity formation.

The Nursing and Midwifery Council (2018) allows up to 600 practice hours to be completed through simulation, reflecting its recognised contribution to safe and effective learning. International standards also provide clear frameworks for quality. The Association for Simulated Practice in Healthcare (ASPiH) sets guidance on simulation fidelity, facilitation, and outcome alignment. The Society in Europe for Simulation Applied to Medicine (SESAM) offers programme-level accreditation, while NHS England promotes simulation faculty development and resources through its Simulation and Immersive Technologies team. Together, these standards support consistent practice and ensure simulation is delivered with pedagogical rigour.

Within simulation, different roles shape the learning experience. Practice supervisors guide and support learners during simulation, while practice assessors evaluate performance against set outcomes. The involvement of experts by experience in co-design and delivery adds authenticity, particularly in scenarios focusing on communication, empathy, or ethical decision-making. Facilitators remain central in leading structured pre-briefing and debriefing, creating psychologically safe spaces for reflection and feedback.

Simulation is not limited to high-fidelity environments. Low-fidelity methods, such as role-play or skills station practice, remain important for building confidence in basic procedures. High-fidelity simulations, including manikins, VR environments, or complex team-based scenarios, allow students to integrate technical and non-technical skills under pressure. Selecting the appropriate approach should always be guided by learning outcomes, available resources, and student readiness, rather than assumptions that more sophisticated technology automatically produces better learning.

A key underpinning concept is fidelity, which refers to the degree of realism achieved. Fidelity may be physical (realism of equipment and environment), psychological (the extent to which learners feel immersed and respond emotionally), or functional (how accurately tasks and processes mirror clinical practice). Effective simulation requires balancing these dimensions to ensure efficiency, authenticity, and relevance.

PEDAGOGICAL FOUNDATIONS FOR IMMERSIVE LEARNING

The effectiveness of immersive technologies depends not only on the realism of the experience but also on their integration into sound pedagogical design. Simulation and digital technologies must be explicitly linked to intended learning outcomes, supported by structured preparation, facilitation, and debriefing.

Several learning theories help explain how immersive technologies contribute to knowledge and skills development. Kolb's experiential learning cycle positions experience, reflection, conceptualisation, and experimentation as core to deep learning. Simulation and VR provide opportunities to move through this cycle repeatedly, reinforcing both technical and non-technical skills.

The Community of Inquiry (CoI) framework highlights the importance of social, cognitive, and teaching presence in online and hybrid learning. Immersive technologies can enhance social presence by strengthening collaboration and communication, while AI-driven avatars and adaptive systems can extend teaching presence by personalising feedback.

Self-determination theory emphasises autonomy, competence, and relatedness as drivers of motivation. Immersive learning environments can promote autonomy by enabling self-paced exploration, competence through scaffolded skill practice, and relatedness via authentic interaction with peers, facilitators, and virtual patients.

Simulation-based learning also benefits from structured approaches such as pre-briefing and debriefing. Pre-briefing ensures learners understand the objectives, expectations, and safe learning environment, while debriefing supports critical reflection, feedback, and integration of theory into practice. Facilitated reflection is consistently identified as one of the most powerful elements of simulation-based education.

Ultimately, immersive learning depends on more than access to new technologies. Effective outcomes are achieved when scenarios are intentionally designed, aligned to curriculum outcomes, and supported by skilled facilitation and structured evaluation.

VIRTUAL TEACHING AND PRACTICE ENVIRONMENTS: FROM SIMULATION TO PRACTICE PLACEMENT

The rise of virtual teaching environments in nursing education has coincided with increased pressure on placement capacity, growing student numbers, and the need for consistent and accessible clinical learning. Immersive approaches offer digitally enabled practice learning that complements, and in some cases partially substitutes, in-person placements.

Virtual practice environments can include immersive simulations delivered through virtual reality, interactive case-based learning modules, structured virtual placements using AI-driven patient avatars, and tailored 360-degree scenarios. These tools can represent a wide range of clinical situations, including complex care pathways, safeguarding conversations, management of the deteriorating patient, and palliative care. Crucially, simulations can be designed to map directly to NMC proficiencies so they contribute meaningfully to practice hours and professional development.

One example is the use of structured virtual placements that deliver thousands of hours of simulated learning across entire cohorts (Hill & Mitchell, 2024). These programmes are typically built on bespoke platforms that guide students through realistic patient journeys, prompt critical decisions, and support reflection through embedded questions, self-assessment, and group debriefs. They are particularly valuable during placement shortfalls or public health emergencies, and they provide an inclusive alternative for learners who face barriers to in-person practice.

Research indicates that when well designed, virtual placements can support confidence, competence, and decision-making to levels comparable with traditional placements (Padilha et al., 2019). Students frequently report that virtual simulations allow them to fail safely, revisit encounters for deeper understanding, and experience scenarios that are rare or logistically difficult in real settings.

The pedagogical effectiveness of virtual practice environments depends on three factors

1. **Alignment with Practice Outcomes and Assessment Criteria**

   Activities should relate directly to professional standards so students can demonstrate proficiency in areas such as communication, prioritisation, safeguarding, and escalation of care. Digital documentation and dashboards can support real-time tracking of progress.

2. **Integration into Curriculum Design**

   Virtual placements should be embedded within module outcomes, assessment strategies, and academic support, rather than offered as optional extras. Educators need preparation to facilitate these experiences with the same rigour as traditional clinical education.

3. **Reflective and Dialogic Learning**

   Critical reflection, peer discussion, and structured debriefing bridge the gap between simulated learning and practice, helping students consolidate insights and apply them with sound clinical judgement.

Virtual environments also support flipped classrooms, asynchronous learning, and interprofessional online

Table 7.1 Features That Support High-quality Virtual Practice Environments in Nursing Education

Feature	Description
Scenario realism	Use of dynamic, branching case scenarios based on authentic clinical pathways.
Learner agency	Opportunities for students to make decisions, receive feedback, and reflect.
Measurable outcomes	Clear mapping to NMC proficiencies and programme learning outcomes.
Digital documentation	Integration of e-portfolios or learning dashboards for progress tracking.
Structured debrief and feedback	Facilitated discussion to consolidate and apply learning.
Equity and accessibility	Accessible formats for all learners, including those with additional learning needs.

collaboration. Platforms such as Microsoft Teams, Moodle, and purpose-built simulation software can host online case conferences, formative quizzes, virtual clinical briefings, and peer-led learning. See Table 7.1 for features that characterise high quality virtual practice environments in nursing education.

ARTIFICIAL INTELLIGENCE AND AUGMENTED REALITY: INNOVATION AND INTEGRATION

AI and AR are increasingly influencing nurse education through innovative simulation tools and interactive learning platforms. These technologies offer new dimensions of teaching and learning, from decision-support training to interactive anatomical visualisation, and are becoming more accessible in both undergraduate and postgraduate curricula.

For example, analytics dashboards can provide educators with insight into patterns of clinical thinking, allowing for targeted feedback or curriculum adjustments. However, ethical considerations around data use, bias, and decision transparency must be actively addressed when integrating AI into educational environments (Topol, 2019).

ARTIFICIAL INTELLIGENCE IN NURSING EDUCATION

AI has emerged as a key enabler of personalised learning experiences in health education. Its applications include intelligent tutoring systems, adaptive learning platforms, and virtual patients that respond to learner input in real time. These systems can analyse learner performance data and offer tailored feedback, helping students refine their clinical reasoning, prioritisation, and communication skills.

In a randomised controlled trial, Padilha et al. (2019) found that students using AI-enabled clinical virtual simulations demonstrated significantly improved knowledge retention and clinical reasoning compared to those participating in traditional simulations. These benefits are particularly evident when AI is used to simulate patient deterioration, diagnostic uncertainty, or ethical decision-making—areas where structured feedback and repetition are essential.

AI-driven simulations also support formative assessment and early identification of learning needs.

AUGMENTED REALITY IN NURSING EDUCATION

AR enhances the physical learning environment by overlaying digital elements, such as 3D anatomical models or procedural guidance, onto the real world. This allows learners to engage with content interactively, supporting the development of spatial awareness, procedural memory, and technical competence.

Applications of AR in nursing education include simulated wound care, visualisation of anatomy, and step-by-step clinical procedure walkthroughs using devices like tablets or AR headsets. A study by Koivisto et al. (2016) showed that AR-based training improved students' confidence and skill performance in basic nursing procedures, particularly in novice learners.

AR is also useful in team-based learning, where groups of students interact with the same augmented scenario, encouraging collaborative decision-making and real-time peer discussion. This aligns well with interprofessional education frameworks and the NMC's emphasis on team-based working and person-centred care.

INNOVATION BOX

Scenario

A 72-year-old person with type 2 diabetes and COPD is admitted with shortness of breath.

Team tasks

Perform an initial assessment, prioritise care, escalate concerns, administer medicines, and begin discharge planning

AR features deteriorating observations, audible wheeze, electronic health record, prescription interactions, a patient avatar with speech

Learning outcomes

- Provide safe, effective, evidence-informed care in a simulated clinical context
- Develop interprofessional communication, delegation, and teamwork
- Apply critical thinking when prioritising care in dynamic environments
- Reflect on attitudes, bias, and decision-making under pressure
- Practise person-centred care while managing social and clinical complexity

Debrief questions

1 What was it like working together in an augmented reality setting?
2 How did the environment influence your communication or decision-making?
3 What were your priorities at the first presentation?
4 How did your team assess and manage the person's condition?
5 Which communication strategies worked well, and which did not?
6 Were there moments of uncertainty, and how did the team respond?
7 How did each profession contribute to decisions?
8 Were there any red flags you missed or recognised late?

Reflections on using AR as a simulation modality

- How did AR help or hinder your assessment of the person and the environment
- Which elements felt most realistic or immersive
- Did the overlays or interactive elements improve your understanding of the scenario, and how
- Did anything about the AR experience distract you from the clinical task

INTEGRATION STRATEGIES FOR AI AND AR

Successful integration of AI and AR into nursing curricula requires careful planning, institutional support, and pedagogical alignment. The following strategies can guide implementation:

- **Curriculum Alignment**: Immersive tools should be mapped to specific learning outcomes and NMC proficiencies. They should not replace, but complement, experiential and practice-based components.
- **Faculty Development**: Educators need structured training and opportunities to explore these tools, with emphasis on pedagogical value rather than technical novelty.
- **Student Preparation**: Orientation sessions can help learners understand the role of immersive technology,

reduce anxiety, and encourage responsible digital citizenship.

- **Infrastructure and Equity**: Institutions must ensure reliable access to hardware, software, and connectivity, addressing digital exclusion and accessibility.

When used with purpose, AI and AR can help nurse educators deliver transformative, learner-centred experiences that build clinical insight, technical skill, and professional confidence. These strategies ensure that students are prepared to practise in increasingly digital clinical environments where technological literacy is recognised as a core competence.

These strategies also prepare students to work in increasingly digital clinical environments where technological literacy is recognised as a core competence.

360 DEGREE VIDEO IN NURSING EDUCATION

360-degree video provides a versatile and accessible approach to immersive learning, particularly valuable for novice users or where resources are limited. Unlike fully interactive VR,

360-degree video uses omnidirectional cameras to capture real-world clinical scenarios, enabling learners to explore environments from multiple perspectives through headsets or standard screens. This creates a strong sense of presence and emotional connection while remaining more cost-effective to produce and distribute than high-fidelity virtual reality.

STRENGTHS

- Affordability and Scalability: Relatively inexpensive to create and easy to share across institutions.

- Authentic Context: Real-world footage supports realism and emotional engagement, especially in areas such as communication, empathy, or ethical decision-making.

- Standardisation: Ensures consistent delivery of scenarios, contributing to equity in learning.

- Safe Rehearsal: Enables learners to observe and reflect on sensitive encounters, such as breaking bad news or dementia care, without risk to patients.

LIMITATIONS AND CONSIDERATIONS

- Limited Interactivity: Learners are primarily observers rather than active participants.

- Production Demands: Effective content requires careful filming, editing, and collaboration between educators and media specialists.

- Pedagogical Alignment: Without clear integration into learning pathways, 360-degree video risks becoming a novelty rather than a meaningful tool.

To maximise its impact, 360-degree video should be embedded within a structured educational design that incorporates debriefing, reflection, and assessment. Park et al. (2024) emphasise that the choice of simulation modality should be driven by pedagogical intent rather than technology alone, ensuring fidelity, facilitation, and faculty readiness remain central to learner experience.

Writing scenarios for AI in nurse education involves creating realistic, person-centred virtual characters that simulate clinical situations to support student learning. Each scenario should include key details such as the character's identity (e.g. age, medical history, presenting complaint), what they know about their condition, and what they want to find out, such as treatment options or medication guidance. Including emotional, social, and psychological context adds depth and realism, helping students to develop clinical reasoning, communication, and empathy. These AI-driven interactions provide safe, repeatable opportunities for students to practise assessment and decision-making, and align with nursing education priorities such as interprofessional teamwork and person-centred care.

ACTIVITY

Try to write your own AI character to use for simulation

1. Who is the patient? (Background Information)

   Describe the character's demographic details and current clinical concern. Include relevant medical history, lifestyle factors, or social context if appropriate.

   Example:

   Freddie is a 40-year-old warehouse worker who presents with pain in his right hip. The pain started three weeks ago and has gradually worsened. He reports that the pain intensifies with rotation and weight-bearing. He has no known allergies and takes no regular medication.

2. What does the patient *know* about their condition?

   Explain the patient's current understanding of their symptoms or health status. This sets the stage for clinical questioning and communication.

   Example:

   Freddie knows that the pain is located in his right hip and worsens when he moves or rotates it. He recalls twisting his leg awkwardly while lifting a heavy box at work, but he did not think much of it at the time. He suspects he may have strained a muscle.

3. What does the patient *want to know*?

   Outline the patient's concerns, questions, and expectations for their care. These guide the student's clinical reasoning and communication skills.

   Example:

   Freddie wants to know what might be causing the pain, whether he should be worried, and if he needs an X-ray or other investigations. He is also asking what kind of pain relief is suitable, how much he can take, and whether he should avoid work or certain movements.

4. (Optional) What emotional or psychological state is the patient in?

   This helps build empathy and person-centred care into the scenario.

   Example:

   Freddie is frustrated and anxious about missing work, as he is the main earner in his household. He is also nervous about taking strong medication, having had a bad reaction to opioids in the past.

ONLINE NURSING EDUCATION: TRENDS AND CHALLENGES

Online learning has become a central feature of contemporary nursing education, particularly following the COVID-19 pandemic. From asynchronous content delivery to synchronous webinars and virtual clinical simulations, online modalities now underpin many undergraduate and postgraduate programmes. While these approaches bring significant flexibility and scalability, they also present challenges that must be carefully managed by educators.

CURRENT TRENDS IN ONLINE NURSING EDUCATION

Online nursing education increasingly incorporates blended approaches that combine virtual content with in-person simulation or placement-based learning. Learning management systems (LMS) such as Moodle and Canvas support structured module delivery, enabling integration of multimedia content, formative assessments, and discussion forums. Web conferencing tools like Microsoft Teams and Zoom are used for interactive lectures, clinical case discussions, and peer-led seminars.

A notable trend is the expansion of virtual simulation into online delivery. These tools offer high-fidelity patient scenarios in fully remote environments, enabling learners to practise assessment, diagnosis, and decision-making from any location (Foronda et al., 2020). Paired with structured debriefing, they can form a powerful component of remote clinical education.

There is also increased attention to online peer collaboration and the use of co-constructed learning spaces where students contribute to resources, lead discussions, or peer-review clinical reasoning. This aligns with constructivist learning principles and supports student engagement in distributed settings.

CHALLENGES IN ONLINE DELIVERY

Despite these innovations, online nurse education is not without challenges. Digital exclusion remains a major concern, with students facing barriers such as inadequate internet access, lack of quiet study space, or unfamiliarity with digital tools (Watermeyer et al., 2021). These issues can disproportionately affect students from underrepresented backgrounds and contribute to attainment gaps.

Maintaining clinical authenticity online is also difficult. Without careful design, online learning may feel disconnected from real-world practice, undermining student confidence and application. As such, it is essential that educators build in authentic scenarios, reflection, and opportunities for dialogue.

Furthermore, sustaining motivation in virtual environments can be challenging. Educators must consider how to design content that is interactive, relevant, and emotionally engaging. Gamification, formative quizzes, breakout groups, and scenario-based learning can all help maintain presence and participation (Koivisto et al., 2016). Table 7.2 highlights examples of immersive and online tools currently used in nurse education, alongside their pedagogical benefits.

Table 7.2 Examples of Immersive and Online Tools Currently Used in Nurse Education, Alongside Their Pedagogical Benefits

Technology/tool	Educational application	Benefits
Virtual Reality (VR)	Simulated clinical environments, such as trauma or ward rounds	Enhances decision-making, reduces anxiety, and offers a safe practice space
Augmented Reality (AR)	Interactive anatomical overlays, procedural step-throughs	Supports psychomotor learning and spatial understanding
Artificial Intelligence (AI)	Adaptive simulations, virtual patients, predictive analytics	Provides real-time feedback, supports personalisation of learning
Learning Management Systems	Module delivery, quizzes, asynchronous content	Enables structured access and learner tracking
Web conferencing (Teams, Zoom)	Interactive teaching, case discussions, group tutorials	Maintains real-time presence and supports collaborative learning
Gamification platforms	Clinical reasoning games, interactive branching scenarios	Boosts motivation and consolidates theoretical knowledge
E-portfolios/dashboards	Tracking of proficiencies, reflection logs, and digital credentials	Supports assessment for learning and evidence collection

CREATING IMMERSIVE LEARNING ENVIRONMENTS: DESIGN, ETHICS, AND STUDENT VOICE

Designing immersive learning environments in nursing education requires more than the application of advanced technology. It involves thoughtful curriculum integration, ethical foresight, and active collaboration with learners. For immersive tools to contribute meaningfully to student development, their design must support inclusivity, authenticity, and reflective engagement.

PRINCIPLES OF IMMERSIVE LEARNING DESIGN

Effective immersive learning environments are intentionally structured to engage students cognitively, emotionally, and practically. They are not simply digital replications of face-to-face teaching, but transformative spaces where learners can test their knowledge, experience consequences, and reflect in a safe and supported manner.

Key design principles include:

- **Authenticity**: Scenarios should reflect real clinical contexts, using standardised documentation, realistic communication challenges, and patient diversity. This supports the development of transferable skills and enhances professional readiness (Cant & Cooper, 2017).

- **Progressive Complexity**: Learning environments should scaffold students' engagement through increasingly complex decision-making and emotional intensity, allowing for consolidation and challenge.

- **Feedback and Reflection**: Embedded debriefs, guided reflections, and feedback mechanisms are critical to help students make sense of their experiences and align them with professional expectations (INACSL Standards Committee, 2021).

- **Accessibility and Inclusivity**: Platforms must support learners with varied needs, including those with sensory, cognitive, or language-related barriers. Design should follow universal design principles, offering alternative formats and supports.

A co-designed approach, where students are consulted or involved in the design of immersive content, can improve relevance, uptake, and engagement. This is particularly important when dealing with sensitive content such as mental health, end-of-life care, or equality-related scenarios. Co-creation empowers learners and reinforces professional values of partnership and collaboration (Bovill et al., 2011).

ETHICAL CONSIDERATIONS IN IMMERSIVE DESIGN

Immersive technologies raise important ethical considerations that educators must address when integrating them into curricula. These include:

- **Informed Consent**: Students should be made aware of the emotional and cognitive demands of immersive scenarios. Content warnings, opt-outs, and emotional safety protocols must be established, especially in trauma-informed education.

- **Data privacy and Digital Surveillance**: Many immersive tools capture user data for analytics or personalisation. Educators must understand and communicate how this data is used, stored, and protected, in line with institutional and legal requirements (Blease et al., 2020).

- **Simulation Fidelity vs. Emotional Realism**: High-fidelity simulation can be emotionally intense. Educators must carefully balance realism with psychological safety, ensuring opportunities for debriefing and support (Dieckmann et al., 2020).

- **Bias and Representation**: If not carefully designed, immersive content may inadvertently reproduce stereotypes or omit marginalised groups. Scenarios should reflect a wide range of patients, conditions, and identities, and must be periodically reviewed for cultural relevance and fairness.

STUDENT VOICE AND CO-CREATION

Involving students in the design and evaluation of immersive learning can support deeper engagement and ensure that content is pedagogically and socially relevant. Student feedback has shown that immersive learning feels most impactful when learners see themselves reflected in the content and feel psychologically safe during participation (McGaghie et al., 2010).

Mechanisms for student voice include:

- Participatory scenario design workshops
- Student-led peer evaluation of immersive tools
- Reflective journals and feedback forms post-simulation
- Focus groups to explore emotional and cognitive impacts

These strategies align with inclusive pedagogy and support the development of shared responsibility for learning. For educators undertaking the PGCAP or similar development routes, embedding student voice in immersive education supports values-based teaching and reflective practice.

GAMIFICATION IN NURSING EDUCATION: PRINCIPLES AND PRACTICE

Gamification, the use of game mechanics and design elements in non-game contexts, is an increasingly popular strategy for enhancing engagement, motivation, and critical thinking in nurse education. When implemented purposefully, gamification can support the development of clinical reasoning, prioritisation, communication, and teamwork in a safe and motivating learning environment.

UNDERSTANDING GAMIFICATION IN HEALTH EDUCATION

Gamification differs from full educational games in that it embeds game-like elements into learning activities rather than relying on complete, standalone games. Examples include point scoring, level progression, badges, timers, leaderboards, and scenario branching. These elements are integrated into simulations, case-based learning, or virtual environments to create structured challenges and reinforce learning through feedback and reward (Deterding et al., 2011).

In nurse education, gamification has been successfully applied in areas such as infection prevention, pharmacology, ethics, communication, and acute care decision-making. Common formats include:

- **Digital branching scenarios**, where learners make choices in clinical cases that lead to multiple outcomes

- **Timed quizzes or simulations**, testing clinical judgement under pressure

- **Narrative-based challenges**, using patient stories to frame tasks and decisions

- **Role-play with scoring mechanisms**, encouraging peer feedback and reflection

These formats mirror real-world complexity and uncertainty while keeping students actively engaged.

PEDAGOGICAL THEORIES SUPPORTING GAMIFICATION

Gamification draws on several well-established learning theories:

- **Self-determination theory** (Deci & Ryan, 1985) supports the idea that learners are more motivated when they experience autonomy, competence, and relatedness—principles embedded in well-designed gamified learning.

- **Constructivist theory** posits that learners build knowledge through active engagement and reflection. Gamified activities often include exploration, feedback, and debriefing to support this process.

- **Cognitive load theory** helps explain why chunked, goal-oriented tasks—like those in gamified learning—can aid memory and skill development by reducing extraneous cognitive burden (Sweller et al., 2011).

The inclusion of immediate feedback, safe failure, and spaced repetition makes gamification particularly suitable for reinforcing difficult or high-risk clinical content.

EXAMPLES IN NURSING EDUCATION PRACTICE

Gamification in nurse education has been implemented through both bespoke simulation platforms and accessible tools like Kahoot!, Twine, or SimX. For example:

- Twine allows educators to create branching clinical stories where students' decisions affect patient outcomes.

- SimX offers VR and gamified patient care scenarios with performance metrics.

- Kahoot! and Quizizz are commonly used for formative assessment in pharmacology or anatomy.

These tools are often well-received by students, who report that gamified elements make content more memorable and enjoyable (Koivisto et al., 2018). However, they are most effective when paired with critical reflection, facilitated discussion, and clear links to curriculum outcomes.

BEST PRACTICE FOR IMPLEMENTATION

To integrate gamification effectively, nurse educators should:

- Ensure clear alignment with learning outcomes and NMC proficiencies

- Avoid over-reliance on competitive elements that may discourage participation

- Include structured debriefing and reflection to reinforce meaning

- Use gamification as a complement, not a substitute, for other pedagogies

- Regularly evaluate impact and student feedback

Gamification should not be viewed as a gimmick or distraction but as a meaningful pedagogical strategy. When implemented thoughtfully, it offers a dynamic way to engage learners in complex clinical concepts, promote decision-making under pressure, and build resilience.

EMBEDDING DIGITAL TRANSFORMATION INTO CURRICULUM DESIGN

Digital transformation in healthcare and education refers to the integration of digital tools, data, and technologies into everyday systems, processes, and practices. For nurse education, this means rethinking not just how students are taught, but how curricula are constructed, delivered, and assessed in response to a rapidly evolving digital landscape.

To prepare digitally fluent nursing graduates, nurse educators must embed digital transformation principles throughout curriculum design—not as isolated digital skills modules, but as an integrated thread across theoretical, clinical, and professional learning.

DEFINING DIGITAL TRANSFORMATION IN NURSE EDUCATION

Digital transformation goes beyond using online platforms or simulation tools; it encompasses a cultural and structural shift toward innovation, adaptability, and data-informed practice (Health Education England [HEE], 2021). It requires educators to align teaching with the realities of digital clinical practice, including electronic patient records, telehealth, decision-support tools, and digital communication platforms.

This shift also demands pedagogical innovation. Curriculum design must reflect how nurses work in digital environments, understand data governance, navigate ethical challenges, and use technology to support person-centred care. These goals are increasingly reflected in strategic documents such as the NHS Long Term Workforce Plan (NHS England, 2023) and HEE's Digital Capabilities Framework (HEE, 2021), both of which highlight digital readiness as a core graduate attribute.

CURRICULUM-LEVEL STRATEGIES FOR INTEGRATION

Effective digital transformation in nurse education begins at the curriculum planning stage. Educators should consider:

- **Digital Fluency as a Curriculum Thread**: Embed digital themes across modules (e.g. safe digital communication in ethics, EHR navigation in documentation, wearable technology in chronic disease management).
- **Mapping to Regulatory and Workforce Frameworks**: Align content with standards such as the NMC (2018) Future Nurse proficiencies and HEE's (2021) digital capability domains, ensuring coherence and relevance.
- **Cross-cutting Themes**: Link digital transformation to wider educational priorities, such as sustainability, inclusion, and health equity. For example, discussions on digital access and digital poverty can connect technological content to the social determinants of health.
- **Practice-based Application**: Provide simulation and placement experiences that reflect the digital realities of healthcare (e.g. using mock EHRs, virtual MDT meetings, or AI-supported clinical tools).
- **Assessment Innovation**: Include digital tools in assessment, such as e-portfolios, digital OSCEs, screencast reflections, or scenario-based tasks using branching logic.

PROFESSIONAL DEVELOPMENT AND CULTURAL CHANGE

Digital transformation also requires a shift in academic culture. Nurse educators need opportunities to develop confidence and competence in using and teaching with technology. This includes protected time for digital CPD, cross-disciplinary collaboration, and support from institutional infrastructure.

Educational leaders should champion a culture of curiosity, experimentation, and feedback, ensuring that digital innovation is inclusive and underpinned by pedagogical reasoning, not simply driven by market trends or platform availability.

Staff development programmes such as the PGCAP, Advance HE fellowship routes, or CPD sessions on immersive technology can all contribute to growing digital leadership among nurse educators.

SUSTAINING CHANGE THROUGH EVALUATION

Embedding digital transformation is not a one-off task—it requires ongoing review and adaptation. Evaluation should explore:

- Student and staff digital confidence
- Learning outcomes linked to digital tools
- Impact on accessibility, equity, and student engagement
- Preparedness for digital clinical environments

Data from module evaluations, student feedback, and digital audits can inform improvements and highlight areas where support is still needed.

By embedding digital transformation strategically, nursing curricula can better prepare learners for future practice, support educator growth, and align higher education with the realities of 21st-century healthcare.

REFLECTIVE PRACTICE, EVALUATION, AND FUTURE DIRECTIONS

As immersive technologies continue to reshape the landscape of nurse education, their sustained impact depends not only on technical innovation but also on the capacity of educators to engage in ongoing reflection, evaluation, and strategic foresight. Embedding immersive and digital approaches requires a culture of critical enquiry, one where pedagogy leads technology, and student learning remains at the heart of every decision.

THE ROLE OF REFLECTIVE PRACTICE IN IMMERSIVE TEACHING

Reflective practice is a cornerstone of nursing and nurse education. For educators integrating immersive technologies, it provides a structured way to assess what works, what challenges arise, and how practice might evolve. Educators should be encouraged to engage in both individual and collective reflection, whether through teaching journals, peer observation, or scholarship of teaching and learning (SoTL) projects.

Critical reflection might include:

- Evaluating student engagement and emotional responses in immersive simulations
- Reflecting on how inclusivity and accessibility were supported in digital environments
- Identifying gaps between simulation and clinical placement experiences
- Considering ethical dilemmas that arise in AI-supported learning

These reflections can feed into programme enhancement, educator CPD, and institutional policy.

EVALUATING IMMERSIVE TECHNOLOGY IN EDUCATION

Evaluation should be embedded at all stages of immersive technology use, from pilot testing to routine delivery. While student satisfaction data is helpful, deeper evaluation considers the impact on learning outcomes, skill development, digital confidence, and preparedness for practice.

Useful methods include:

- Pre/post intervention surveys
- Competency tracking dashboards
- Student focus groups
- Educator reflective reports
- Practice partner feedback on student readiness

Mixed-method approaches are particularly useful for capturing both measurable outcomes and the qualitative richness of immersive learning (Foronda et al., 2020).

Educators undertaking PGCAP or formal academic development can also use these evaluations to build case studies, submit for Advance HE fellowship recognition, or contribute to practice-based research outputs.

LOOKING AHEAD: THE FUTURE OF IMMERSIVE EDUCATION

The next phase of digital transformation in nurse education will likely include:

- Increased personalisation through adaptive learning pathways and AI

- Cross-institutional collaboration using shared simulation repositories

- Enhanced student co-design, especially in scenario development and assessment

- Greater integration of global health and sustainability themes into immersive learning

- Expansion of immersive technologies into community and primary care scenarios, not just acute settings

- Future directions are also likely to see the development of cross-institutional simulation repositories, greater emphasis on student co-design of scenarios and assessments, and the integration of sustainability and global health themes into immersive curricula.

Educators will play a pivotal role in leading these developments, advocating for ethical, inclusive, and learner-centred uses of technology. Those involved in academic practice development are ideally placed to model critical engagement, publish educational research, and influence national and institutional strategies.

CONCLUSION

Digital and immersive technologies are now a central feature of nursing education. Simulation, virtual practice environments, AI, AR, and 360-degree video each provide opportunities to extend traditional learning, strengthen clinical reasoning, and support professional identity formation in safe and structured ways.

The evidence shows that when these approaches are designed with clear pedagogical intent, mapped to professional standards, and supported through facilitation and debriefing, they can offer learning experiences comparable to traditional practice placements. They also contribute to addressing capacity pressures and widening access to complex scenarios that may be difficult to encounter in clinical settings.

Challenges remain, including variation in resources, the need for faculty development, and ongoing debates about fidelity, assessment, and equity of access. Successful integration requires alignment with NMC standards, collaboration with simulation networks, and institutional investment in digital infrastructure.

Looking ahead, immersive technologies should not be seen as a replacement for practice learning, but as a complementary set of tools that enrich curricula and prepare students for the realities of a digitally enabled healthcare system. Nurse educators play a crucial role in ensuring that their use remains person centred, evidence informed, and grounded in the principles of safe and effective practice.

TAKE-HOME POINTS

1. Immersive technologies like VR, AR, and AI offer powerful opportunities to enhance experiential learning, clinical reasoning, and student engagement, but must be underpinned by strong pedagogy and critical reflection.

2. Digital transformation should be embedded across curricula, aligning with regulatory standards, professional values, and workforce expectations.

3. Nurse educators are not passive adopters of technology but strategic leaders who shape the future of healthcare education through co-design, scholarship, and reflective teaching.

CPD REFLECTIVE QUESTIONS

1. How do you currently use digital or immersive tools in your teaching, and how could these be more closely aligned with learning outcomes or NMC proficiencies?

2. What steps could you take to embed co-design and student voice in the development of simulation or immersive activities within your programme or module?

3. In what ways can you contribute to the wider conversation on digital transformation in nurse education, through publication, presentation, or institutional leadership?

REFERENCES

Azher, S., Cervantes, A., Marchionni, C., Grewal, K., Marchand, H., & Harley, J. M. (2023). Virtual simulation in nursing education: headset virtual reality and screen-based virtual simulation offer a comparable experience. *Clinical Simulation in Nursing*, 79, 61–74. https://doi.org/10.1016/j.ecns.2023.02.009.

Blease, C., Kaptchuk, T. J., Bernstein, M. H., Mandl, K. D., Halamka, J. D., & DesRoches, C. M. (2020). Artificial intelligence and the future of primary care: exploratory qualitative study of UK general practitioners' views. *Journal of Medical Internet Research*, 22(3), e12802. https://doi.org/10.2196/12802.

Bovill, C., Cook-Sather, A., & Felten, P. (2011). Students as co-creators of teaching approaches, course design, and curricula: implications for academic developers. *International Journal for Academic Development*, 16(2), 133–145. https://doi.org/10.1080/1360144X.2011.568690.

Cant, R. P., & Cooper, S. J. (2017). Simulation in the internet age: the place of web-based simulation in nursing education. An integrative review. *Nurse Education Today*, 49, 63–71.

Deci, E. L., & Ryan, R. M. (1985). *Intrinsic Motivation and Self-determination in Human Behavior*. Springer. https://doi.org/10.1007/978-1-4899-2271-7.

Deterding, S., Dixon, D., Khaled, R., & Nacke, L. (2011). From game design elements to gamefulness: defining "gamification." *Proceedings of the 15th International Academic MindTrek Conference* (pp. 9–15). ACM.

Dieckmann, P., Gaba, D., & Rall, M. (2020). Deepening the theoretical foundations of patient simulation as social practice. *Simulation in Healthcare*, 12(3), 183–193.

Foronda, C., Fernandez-Burgos, M., Nadeau, C., Kelley, C. N., & Henry, M. N. (2020). Virtual simulation in nursing education: a systematic review spanning 1996 to 2018. *Simulation in Healthcare*, 15(1), 46–54. https://doi.org/10.1097/SIH.0000000000000411.

Health Education England (2021). *Digital capabilities framework*. London: Health Education England. https://digital-transformation.hee.nhs.uk/binaries/content/assets/digital-transformation/nhs-digital-academy/digital-literacy-capability-framework-2018.pdf. Accessed: (9 December 2025).

Hill, B., & Mitchell, A. (2024). Virtual placements in nursing education. *British Journal of Nursing*, 33(12). https://doi.org/10.12968/bjon.2024.0183.

INACSL Standards Committee (2021). INACSL standards of best practice: simulation design. *Clinical Simulation in Nursing*, 58, 1–8.

Koivisto, J., Haavisto, E., Niemi, H., Katajisto, J., & Multisilta, J. (2018). Elements explaining learning outcomes in health care simulation games: case: a simulation game for teaching interpersonal communication and empathy. *Nurse Education Today*, 62, 90–96.

Koivisto, J. M., Multisilta, J., Niemi, H., Katajisto, J., & Eriksson, E. (2016). Learning by playing: a cross-sectional descriptive study of nursing students' experiences of learning clinical reasoning. *Nurse Education Today*, 45, 22–28. https://doi.org/10.1016/j.nedt.2016.06.009.

McGaghie, W. C., Issenberg, S. B., Petrusa, E. R., & Scalese, R. J. (2010). A critical review of simulation-based medical education research: 2003–2009. *Medical Education*, 44(1), 50–63.

NHS England (2023). *NHS long term workforce plan*. https://www.england.nhs.uk/publication/nhs-long-term-workforce-plan/. Accessed: (9 December 2025).

NHS England (2024). *Definitions of simulation and immersive technologies*. Simulation and Immersive Technologies Team. https://www.england.nhs.uk/ourwork/innovation/

Nursing and Midwifery Council (2018). *Future nurse: standards of proficiency for registered nurses*. https://www.nmc.org.uk/standards/standards-for-nurses/future-nurse-standards/. Accessed: (9 December 2025).

Padilha, J. M., Machado, P. P., Ribeiro, A., Ramos, J., & Costa, P. (2019). Clinical virtual simulation in nursing education: randomized controlled trial. *Journal of Medical Internet Research*, 21(3), e11529. https://doi.org/10.2196/11529.

Park, L. J., Ford, C., & Melling, A. C. (2024). Using virtual reality to teach nursing students communication skills when breaking bad news: a focus group exploration of participant experiences. *Journal of Applied Learning and Teaching*, 6(S1), 1–10. https://doi.org/10.37074/jalt.2023.6.S1.16.

Sweller, J., Ayres, P., & Kalyuga, S. (2011). *Cognitive Load Theory*. Springer.

Topol, E. (2019). *Deep Medicine: How Artificial Intelligence Can Make Healthcare Human Again*. Basic Books.

Watermeyer, R., Crick, T., Knight, C., & Goodall, J. (2021). COVID-19 and digital disruption in UK universities: afflictions and affordances of emergency online migration. *Higher Education*, 81, 623–641. https://doi.org/10.1007/s10734-020-00561-y.

Embedding Global Health Perspectives in Nursing Education

CHAPTER 8

Jacqui Bolton

Florence Nightingale Faculty of Nursing, Midwifery and Palliative Care, Department of Adult Nursing, King's College London, UK

AIM

This chapter aims to explore how global health perspectives can be embedded within nursing education through inclusive, culturally responsive, and innovative teaching approaches. The Virtual International Elective (VIE) is used as a central case study to show how digital learning can support equity, strengthen cultural competence, and build global insight.

LEARNING OUTCOMES

After engaging with this chapter, readers will be able to:

1. Explain the importance of global health perspectives in nursing education and practice.

2. Identify approaches for developing cultural competence and global awareness without international travel.

3. Evaluate the role of digital innovation and virtual electives in widening participation and promoting equity.

4. Reflect on the transferable skills gained through immersive global health education experiences.

INTRODUCTION

Global health is increasingly recognised as a core component of nursing education, reflecting the interconnectedness of health systems, populations, and policy challenges worldwide. This chapter explores definitions and frameworks of global health, its relevance to nursing curricula, and practical strategies for embedding it through both theoretical and experiential learning. Central to the discussion is the case study of the Virtual International Elective (VIE), developed during the COVID-19 pandemic and subsequently recognised for its innovative, inclusive approach.

For nurse academics undertaking a Postgraduate Certificate in Academic Practice (PGCAP), the discussion is situated within the broader purpose of transformative

education. Embedding global health perspectives involves more than introducing new content; it requires designing learning experiences that challenge assumptions, foster critical reflection, and prepare students to engage ethically with a complex and diverse world. The VIE illustrates how digital innovation, inclusivity, and collaboration can be harnessed to enhance transformative learning.

In addition, this chapter reflects on wider themes of sustainability, digital pedagogy, and the ethical dimensions of international educational collaboration. The lessons drawn from the VIE are transferable across a range of nursing education contexts and contribute to the preparation of nurses as globally informed practitioners.

Transformative Nursing Education, First Edition. Edited by Aby Mitchell and Barry Hill.

WHAT DO WE MEAN BY A GLOBAL HEALTH PERSPECTIVE?

There is broad agreement on the importance of embedding global health perspectives within undergraduate nursing curricula (Clark et al., 2016; Dawson et al., 2016). However, there is less consensus on what is meant by the term *global health*. A systematic review by Salm et al. (2021) highlighted the variety of definitions proposed between 2009 and 2019, concluding that no single definition dominates, and that the meaning often depends on the agenda of the institution or author adopting it.

One of the most widely cited definitions is offered by Koplan et al. (2009), who describe global health as *'an area of study, research, and practice that places a priority on improving health and achieving equity in health for all people worldwide'* (p. 1995). This emphasis on health equity provides a useful starting point for nursing education.

However, to determine what a global health perspective should incorporate, it is helpful to consider how the field has developed more recently.

Emerging frameworks such as planetary health, health justice, and the decolonisation of global health education have shifted attention towards the structural and environmental factors that shape health outcomes (Salm et al., 2021). These perspectives challenge traditional power dynamics in global partnerships and highlight the importance of sustainability, mutual learning, and ethical co-production of knowledge. Embedding these critical perspectives within nurse education enables students to examine not only health inequalities but also the global systems and structures that reproduce them.

KEY ELEMENTS OF A GLOBAL HEALTH PERSPECTIVE

Just as there is no single agreed definition of global health, there is also little consensus on what it should encompass within nursing education. Clark et al.'s (2016) systematic review in *Nurse Education Today* examined 25 studies to identify core competencies in global health for nurses. From this work, 12 competencies were outlined, ranging from understanding global disease burdens to developing skills in cultural competence and advocacy.

Importantly, global health education should not only reflect institutional or professional priorities but also take into account the student perspective. Students frequently identify the need for practical, relevant insights that connect global challenges with local practice. Embedding global health into curricula should therefore balance theoretical knowledge with opportunities for applied learning, ensuring that competencies translate into practice.

GLOBAL HEALTH POLICY CONTEXT

The embedding of global health perspectives in nurse education is not only a pedagogical choice but also a response to the wider policy environment that shapes healthcare practice and professional development. International and national policy frameworks emphasise the importance of preparing nurses to respond to diverse populations, health inequalities, and transnational challenges such as pandemics and climate change. Understanding this policy context provides an essential rationale for innovations such as the Virtual International Elective (VIE) and highlights why global health content should be considered a core component of the nursing curriculum rather than an optional supplement.

WORLD HEALTH ORGANIZATION

The World Health Organization (WHO) plays a central role in setting global priorities for nursing and health education. The *Global Strategic Directions for Nursing and Midwifery 2021–2025* (WHO, 2021) identifies four key areas for action: education, jobs, leadership, and service delivery. The report emphasises that nurses are critical to achieving Universal Health Coverage (UHC) and the Sustainable Development Goals, and it calls on countries to strengthen nursing education to meet both local and global health demands. A strong emphasis is placed on preparing nurses to lead, influence policy, and contribute to international health systems. This framework situates nurse education firmly within a global agenda, positioning students not just as future practitioners but also as potential leaders in health improvement worldwide.

UNITED NATIONS SUSTAINABLE DEVELOPMENT GOALS

The United Nations Sustainable Development Goals (SDGs; United Nations, 2015) provide another influential backdrop. While SDG 3 focuses specifically on ensuring healthy lives and promoting wellbeing, other goals are closely interlinked with health outcomes. For example, SDG 4 (quality education) underpins the delivery of equitable healthcare, while SDG 5 (gender equality) and SDG 10 (reduced inequalities) connect directly to social determinants of health. SDG 13 (climate action) also underscores the need for health professionals to address the impacts of environmental change on health. For nursing education, this interconnected agenda highlights the need to prepare students for complex, interrelated global health challenges that extend beyond clinical expertise to include advocacy, systems thinking, and sustainability.

INTERNATIONAL COUNCIL OF NURSES

The International Council of Nurses (ICN) further reinforces the global mandate for nursing engagement in health leadership and education. Its policy statements emphasise the nurse's role in advancing health equity, tackling workforce shortages, and contributing to international health priorities (International Council of Nurses, 2021a). The ICN has consistently highlighted the importance of cultural competence, ethical practice, and advocacy for vulnerable populations, stressing that these must be embedded within curricula. By promoting international collaboration and professional solidarity, the ICN provides an important platform through which nurses can shape global health agendas. Its calls for investment in education and leadership development echo directly into the work of higher education institutions, training the future workforce.

UK POLICY CONTEXT

In the UK, national policy drivers align closely with these international agendas. The *Future Nurse: Standards of Proficiency for Registered Nurses* (NMC, 2018) emphasises holistic, person-centred care, cultural competence, and preparedness to work with diverse populations. The Nursing and Midwifery Council highlights the importance of critical reflection and responsiveness to wider determinants of health, ensuring that newly qualified nurses are equipped to practise in an increasingly interconnected world.

At a strategic level, the NHS has also demonstrated commitment to global health through initiatives such as the NHS Global Health Exchange and international fellowship programmes. These schemes highlight the value placed on cross-border collaboration and the reciprocal learning that arises from sharing expertise internationally. The Department of Health and Social Care has further acknowledged the need for sustainable global partnerships, recognising that global health priorities, whether migration, pandemics, or climate change, have direct consequences for UK health services and must therefore be reflected in professional training.

Consequently, the current policy landscape demonstrates that global health education is a professional and ethical necessity. Nurses are increasingly called upon to understand health challenges beyond national borders, to practise with cultural competence, and to contribute to the achievement of global goals for health and equity. Embedding global health perspectives within curricula is therefore not a matter of choice but of alignment with international and national mandates. In this context, initiatives such as the VIE represent not only innovative pedagogical practice but also a direct response to policy imperatives. The following section explores the theoretical underpinnings that inform how such approaches can be effectively delivered in.

THEORETICAL FOUNDATIONS OF GLOBAL HEALTH EDUCATION

Embedding global health perspectives into nursing curricula benefits from being grounded in established educational theory. For nurse academics undertaking a Postgraduate Certificate in Academic Practice (PGCAP), these frameworks help explain not only *why* such initiatives matter but also *how* they support transformative teaching and learning.

TRANSFORMATIVE LEARNING THEORY

Mezirow's (1991) theory of transformative learning is particularly relevant. It emphasises how learners undergo deep shifts in perspective through critical reflection and exposure to new or challenging experiences. The Virtual International Elective (VIE), by presenting students with diverse health systems, cultural practices, and ethical dilemmas, creates opportunities for them to reassess assumptions and develop a more global outlook. Structured activities such as travel logs, book clubs, and debriefs are deliberately designed to foster this kind of perspective transformation.

EXPERIENTIAL LEARNING THEORY

Kolb's (1984) experiential learning cycle offers another valuable lens. His model identifies four stages: concrete experience, reflective observation, abstract conceptualisation, and active experimentation. The design of the VIE aligns closely with this process. Students engage in virtual placements (experience), reflect through group discussions and travel logs (observation), explore wider issues via reading and film discussions (conceptualisation), and apply insights in clinical practice or subsequent sessions (experimentation).

CULTURAL COMPETENCE MODELS

Developing cultural competence is central to global health education. Campinha-Bacote's (2002) model identifies five interrelated constructs: cultural awareness, knowledge, skill, encounters, and desire. The VIE facilitates each of these, offering structured exposure to different healthcare practices while encouraging students to reflect on their own biases and assumptions.

GLOBAL CITIZENSHIP EDUCATION

UNESCO's (2015) framework for global citizenship education underpins the VIE's focus on inclusion, equity, and sustainability. By positioning students as members of a global community, it promotes solidarity, empathy, and collective responsibility. The accessible, non-travel format of the VIE exemplifies this, enabling participation from students who may otherwise face financial or logistical barriers.

CRITICAL PEDAGOGY

Finally, Freire's (1970) critical pedagogy highlights the importance of dialogue, co-creation, and shared power in education. Rather than positioning international partners as passive recipients of Western knowledge, the VIE fosters horizontal exchange in which all participants are both learners and teachers. This approach helps to resist reproducing colonial dynamics within global health education.

Together, these theoretical perspectives provide a robust rationale for embedding global health into nursing curricula. They offer a shared vocabulary for academics designing curricula and demonstrate how digital innovation, cultural competence, and critical reflection can combine to create transformative educational experiences.

APPLYING LEARNING FRAMEWORKS TO THE VIRTUAL INTERNATIONAL ELECTIVE

The value of learning theories lies in their application. Within the Virtual International Elective (VIE), principles from Kolb, Mezirow, Campinha-Bacote, and Freire were not only consciously embedded in the design but also emerged naturally during delivery. Together, they created a rich and authentic learning environment.

KOLB'S EXPERIENTIAL LEARNING CYCLE

Kolb's (1984) model was evident in the sequential stages of the VIE. Students' *concrete experience* came not from staged simulations but from authentic interactions with international peers. Participation in cross-continental group work required adapting communication styles, collaborating on unfamiliar problems, and managing challenges such as unstable internet connections. Structured debriefs provided opportunities for *reflective observation*, enabling students to consider what had surprised them and how cultural contexts shaped decision making. This was followed by *abstract conceptualisation*, where learners linked reflections to theoretical models such as teamwork frameworks, global health inequalities, or patient safety principles. Finally, *active experimentation* occurred when students applied these insights in later sessions or clinical placements, for example, by consciously adapting communication styles or checking cultural appropriateness before making decisions.

MEZIROW'S TRANSFORMATIVE LEARNING

Mezirow's (1991) theory came to life when students encountered 'disorienting dilemmas'. Many UK participants initially assumed that local practice represented a global gold standard.

When exposed to innovative approaches in low-resource settings, this view was challenged, while international students were often surprised by bureaucratic barriers in the UK. Facilitated reflection helped students critically reassess assumptions, leading to evidence of perspective transformation. Post-session reflections frequently included references to a growing sense of global citizenship and a redefined professional identity.

CAMPINHA-BACOTE'S MODEL OF CULTURAL COMPETENCE

The VIE also demonstrated the dynamic, ongoing process described in Campinha-Bacote's (2002) model. Students developed *awareness* by identifying their own biases, gained *knowledge* from exposure to diverse practices, and built *skills* through cross-cultural communication. The authentic *encounters* were particularly powerful, encouraging meaningful dialogue with peers from different contexts. Most significantly, the programme nurtured *cultural desire* by fostering curiosity, respect, and willingness to engage across difference.

FREIRE'S CRITICAL PEDAGOGY

Finally, the VIE reflected Freire's (1970) emphasis on dialogue and reciprocity. Learning was positioned as a shared endeavour: participants explored case studies, challenged assumptions, and co-created solutions. International peers were valued as equal partners, not as case examples or passive recipients of knowledge. Evaluations reinforced this approach, with students describing the experience as 'learning with, rather than about, others'.

SUMMARY

Taken together, these frameworks show that the VIE was more than an innovative teaching activity. It functioned as a living example of multiple educational theories in action, blending experiential processes, transformative reflection, cultural competence, and critical pedagogy. This convergence provided a powerful model of how theory-informed curriculum design can enhance student learning in global health.

WHY EMBED GLOBAL HEALTH IN NURSING CURRICULA?

Calls to reshape health professional education in response to an increasingly globalised world have been consistent for more than a decade. Richardson et al. (2017) argued that the content, context, and conditions of education must adapt to prepare nurses for interconnected health challenges. The United Nations' Sustainable Development Goals (SDGs) (2015) reinforced this agenda by recognising the shared responsibility of all nations in addressing health inequalities.

Despite this, global health is sometimes still viewed as a niche area relevant only to those planning to work overseas. Recent epidemics and pandemics, including Ebola and COVID-19, have shown this to be a narrow perspective (Boulton, 2015; CDC, 2020). The phrase 'no one is safe until everyone is safe' captured how local health challenges quickly become global threats.

Embedding global health into nursing curricula enables students to understand the social, cultural, and structural factors shaping health outcomes. This is particularly relevant in the UK, where increasingly diverse populations require nurses to provide culturally safe and person-centred care.

Global health perspectives also align with regulatory and quality benchmarks. The Nursing and Midwifery Council's *Future Nurse: Standards of Proficiency* (2018) highlights cultural competence, leadership, and public health, while the Quality Assurance Agency benchmarks call for graduates to engage with international perspectives and health inequalities. Including global health content, therefore, supports compliance while strengthening preparedness for contemporary practice.

EMBEDDING GLOBAL CITIZENSHIP IN NURSING EDUCATION

Global citizenship reflects an awareness of interconnectedness across cultures, nations, and communities, alongside a commitment to contribute to a more equitable and sustainable world. In nursing education, this aligns closely with the Nursing and Midwifery Council's (2018) standards, which emphasise equality, human rights, and culturally safe practice.

Introducing global citizenship can begin with foundational discussions on health equity, climate justice, and the social determinants of health. These discussions are most effective when situated in real-world scenarios. For example, students might explore how the health of asylum seekers in the UK illustrates wider global injustices, or how climate change contributes to health inequalities in both high- and low-income countries.

Active pedagogies help embed these principles. Structured debates, ethical dilemmas, and role play allow students to reflect on their responsibilities as nurses within a global society. Placement preparation can also incorporate global citizenship, encouraging students to consider their roles within diverse communities and their responses to moral dilemmas involving privilege, access, or sustainability.

Crucially, global citizenship does not depend on international travel. Rather, it encourages students to act locally with global awareness. This approach fosters an ethical mindset and strengthens cultural competence, enabling nurses to provide inclusive, person-centred care across all healthcare settings.

APPROACHES TO EMBEDDING GLOBAL HEALTH IN NURSING CURRICULA

THEORETICAL PERSPECTIVES

Embedding global health requires a solid theoretical foundation. Core concepts can be delivered through stand-alone modules or embedded as a 'golden thread' across the programme. Whichever approach is chosen, the aim should be to ensure that global health learning fosters lifelong skills, enabling students to provide culturally competent, person-centred care in increasingly diverse societies.

ELECTIVES AND EXCHANGES

Experiential learning is a powerful way of deepening global health understanding. International electives and exchanges have traditionally enabled nursing students to work alongside healthcare professionals in other contexts, offering first-hand exposure to the social, cultural, and organisational factors shaping practice. Such placements often lead to lasting insights into health inequalities and the development of cultural competence (McInally et al., 2015; Sims, 2016).

Between 2015 and 2023, the author coordinated electives and exchanges for undergraduate nursing and midwifery students at King's College London (KCL). These experiences demonstrated the value of immersion in diverse healthcare environments, but they also highlighted the challenges of access. Opportunities were often constrained by governance processes, funding, institutional contacts, and, ultimately, student circumstances.

The COVID-19 pandemic brought these issues into sharp focus. In March 2020, 84 KCL students were preparing for one-month international electives when border closures and lockdowns forced cancellation. A two-week summer school, developed in partnership with Manipal Academy of Higher Education (MAHE) through UKIERI funding, was also postponed. Students expressed profound disappointment, not only because of financial loss but also because of missed opportunities for professional and personal growth.

These circumstances created the conditions for innovation. With in-person electives no longer feasible, new approaches were needed to ensure students could continue to benefit from global perspectives. Out of this necessity, the concept of a Virtual International Elective (VIE) began to take shape.

CASE STUDY: AROUND THE WORLD IN SIX WHO REGIONS

BACKGROUND

Plato's maxim that 'necessity is the mother of invention' (Plato, 2000) captures the origins of the Virtual International Elective (VIE). The COVID-19 pandemic disrupted education and healthcare worldwide, halting international travel and placements. At King's College London (KCL), 84 students preparing for one-month electives saw their plans cancelled in March 2020, just days before departure. Summer schools and reciprocal exchanges were also postponed indefinitely.

As disappointment grew among students, and with future electives looking increasingly uncertain, the idea of a virtual elective began to emerge. At first dismissed as unrealistic, the concept gained traction as colleagues pooled international contacts, explored digital platforms, and considered how core aims of an elective—immersion, cultural learning, and critical reflection—might be replicated online. Out of these discussions, the VIE model was developed.

ADAPTING AIMS AND OBJECTIVES

The VIE was designed to mirror the aims of in-person electives while adapting them for a virtual environment. Key objectives included

- providing opportunities to experience nursing and midwifery in different cultural and organisational contexts

- fostering critical thinking about global challenges and healthcare systems

- developing cultural competence that could be applied in practice

- creating a cohesive, supportive community of learners during a time of isolation

Two additional aims were shaped by the pandemic context: to maintain educational standards despite reduced placement capacity, and to support students who were unable to continue in practice due to co-morbidities, caring responsibilities, or bereavement.

DEVELOPING A STRUCTURE

The VIE was scheduled for four weeks in March, aligning with the existing placement calendar. Its structure was based on the six WHO regions (WHO, 2025). Students travelled virtually, making sequential visits to partner institutions, healthcare professionals, and researchers across 20 countries.

The selection of host countries was guided by existing faculty and institutional partnerships. Each host was asked to identify one or two key challenges in their healthcare system and to share innovative approaches to addressing them. Importantly, hosts retained control over the style and format of their sessions, ensuring cultural authenticity.

PARTICIPANT SELECTION

Eligible participants included undergraduate nursing students from adult, child, and mental health branches at KCL whose electives had been cancelled. Interested students were invited to apply by submitting a short rationale for their participation. This process reinforced the expectation that engagement would be active and sustained.

CONTENT AND DELIVERY

The VIE combined synchronous and asynchronous learning to equate to 150 practice hours. Synchronous sessions included interactive visits with international hosts, live

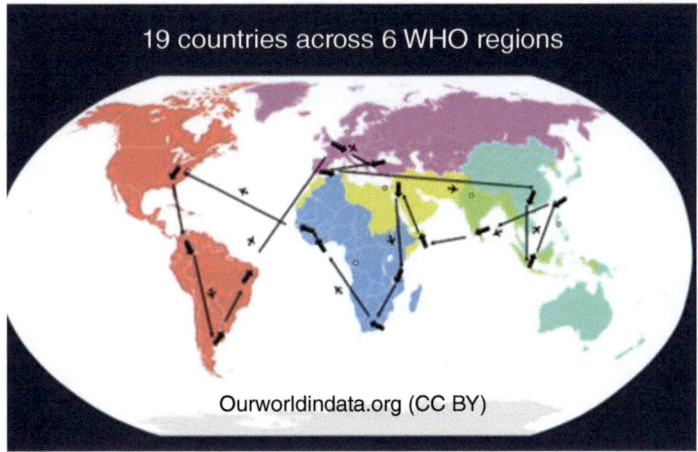

FIGURE 8.1 'Where did we travel?' *Source:* Adapted from Our World in Data (2021)

presentations, and group discussions. These totalled 68 hours. To support deeper learning, additional activities included pre-visit research tasks, quizzes, reflective travel logs, book and film clubs, and group projects.

Students began their journey in the UK, preparing by reviewing WHO resources and reflecting on their expectations. Over the next four weeks, they travelled virtually through Europe, the Western Pacific, the Eastern Mediterranean, South-East Asia, Africa, and the Americas. Encounters ranged from formal presentations in India to student-produced films in Colombia, with unplanned interruptions, such as power cuts in Sudan, reinforcing the sense of 'being there'.

The sequence of visits is illustrated in Figure 8.1, which maps the 20 host countries visited across the six WHO regions. This visual representation helped students situate each session geographically and reinforced the sense of global scope.

Time zone differences posed challenges, requiring careful scheduling and occasional last-minute adjustments. For example, one visit to the United States had to be rescheduled after an error in calculating time differences. These moments reinforced the need for flexibility, mirroring the unpredictability of in-person electives.

IMPLEMENTING THE OBJECTIVES AND CREATING A SENSE OF 'BEING THERE'

A central aim of the VIE was to replicate the immersive quality of an international placement by fostering a genuine sense of 'being there'. Achieving this required careful design of both the learning activities and the language used throughout the programme.

SYNCHRONISED EXPERIENCES

Synchronous participation was essential for creating immediacy and authenticity. The unpredictability of real-world conditions reinforced this. For example, students experienced a power cut during a session in Sudan and an earthquake tremor during a visit to Greece. While disruptive, such incidents enhanced the realism of the experience and prompted reflection on resilience and resourcefulness in different healthcare contexts.

LANGUAGE AND COMMUNICATION

The sense of travel was further supported through the way communications were framed. Emails and timetables were styled as travel itineraries, and updates were written as if students were journeying together. This narrative approach strengthened engagement and helped sustain motivation over the four-week period.

CULTURAL EXPRESSION AND DIVERSITY

Hosts were encouraged to present sessions in a manner that reflected their own cultural practices. In India, this resulted in a formal programme with a master of ceremonies, pre-set questions, and structured timings, while in Colombia, students created short films showcasing aspects of nursing and local culture. These contrasting styles not only enhanced

Table 8.1   Examples of Student Feedback on the VIE Experience

Adapting communications to embed a sense of "being there"
Welcome to the VIE! I look forward to meeting you in the departure lounge prior to check-in at 10 am. Please do not be late, or you will miss your flight!
After a fascinating day learning about the role of saunas in Finnish healthcare, and exploring one of the models used for a Syrian refugee camp in Greece, we will be travelling overnight to China.
I hope you had a lovely weekend and a safe flight into the Eastern Mediterranean region.
Good evening, fellow travellers! I hope you have all kept well over the weekend and have had the opportunity to explore the South-East Asia region further. Tomorrow we transfer to Nepal for the final visit of this week. The travel log for Week 3 has now been posted, so please make sure you 'know before you go'. We will then travel overnight to the WHO Africa region, arriving in Tanzania.
Good morning! I hope you had a smooth journey across to the USA and perhaps even found some time for a little sightseeing over the weekend.
As we make our way back to the UK and prepare to go into quarantine, it is time to reflect on our momentous journey over the last month. Many of you have expressed envy at the ceremonies enjoyed by students in other faculties we have visited. We will therefore finish with our own closing ceremony (with thanks to a video from Hospital Británico, Argentina), followed by a virtual drinks and nibbles reception. Now sit back and enjoy the last leg of your journey.

cultural insight but also reminded participants that there is no single 'correct' way to share knowledge.

STUDENT REFLECTIONS

Student feedback indicated that these design features were successful in generating immersion. Many participants commented that, despite being online, the experience felt like 'real travel' and created lasting impressions. Examples of this feedback are presented in Table 8.1, which illustrates how students perceived the value of the VIE in enhancing their cultural awareness and professional growth.

ENHANCING CULTURAL COMPETENCE

Developing cultural competence was a core objective of the VIE. To support this, each host partner was encouraged to design and deliver their session in a culturally authentic way. While pre-session discussions provided a framework, facilitators avoided imposing a standardised format. This allowed students to experience genuine diversity in communication styles, teaching methods, and cultural expression.

CONTRASTING APPROACHES

The contrasts between sessions illustrated the importance of cultural context. In India, the programme was carefully choreographed, with a master of ceremonies, formal introductions, pre-set questions, and structured timings, ending with a vote of thanks. By contrast, hosts in Colombia gave their students ownership of the session, producing short films about nursing and local culture and sharing a colourful welcome flyer. These very different approaches emphasised that no single teaching style is 'correct' and that professional practice is always embedded within culture.

LANGUAGE AND COMMUNICATION

Language also provided opportunities for cultural learning. While most sessions were conducted in English, the visit to Argentina was delivered in Spanish. Rather than pre-translating the materials, a bilingual colleague provided live translation in the chat and later produced a transcript. This encouraged participants to attend closely to non-verbal cues—such as tone, gesture, and expression—reinforcing the importance of communication beyond words.

HUMOUR AND MISUNDERSTANDING

Cultural differences also became apparent through language. During a session in Ghana, the carbohydrate-rich staple food *fufu* was discussed in relation to diabetes. In an earlier visit to Nepal, however, students had learned that *fufu* (फुफु) means 'aunt' in Nepali. This prompted one participant to joke about 'not eating your aunt', a light-hearted moment that reinforced the need for sensitivity when navigating cross-cultural dialogue.

Table 8.2   Student Reflections on Developing Cultural Competence

Key learning point	Student reflection
Importance of cultural context	*'I have learned that it is important to understand the cultural context in which the patient views their condition and treatments'.*
Asking questions	*'It is important to have the courage to ask questions when there is a lack of understanding or clarity as a health provider'.*
Person-centred care	*'We cannot expect to know everything about every culture, but being person-centred means making the effort to understand our patients' cultural viewpoints'.*
Avoiding assumptions	*'Never assume, generalise, or stereotype'.*

STUDENT REFLECTION

At the mid-point interview, students reflected on the different approaches they had experienced and the cultural insights these provided. Evaluations carried out through online polling and interactive whiteboards highlighted the impact of these encounters. Students consistently described the programme as a 'unique opportunity' to gain first-hand cultural insight, creating lasting impressions and lessons for lifelong learning.

As part of this process, students were also asked to consider what they had learned so far that had improved their cultural competence. Their reflections captured both the challenges and responsibilities of person-centred care in diverse contexts. Key themes are shown in Table 8.2, which highlights the importance of cultural context, curiosity, person-centred practice, and avoiding stereotypes.

CEREMONY AND MEANING

The significance of ceremony in different cultures also left a strong impression. Inspired by international examples, the VIE concluded with a closing ceremony that included a video from Hospital Británico, Argentina, showing students carrying lamps in tribute to Florence Nightingale. For many, this prompted a new appreciation of the privilege of studying at the Florence Nightingale Faculty. One student, who had begun her training in India, shared photographs of end-of-year ceremonies where students honoured their lecturers, further reinforcing the value of cultural rituals in education.

ENHANCING THE STUDENT EXPERIENCE THROUGH INNOVATIVE PRACTICE

VERIFYING PRACTICE HOURS

The Nursing and Midwifery Council's (2020) emergency standards, introduced during the COVID-19 pandemic, created greater flexibility in how practice hours could be achieved. This flexibility made it possible to design a 150-hour Virtual International Elective (VIE), offering a vital alternative for students with co-morbidities while easing pressure on practice partners. However, it also raised important questions about maintaining standards, evidencing attendance, and ensuring alignment with learning outcomes.

To address these challenges, a dedicated Practice Assessment Document was created for the VIE. Renamed the *VIE Travel Log* to reinforce the sense of 'being there', it provided a structured record of learning, certified attendance, and demonstrated how objectives had been met. The Travel Log also guided students through the experience, incorporating tasks such as pre-session research, reflective entries, and post-session consolidation.

Monitoring attendance during synchronous sessions was relatively straightforward, but verifying active participation required additional safeguards. To promote accountability, VIE hosts were asked to provide three questions during their sessions, which students were required to answer in their Travel Logs. This not only evidenced engagement but also encouraged focused listening and critical reflection.

All visits were recorded and edited, but recordings were withheld until practice hours had been confirmed. This replicated the accountability of in-person placements, ensuring students engaged in real time. Recordings were later repurposed as teaching resources in other programmes, extending the impact of the VIE beyond its original context.

CREATING A COHESIVE GROUP OF TRAVELLERS

As with in-person electives, the VIE was designed to equate to 150 placement hours. However, spending seven and a half hours a day on Microsoft Teams calls for four consecutive weeks was neither desirable nor realistic. Instead, synchronous visits with the 20 VIE hosts constituted 86 hours of activity. The remaining hours were achieved through carefully designed asynchronous tasks that encouraged independent study, critical reflection, and peer collaboration.

In addition to the pre-visit quizzes and research requirements outlined earlier, innovative approaches were introduced to promote deep learning and strengthen group cohesion. Two new pedagogical strategies were adopted: *learning through film* and a *book club*. All VIE participants were required to take part in both activities.

THE BOOK CLUB

Each student was asked to choose one of four pre-selected books, all written by healthcare professionals with first-hand experience of working in diverse cultural or global contexts. The books were chosen for their ability to convey a strong 'sense of being there' while providing insights into health and healthcare in different environments. On the first day of the VIE, participants were introduced to the book options and asked to indicate their preference. Reading time was built into the elective, and students were encouraged to record six key points from their chosen book, with page references, in their Travel Log.

These notes formed the basis of small-group online discussions, in which three or four students who had read the same book compared their reflections. The discussions were lively, with participants drawing connections between the narratives and the healthcare challenges they were learning about through the VIE. For many, the book club provided a powerful opportunity to link lived experiences from the field with theoretical perspectives.

LEARNING THROUGH FILM

The film strand of the programme complemented the book club. Students were asked to select one of four films, each chosen for its relevance to global health themes and accessibility via university resources. After watching, they wrote a short reflection in their Travel Log. In small-group meetings, each student explained the storyline and key insights from their chosen film, encouraging reciprocal learning across different topics.

This activity proved extremely popular. Students commented that hearing their peers' interpretations of films they had not watched was as valuable as their own viewing. Many highlighted that the combination of books and films deepened their empathy, widened their perspectives, and gave them new ways of engaging with global health issues.

COHESION AND COMMUNITY

Both the book club and film activities contributed significantly to building a sense of camaraderie among participants. Students began to form strong peer connections, often continuing discussions informally after scheduled sessions. For some, the group cohesion became a source of support during an otherwise isolating time in the pandemic. Staff observed that quieter students gained confidence in these smaller, themed discussions, which encouraged more equal participation.

This combination of structured academic tasks and informal peer interaction ensured that the VIE was not experienced simply as a series of online lectures. Instead, it became a shared journey, one that fostered community, encouraged creativity, and enhanced the learning experience for all participants.

STUDENT VOICE AND CO-CREATION IN GLOBAL HEALTH CURRICULUM DESIGN

While student evaluations are well established in most programmes, co-creation goes further by actively involving students in curriculum development. Within global health education, this approach not only enhances relevance but also strengthens engagement and fosters more inclusive learning environments.

MOVING BEYOND EVALUATION

Traditional module evaluations often focus on feedback after delivery, providing staff with useful information for future iterations. Co-creation, however, invites students into the design process itself, positioning them as partners rather than passive recipients. This helps to ensure that global health curricula remain dynamic and responsive to student needs, as well as to evolving global contexts.

EXAMPLES OF CO-CREATION

The VIE demonstrated the value of student involvement in shaping educational experiences. Several activities emerged from student suggestions, including themed discussion groups, peer-led reflective tasks, and the development of virtual 'thank you' gifts for host partners. Looking ahead, there are many opportunities to deepen this model of partnership. Examples might include

- inviting former VIE participants to co-facilitate pre-departure briefings for new cohorts
- creating student-led seminars on global issues of personal or professional interest
- establishing reflective portfolios that feed directly into the ongoing design of modules

BENEFITS OF PARTNERSHIP

Engaging students as co-creators brings multiple benefits. It empowers students to develop leadership and facilitation skills, ensures the curriculum remains relevant and inclusive, and models the collaborative ethos central to global health itself. Co-creation also enhances students' sense of ownership and responsibility for their learning, encouraging deeper reflection and sustained engagement.

ALIGNMENT WITH POLICY

This approach reflects a wider shift in UK higher education, where student-staff partnerships are increasingly recognised as markers of quality and innovation. In global health education, the commitment to reciprocity and inclusivity aligns closely with these policy directions, further strengthening the case for embedding co-creation into programme design.

ADDITIONAL KEY CONSIDERATIONS

Embedding global health perspectives in nursing education requires attention to wider issues that extend beyond curriculum content. The development and delivery of the VIE highlighted several cross-cutting considerations that are central to designing inclusive, sustainable, and effective programmes.

SUSTAINABILITY

No study of global health is complete without reference to the United Nations Sustainable Development Goals (SDGs) (United Nations, 2015). While Goal 3 focuses explicitly on health and well-being, the interconnections across all 17 goals highlight the broader relationship between sustainability and global health outcomes. The VIE engaged directly with these priorities by offering an international learning experience without the environmental impact of air travel. Students described it as a 'once-in-a-lifetime experience' that combined the benefits of international exposure with a sustainable, home-based approach.

EMBRACING TECHNOLOGY

The rapid pivot to online learning during the COVID-19 pandemic exposed both opportunities and challenges for higher education (Watermeyer et al., 2021). For the VIE, platforms such as Microsoft Teams became essential tools for synchronous engagement, breakout discussions, and collaborative whiteboards. Concerns about internet bandwidth, particularly in low-resource contexts such as Sierra Leone and Somalia, were addressed through careful planning and the lower data requirements of Teams compared with other platforms such as Zoom. Technical problems were relatively few, and the chat function quickly developed into a lively peer-support space, with students often helping each other troubleshoot IT difficulties. This not only strengthened group cohesion but also enhanced participants' digital skills.

DIGITAL PEDAGOGIES AND INNOVATION IN GLOBAL HEALTH EDUCATION

While the Virtual International Elective (VIE) highlighted the benefits of mainstream platforms such as Microsoft Teams, the digital landscape in higher education continues to expand rapidly, offering new ways to engage students in global health learning. Digital pedagogy, broadly defined as the critical and creative use of technology to support learning, is increasingly recognised as central to health professions education. Moving beyond the emergency adaptations prompted by the COVID-19 pandemic, educators are now exploring how to integrate digital tools into curricula in a sustainable and pedagogically robust manner.

VIRTUAL AND AUGMENTED REALITY

Immersive technologies such as virtual reality (VR) and augmented reality (AR) are beginning to transform health education. For global health, VR simulations can recreate the experience of working in resource-limited settings, disaster zones, or culturally distinct communities, providing learners with a sense of 'being there' without the need for travel. For example, nursing students might engage in a VR-based maternal health scenario in sub-Saharan Africa, managing obstetric emergencies with limited resources and cultural considerations. These experiences align with experiential learning theory, offering concrete experiences that can be reflected upon and applied in practice. Early research indicates that such simulations enhance empathy, situational awareness, and decision-making skills (Foronda et al., 2020).

MASSIVE OPEN ONLINE COURSES (MOOCS) AND OPEN ACCESS LEARNING

Another area of innovation is the use of MOOCs and open-access learning resources. Platforms such as FutureLearn and Coursera now host global health courses developed by international universities, enabling nursing students to access expertise beyond their own institution. Integrating these into curricula not only broadens students' exposure to global perspectives but also promotes self-directed learning and professional networking. Importantly, many of these resources are free, thereby aligning with commitments to equity and widening participation. The challenge for educators is to scaffold this learning so that it complements, rather than duplicates, core teaching.

ARTIFICIAL INTELLIGENCE AND TRANSLATION TOOLS

The integration of artificial intelligence (AI) into global health education is an emerging frontier. AI-driven translation applications now allow real-time communication across languages, supporting inclusive engagement with international partners. Similarly, AI-powered learning analytics can help educators monitor student progress in large, digitally enabled cohorts, enabling more personalised feedback. Ethical considerations remain significant, particularly around data privacy and equity of access, but AI offers considerable potential for strengthening intercultural dialogue and reflective learning.

SERIOUS GAMES AND GAMIFICATION

Game-based learning approaches, often referred to as 'serious games', are also gaining traction. These use game mechanics such as challenges, rewards, and role-play to engage learners in complex problem-solving. In global health, scenarios might include managing limited resources during a disease outbreak or negotiating health policy in a simulated international forum. Such approaches not only increase motivation and engagement but also provide a safe space for learners to test different strategies and reflect on ethical dilemmas.

OPPORTUNITIES AND CHALLENGES

The expansion of digital pedagogies presents both opportunities and challenges. On the one hand, they offer scalable, sustainable, and engaging ways of embedding global health into nursing curricula. They can reduce costs, widen participation, and enhance intercultural competence by creating interactive and authentic learning opportunities. On the other hand, challenges include digital poverty, variable internet access, and the risk of overemphasising technology at the expense of relational and reflective aspects of learning. Educators must remain alert to these risks, ensuring that technology serves pedagogy rather than driving it.

FUTURE DIRECTIONS

Looking ahead, digital innovation will continue to shape how global health is taught and learned. As universities invest in digital transformation strategies, nurse educators are well placed to experiment with emerging technologies and evaluate their impact on student learning. Partnerships between institutions, including those in low- and middle-income countries, will be vital to ensure that innovations are equitable, culturally appropriate, and contextually relevant. By embracing digital pedagogy critically and creatively, nursing education can move beyond emergency adaptations to establish enduring models of global health learning that are inclusive, sustainable, and transformative.

EQUALITY, DIVERSITY, AND INCLUSION

Equity was one of the VIE's greatest strengths. Traditional international electives are often constrained by financial cost, family responsibilities, health conditions, or lack of overseas contacts. By removing these barriers, the VIE widened participation and enabled students from a range of backgrounds to access global learning. The diversity of King's student population was reflected in the programme, with many participants drawing on their own cultural knowledge to enrich discussions. Several quieter students gained confidence when the group visited countries with which they had personal connections, sharing insights that affirmed both their identity and expertise. Care was also taken to ensure that all resources, including films and books, were freely accessible through the university library or open platforms such as Kanopy, maintaining financial equity across the cohort.

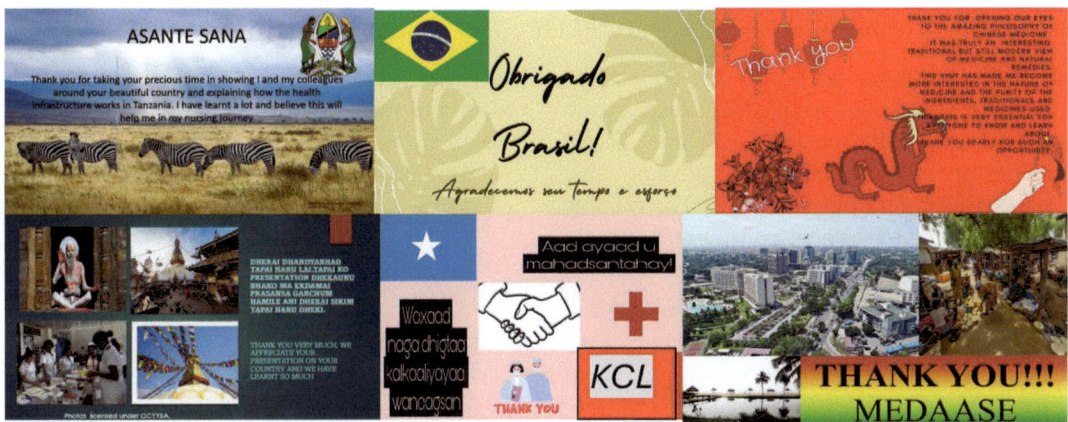

FIGURE 8.2   Tokens of thanks devised by VIE participants and sent to VIE hosts

RECIPROCITY

The principle of reciprocity was central to the VIE. Host partners from 20 countries generously contributed their time and expertise, often in challenging pandemic circumstances. In return, VIE participants created digital 'thank you' gifts, including short films, annotated presentations, creative posters, and postcards designed for each host country. One group produced a video titled *A Day in the Life of a UK Student Nurse*, which was later shared at conferences with their permission. These gestures fostered mutual respect and reinforced the idea of global learning as a two-way exchange. Certificates of contribution were also provided to individual hosts, recognising their role in the elective.

Examples of these tokens of thanks are shown in Figure 8.2, which illustrates the imaginative ways students expressed their appreciation for VIE hosts.

MEETING THE ADAPTED LEARNING AIMS AND OBJECTIVES

Extensive evaluations were carried out using anonymised online platforms. Responses were collated and mapped against the initial aims and objectives that shaped the VIE's development. Without exception, they demonstrated the positive impact of the elective on the overall student experience and confirmed that the intended outcomes were achieved (see Table 8.3). In addition, the VIE enabled students who were unable to continue in practice placements during COVID-19 to be awarded 150 practice hours towards programme completion.

Table 8.3   Student Reported Learning from the Virtual Global Learning Experience

1. Deep learning through contextual immersion: creating a sense of 'being there'

   'Even though the experience was virtual, it felt like real life'.

2. First-hand insight into the challenges experienced by nurses and other healthcare professionals in non-UK settings

   'The stories of nurses and medics across the globe illustrate that, even in the most dire of circumstances, there is always hope'.

3. Development of cultural competence that translates into practice

   (see Figure 8.2)

4. Equality, inclusion, and diversity

   'We would never have been able to afford to travel to 20 different countries and gain all the knowledge we've gained in four weeks'.

5. Learning through innovative practice

   'Character building, mind-expanding, and so much fun! Its transcultural teaching approaches were exciting and engaging'. (STNA judging panel)

6. Creating a cohesive and enjoyable group of fellow travellers

   'This virtual adventure has been fast, action-packed, and fun, generating a warm and lively atmosphere of camaraderie. Each visit has whetted our appetite, enticing us to learn more. We may have reached the end of this trip, but this is just the start of our cultural exploration, in a journey that will be life-long'.

INTERPROFESSIONAL LEARNING IN GLOBAL HEALTH

Global health challenges rarely fall within the boundaries of a single profession. Issues such as infectious disease outbreaks, climate-related health emergencies, and health system inequalities demand collaborative approaches that draw on the expertise of multiple disciplines. For nursing students, engaging in interprofessional learning (IPL) within a global health context provides opportunities to develop the teamwork, communication, and systems-thinking skills that are increasingly essential in contemporary practice.

RATIONALE FOR INTERPROFESSIONAL LEARNING

Interprofessional education (IPE) is defined as students from two or more professions learning about, from, and with each other to enable effective collaboration and improve health outcomes (WHO, 2010). Embedding IPL in global health learning helps students recognise that healthcare is a shared endeavour, where solutions depend on cooperation across professional and cultural boundaries. For example, tackling antimicrobial resistance requires not only nursing and medical expertise but also insights from pharmacy, veterinary science, and public health. Nursing students who experience interprofessional collaboration early in their training are better prepared to advocate for patients in multidisciplinary settings and contribute meaningfully to global initiatives.

EXAMPLES OF INTERPROFESSIONAL GLOBAL HEALTH LEARNING

Several models demonstrate how IPL can be integrated into global health education. In some universities, joint modules bring together students from nursing, medicine, midwifery, and pharmacy to explore global themes such as maternal health or disaster preparedness. Simulation-based IPL has also been used, for example, recreating the response to an Ebola outbreak with students role-playing different professional perspectives. Beyond higher education, international projects frequently require collaboration across professional groups, from humanitarian relief teams to policy forums, illustrating the relevance of interprofessional skills for nurses working in global health contexts.

BARRIERS AND CHALLENGES

Despite its benefits, embedding IPL in curricula is not without challenges. Differences in academic calendars, professional requirements, and assessment strategies can make collaboration between faculties difficult. Professional silos remain entrenched in many institutions, with nursing students often taught separately from peers in medicine or allied health professions. Logistical issues such as time-tabling and resource allocation may also act as barriers.

However, these challenges can be mitigated through careful planning, strong institutional support, and a shared vision of the value of interprofessional learning.

STRATEGIES FOR EFFECTIVE IMPLEMENTATION

To integrate IPL meaningfully into global health education, several strategies can be considered:

- **Shared Case Studies**: Using global health scenarios that cut across professional boundaries encourages students to see problems from multiple perspectives.

- **Joint Simulations**: Interprofessional disaster or outbreak simulations provide authentic opportunities for collaboration and highlight the importance of clear communication and role delineation.

- **Digital Collaboration**: Virtual platforms can connect nursing students with peers from other professions globally, overcoming logistical challenges and broadening perspectives.

- **Facilitated Reflection**: Structured debriefs help students process interprofessional experiences, acknowledge professional stereotypes, and build respect for other disciplines.

BENEFITS FOR NURSING STUDENTS

For nursing students, IPL in global health fosters confidence in communicating across professional hierarchies, enhances appreciation of the nurse's unique contribution, and builds leadership potential. It also develops flexibility and adaptability, qualities that are critical when working in resource-limited or rapidly changing environments. Exposure to interprofessional collaboration during training prepares students for the realities of healthcare delivery, where success depends on partnership rather than isolated expertise.

Consequently, embedding interprofessional learning into global health education aligns with broader policy and workforce priorities. The WHO Framework for Action on Interprofessional Education and Collaborative Practice (2010) identifies IPL as a critical step toward strengthening health systems and improving patient outcomes. Within nursing education, it provides a platform for developing the collaborative mindset needed to address complex global health challenges. By experiencing global health learning alongside other professional groups, nursing students are not only better prepared for future practice but also positioned to take leadership roles in shaping equitable and effective health systems.

LEADERSHIP FOR GLOBAL HEALTH IN NURSING

Nurses are widely recognised as the largest segment of the global healthcare workforce, yet their potential to lead global health initiatives is less frequently realised or addressed within undergraduate education. As highlighted by the World Health Organization (2020) and the International Council of Nurses (2021b), nurses are pivotal to achieving universal health coverage and the Sustainable Development Goals.

Nurses can act as change agents both locally and internationally. Leadership for global health may include policy advocacy, research into cross-border health challenges, and participation in humanitarian response, disaster preparedness, or planetary health initiatives. UK-based examples include nurse participation in NHS Global Fellowships, international placements funded by charitable trusts, and involvement in transnational networks such as the Nightingale Challenge or the Tropical Health and Education Trust (THET).

Incorporating this focus into the nursing curriculum can be achieved through case studies of nurse-led global health projects and facilitated discussions on advocacy and social justice. Assessments might include the development of a position statement on a global health issue or reflective assignments exploring the nurse's role in promoting equity during times of crisis. Embedding leadership for global health within nurse education cultivates confidence, policy literacy, and the professional vision necessary for nurses to act beyond the bedside.

POTENTIAL TO INFLUENCE NURSE EDUCATION

The VIE model demonstrates a pedagogical approach that is both replicable and adaptable for embedding global health perspectives into nursing curricula. While originally designed to replicate the enriching experience of international electives during the pandemic, the model can be tailored to explore cross-cutting approaches across many specialisms. What began as a pragmatic response to necessity has since become a vehicle for lifelong learning that is being embedded into lifelong practice.

The VIE has also showcased international research collaborations, strengthened existing partnerships, and created new connections across faculties worldwide. Participants reported improved IT skills, developed through intensive immersion and mutual support. Collaboration and co-creation deepened, new pedagogies were introduced into the curriculum, and an extensive repository of teaching materials and recordings was collated for use in other modules and programmes.

REFLECTIONS AND DISSEMINATION

This innovative approach was recognised with the Student Nursing Times Award for Teaching Innovation of the Year. It has been endorsed by students, peer reviewers, and collaborating institutions as a significant contribution to developing cultural competence, global insight, and lasting educational benefits. The introduction of novel approaches such as the book and film clubs has proven to be both sustainable and transferable. Beyond embedding cultural competence and global insight, the VIE also alleviated feelings of isolation at the height of the pandemic. Unanticipated benefits included improved IT literacy, widening participation, and strengthened equality, diversity, and inclusion.

The impact of the programme has been widely disseminated, both within the UK and internationally. Presentations and consultancy work have taken place at King's Teaching Excellence Conference (2021), the Philippines Health Conference (2021), the Council of Deans of Healthcare Conference: Innovation (2022), the Royal College of Nursing Conference (2022), the Consortium of Universities for Global Health Conference (2024), Norfolk and Waverley CCG, the University of Surrey, and De Montfort University.

The VIE has also been profiled in internal communications and on the websites of many of the international hosts who made the programme possible. Collaboration remains at the heart of this work, and the continued willingness, generosity, and enthusiasm of partner institutions worldwide have been fundamental to its success.

ETHICAL DIMENSIONS OF GLOBAL HEALTH EDUCATION

Embedding global health perspectives into nursing education is not only a pedagogical or policy choice, but also an ethical responsibility. The way students learn about global health has direct consequences for how they practise as professionals, how they view health inequalities, and how they engage with patients and communities across cultural and national boundaries. A clear focus on ethics helps to ensure that global health education fosters respect, reciprocity, and responsibility rather than reinforcing stereotypes or power imbalances.

EQUITY AND ACCESS

One of the central ethical considerations in global health education is ensuring that all students have fair access to learning opportunities. Traditional overseas electives have often been available only to those who could afford the costs or who did not have caring responsibilities. This raises questions of fairness, since access to international learning should not depend on financial privilege. Programmes such as the VIE demonstrate how digital innovation can widen access, but even here, equity requires attention to issues such as digital poverty, accessibility needs, and time-zone differences when working with international partners.

RECIPROCITY AND PARTNERSHIP

Global health education also raises questions about reciprocity. Too often, international electives have been criticised for a 'parachute' model, where students from high-income countries visit low- or middle-income settings for their own learning benefit, without contributing meaningfully to the host community. Ethical practice requires moving away from one-way knowledge transfer towards genuine partnership and mutual exchange. This includes recognising the expertise of local practitioners, ensuring that students contribute in ways that are valuable to hosts, and maintaining partnerships that are sustainable and respectful.

REPRESENTATION AND CULTURAL SENSITIVITY

Another key dimension is how cultures and communities are represented in teaching materials. There is a risk of perpetuating stereotypes if global health is presented as a story of 'developed' countries helping 'developing' ones. Ethical global health education instead seeks to highlight strengths and innovations from all contexts, encouraging students to see knowledge as diverse and context-dependent. Case studies and examples should be carefully chosen to reflect complexity, avoid deficit narratives, and promote cultural humility.

PROFESSIONAL RESPONSIBILITY

Nursing is built on values of care, advocacy, and respect for human dignity. These values extend beyond local settings into global practice. Embedding ethics into global health education means encouraging students to reflect on their responsibilities not only to individual patients but also to global communities. This includes awareness of environmental sustainability, social justice, and the health impacts of structural inequalities. Reflective activities, such as discussing ethical dilemmas from global case studies, can help students develop the moral reasoning skills needed for professional practice in a globalised world.

ACTIVITY BOX

Think about the nursing session or module you are currently delivering or planning. Begin by identifying the core learning outcomes. Consider how these outcomes relate to healthcare globally, whether through themes of health equity, climate-related health challenges, or the realities of cultural diversity.

The following guiding questions may be used to design an activity or learning moment that embeds global citizenship into your teaching:

- What global health challenge could be included or referenced in your session (for example, antibiotic resistance, maternal health disparities, or pandemic preparedness)?
- How can you encourage students to reflect on their role as global citizens and health advocates?

- Could a diverse patient scenario or international case study be integrated to highlight cultural competence and inclusivity?
- How might you support students to think critically about health inequalities, structural determinants of health, or culturally sensitive care?

This approach does not necessarily require major curriculum redesign. Small adjustments, such as the inclusion of an international case study, or a reflective exercise linking local practice to global determinants of health, can create transformative learning moments that align with wider global health competencies.

The design of activities that embed global health perspectives into everyday teaching raises important questions about access and sustainability. While innovative approaches such as the VIE can widen participation and reduce barriers, traditional models of international electives continue to be associated with significant costs. These financial considerations affect not only individual students but also universities and their international partners. To fully understand the opportunities and challenges of embedding global health into nursing curricula, it is therefore important to examine the economic dimensions of global health education.

THE ECONOMICS OF GLOBAL HEALTH EDUCATION

Embedding global health perspectives into nursing curricula is often framed in terms of ethics, equity, and pedagogy. However, it is equally important to consider the economic dimensions of global health education. Questions of cost, funding, and sustainability shape what opportunities are available to students and institutions, and ultimately influence who is able to participate in global health learning. A critical examination of the economics of global health education highlights both the barriers associated with traditional models and the potential of innovative approaches such as virtual electives to address them.

THE COST OF TRADITIONAL ELECTIVES

Conventional international electives have long been valued for their immersive, experiential learning benefits. Yet, the financial costs associated with overseas placements are considerable. Students typically bear expenses for flights, accommodation, insurance, vaccinations, and visas. Additional hidden costs, such as lost income from employment or disruption to caring responsibilities, further exacerbate inequities. These financial barriers mean that participation in international electives has often been limited to students with the resources or support networks to fund such experiences. As a result, traditional electives risk reproducing structural inequalities rather than widening access.

INSTITUTIONAL AND SYSTEM-LEVEL COSTS

The financial implications are not limited to students. For universities, international electives require significant investment in staff time, risk management, and partnership maintenance. Institutions must provide pre-departure training, negotiate memoranda of understanding, and ensure compliance with safeguarding and legal requirements. Host institutions, particularly in low- and middle-income countries, also carry costs, including supervision, accommodation, and administrative support, which may not always be adequately reimbursed. These costs can place strain on partnerships and raise ethical questions about reciprocity and fairness.

COST-EFFECTIVENESS OF VIRTUAL MODELS

Virtual electives, such as the VIE, present an alternative model that is more cost-effective and equitable. By removing travel and accommodation expenses, virtual programmes dramatically reduce the financial burden on students. They also minimise the environmental costs associated with air travel, aligning with broader sustainability goals. While virtual models require investment in digital infrastructure and faculty time, these costs are relatively modest compared with the expenses of overseas placements. Moreover, once developed, digital resources can be reused and adapted, creating long-term value and scalability.

FUNDING MODELS AND SUSTAINABILITY

The question of how global health education should be funded remains central. Some universities subsidise international electives through scholarships or bursaries, while others rely on student self-funding. Charitable foundations and governmental organisations have occasionally provided support, but funding is often short-term or competitive. For virtual models, sustainability depends on institutional recognition of their value and integration into mainstream curricula. Embedding virtual electives as assessed modules rather than optional add-ons can secure funding through standard teaching budgets. In addition, collaborations with international partners may open access to shared resources and reduce duplication of effort.

EQUITY AND ECONOMIC JUSTICE

The economics of global health education cannot be separated from questions of equity and justice. If participation depends on financial privilege, the result is a narrow pool of students gaining international perspectives, which runs counter to the values of inclusivity and diversity. Virtual models help redress this imbalance by widening access, but they also raise questions about equity for partner institutions. For example, the cost of internet access or digital infrastructure in low-resource settings may still act as a barrier. Ensuring fair distribution of costs and benefits remains a core ethical consideration.

BROADER GLOBAL HEALTH TRENDS AND FUTURE IMPLICATIONS FOR NURSING EDUCATION

While this chapter has focused primarily on pedagogical innovation through the Virtual International Elective (VIE), it is essential to position nursing education within the wider landscape of global health challenges. These global trends have direct implications for how nursing students are taught, prepared, and supported to practise both in the UK and in international contexts.

CLIMATE CHANGE AND HEALTH

The health consequences of climate change are increasingly well documented. Rising temperatures, extreme weather events, food insecurity, and water scarcity all impact health, leading to the spread of vector-borne diseases, deterioration in mental health, population displacement, and the disruption of healthcare infrastructure (Romanello et al., 2021). Nurses must be equipped to understand and respond to these complex, cross-border determinants of health. Embedding climate resilience, planetary health, and environmental sustainability within curricula helps prepare students to engage in advocacy, service redesign, and leadership in this rapidly evolving area.

MIGRATION, DISPLACEMENT, AND REFUGEE HEALTH

Conflict, persecution, and economic instability drive global population movements. The health needs of displaced persons are multifaceted and often exacerbated by trauma, poor living conditions, and barriers to accessing healthcare. For UK-based nurses, this increasingly translates into caring for patients with diverse health beliefs, unfamiliar disease profiles, and potential language barriers. Nurse educators therefore have a duty to prepare students to provide care that is both compassionate and culturally responsive.

HEALTH SYSTEMS STRENGTHENING AND WORKFORCE CAPACITY

Many low- and middle-income countries face chronic shortages of healthcare workers and underfunded health systems. The World Health Organization (2023) continues to highlight the importance of international solidarity in training, supporting, and ensuring fair mobility of health professionals. UK nurse education must prepare students to understand both the global nursing workforce landscape and the ethical considerations of international recruitment. This includes encouraging critical reflection on issues of sustainability, reciprocity, and the distribution of healthcare resources.

GLOBAL PANDEMICS AND CROSS-BORDER COLLABORATION

The COVID-19 pandemic reaffirmed the essential role of nurses in global health emergencies, but it was not the first, nor will it be the last. From HIV to Ebola, and from SARS to Zika, nurses have consistently contributed to pandemic preparedness and response. Preparing future nurses requires an understanding of global cooperation mechanisms, surveillance systems, ethical practice, and interprofessional collaboration during crises.

DECOLONISING GLOBAL HEALTH IN NURSE EDUCATION

Global health has historically been dominated by perspectives from the Global North, often perpetuating power imbalances and one-way knowledge transfer. There is now growing momentum to 'decolonise' global health, a movement that challenges these traditional hierarchies and promotes more equitable, reciprocal, and context-sensitive partnerships (Abimbola et al., 2021). Nurse education must equip students to critically examine whose voices are heard in global health discourse, whose knowledge is valued, and how they themselves can contribute to more equitable collaborations in practice.

INNOVATION BOX

Voices from the Field: A Simulation-based Global Health Experience

An illustrative model of applied pedagogy is 'Voices from the Field: A Simulation-Based Global Health Experience for Healthcare Students'.

Learning Objectives

- Develop an understanding of social determinants of health in global contexts
- Demonstrate culturally responsive care in diverse healthcare environments

- Identify barriers to healthcare access and delivery in resource-limited settings
- Apply global health principles to patient care, including advocacy and interprofessional collaboration

Simulation Scenarios

1. **Maternal Care in Rural Uganda**

   Learners manage a postpartum haemorrhage with limited resources in a rural clinic. They must prioritise care, communicate with a midwife, and support the patient and her family while navigating cultural beliefs and lack of transport.

2. **Cholera Outbreak in an Urban Slum in Bangladesh**

   Students triage patients during an outbreak in a field hospital, balancing infection control, hydration management, and ethical resource allocation under extreme pressure.

3. **Climate Crisis Response in the Philippines**

   Following a typhoon, learners assist in setting up a temporary clinic, manage trauma and dehydration cases, and work within a local disaster response team to identify ongoing health needs and community engagement strategies.

Simulation Modality
Delivered using simulated patients and actors, the scenarios highlight language barriers, emotional stress, and the consequences of decision-making under pressure.

Debrief and Reflection
Structured group debriefing encourages reflection on ethical dilemmas, cultural awareness, emotional response, and lessons for professional practice. Students are prompted to ask themselves, *'How did this scenario challenge my assumptions about health equity'?*

EDUCATOR TOOLKIT: PRACTICAL STRATEGIES FOR EMBEDDING GLOBAL PERSPECTIVES

For nurse academics undertaking a PGCAP, the following adaptable strategies provide practical methods for integrating global perspectives across diverse modules and sessions:

- **Critical incident reflections** – Ask students to examine a clinical case through both local and global lenses, encouraging recognition of health inequalities and differing cultural contexts.
- **Diverse patient scenarios** – Integrate case studies or simulation activities that reflect varied cultural, social, and global determinants of health.
- **Media and narrative resources** – Use film, literature, podcasts, or first-person accounts from different regions to stimulate empathy, critical thinking, and cross-cultural dialogue.
- **Student-led inquiry** – Invite students to identify a global health issue and facilitate a discussion linking their findings back to UK practice.
- **Structured dialogue** – Create opportunities for peer exchange, either through digital platforms with international partners or simulated intercultural role play.
- **Ethical reflection** – Encourage students to reflect on equity, sustainability, and power in everyday nursing practice and professional decision-making.

These strategies are intended as prompts rather than prescriptions. Even small changes in session design can encourage critical reflection, inclusivity, and global awareness, ensuring that the principles of equity, reciprocity, and cultural competence underpin learning across the curriculum.

SUMMARY AND IMPLICATIONS FOR PRACTICE

This chapter has outlined how global health perspectives can be embedded meaningfully in nursing education through theory-informed, inclusive, and innovative pedagogies. Using the Virtual International Elective (VIE) as a case study, it has shown how digital approaches can overcome physical, financial, and structural barriers to international experience. Global health competencies, such as cultural understanding, systems thinking, and global citizenship, are transferable across contexts and vital to person-centred care in today's multicultural health systems.

For nurse academics undertaking a PGCAP, the implications extend beyond global health alone. The VIE illustrates how transformative pedagogy can be achieved through deliberate design, challenging assumptions, creating space for reflection, and encouraging students to act as socially responsible practitioners. The principles of co-creation, reciprocity, inclusivity, and critical pedagogy are transferable to a wide range of teaching contexts. Whether designing a seminar, structuring a simulation, or planning an assessment, the key question is how the activity will enable students to engage critically, develop broader perspectives, and carry these insights into professional practice.

Embedding global health perspectives is therefore both an example of, and a metaphor for, the wider task of transformative nurse education.

FUTURE DIRECTIONS AND RESEARCH IN GLOBAL HEALTH NURSING EDUCATION

As this chapter has shown, embedding global health perspectives into nursing education has immediate benefits for students, educators, and wider health systems. Yet the field is dynamic, and new opportunities and challenges continue to emerge. Looking ahead, both practice and research have a crucial role to play in shaping how global health education evolves within nursing curricula.

STRENGTHENING EVIDENCE ON IMPACT

Although innovative approaches such as the VIE have demonstrated positive student experiences, there remains a need for more robust research on long-term outcomes. Questions such as whether global health education influences graduates' career trajectories, enhances cultural competence in practice, or improves patient outcomes are not yet fully answered. Longitudinal studies tracking students from education into professional roles could provide valuable insights. Similarly, comparative studies between virtual and in-person electives would deepen understanding of what kinds of learning experiences have the greatest impact and for whom.

EXPANDING PEDAGOGICAL MODELS

Future directions will also involve the development of diverse pedagogical models. While digital tools such as VR, simulation, and MOOCs are promising, they should not be seen as one-size-fits-all solutions. Research should explore how different modalities work for varied student populations, and how they can be integrated into curricula in ways that enhance, rather than replace, relational learning. There is also scope for greater use of co-created pedagogies, where students and international partners are directly involved in designing and delivering global health content.

DECOLONISING GLOBAL HEALTH EDUCATION

One of the most important emerging trends is the movement to decolonise global health. This involves questioning whose knowledge is prioritised, how global partnerships are structured, and whether education perpetuates or challenges global inequities. Future research could examine how nursing curricula can foreground perspectives from the Global South, integrate indigenous knowledge systems, and ensure reciprocity in collaborations. For educators, this means moving beyond representation to critical engagement with power, privilege, and history in shaping global health discourse.

INTEGRATING GLOBAL HEALTH ACROSS THE CURRICULUM

At present, global health in nursing education is often positioned as an elective or supplementary component. A future direction is to embed global health principles across all aspects of curricula, from foundational sciences to advanced practice. This would align with the recognition that health systems are globally interconnected, and that every nurse, regardless of role or location, benefits from a global perspective. Research could explore practical models for integration, including curriculum mapping, shared learning outcomes, and interprofessional teaching strategies.

POLICY AND WORKFORCE ALIGNMENT

The global nursing workforce is facing critical challenges, including shortages, migration, and increasing demands from ageing populations and climate change. Research is needed to examine how nurse education can best align with these workforce priorities, preparing graduates to contribute to both national and international health goals. Partnerships with professional bodies such as the ICN, as well as alignment with policy frameworks like the WHO Global Strategic Directions for Nursing and Midwifery, will be vital in this respect.

SUSTAINABILITY AND DIGITAL EQUITY

As education becomes increasingly digitised, sustainability and digital equity must remain central. Research can help evaluate the environmental benefits of virtual electives, the digital divide affecting student access, and the pedagogical implications of new technologies. Ethical frameworks will be needed to guide the use of AI, VR, and other tools in ways that are inclusive, equitable, and culturally sensitive.

BUILDING RESEARCH CAPACITY

Finally, there is a need to build capacity for research in global health nursing education itself. This includes supporting early-career nurse researchers, encouraging international collaboration, and securing funding streams dedicated to education-focused studies. Strengthening research networks across institutions and countries will ensure that innovation is shared and adapted to diverse contexts, rather than confined to isolated case studies.

CONCLUSION

The future of global health nursing education lies in expanding both practice and research. By strengthening evidence, diversifying pedagogies, decolonising curricula, and aligning with policy and workforce priorities, educators can prepare nurses who are globally aware, ethically grounded, and professionally agile. Research will be central in this process, providing the evidence base needed to guide innovation and ensure that global health education remains responsive to evolving challenges. In this way, global health nursing education can continue to equip future generations of nurses with the knowledge, skills, and values required to contribute to health equity, locally and globally.

KEY TAKE-HOME POINTS

- Embedding global health perspectives into nursing curricula promotes equity, cultural competence, and person-centred care.

- Virtual electives such as the VIE provide innovative and sustainable alternatives to traditional international placements.

- Collaborative, reflective, and inclusive approaches are key to transformative global health education.

CPD REFLECTIVE QUESTIONS

1. How can you support students to develop global awareness and cultural competence within your current teaching or practice setting?

2. What barriers exist to delivering global health content, and how might digital innovation help overcome them?

3. In what ways could your team adopt reciprocity and ethical collaboration in future global education partnerships?

REFERENCES

Abimbola, S., Asthana, S., Montenegro, C., Guinto, R. R., Jumbam, D. T., Louskieter, L., Mwisongo, A., & Pai, M. (2021). Addressing power asymmetries in global health: imperatives in the wake of the COVID-19 pandemic. *PLoS Medicine*, 18(4), e1003604. https://doi.org/10.1371/journal.pmed.1003604.

Boulton, J. (2015). Ebola: where did it come from and where might it go? *British Journal of Nursing*, 23(18), 988–991. https://doi.org/10.12968/bjon.2014.23.18.988.

Campinha-Bacote, J. (2002). The process of cultural competence in the delivery of healthcare services: a model of care. *Journal of Transcultural Nursing*, 13(3), 181–184. https://doi.org/10.1177/10459602013003003.

Centre for Disease Control and Prevention (2020). *CDC Museum COVID-19 Timeline*. https://www.cdc.gov/museum/timeline/covid19.html

Clark, M., Raffray, M., Hendricks, K., & Gagnon, A. J. (2016). Global and public health core competencies for nursing education: a systematic review of essential competencies. *Nurse Education Today*, 40, 173–180. https://doi.org/10.1016/j.nedt.2016.02.026.

Dawson, M., Gakumo, C., Phillips, J., & Wilson, L. (2016). Process for mapping global health competencies in undergraduate and graduate nursing curricula. *Nurse Educator*, 41(1), 37–40. https://doi.org/10.1097/NNE.0000000000000199.

Foronda, C., Fernandez-Burgos, M., Nadeau, C., Kelley, C. N., & Henry, M. N. (2020). Virtual simulation in nursing education: a systematic review spanning 1996 to 2018. *Simulation in Healthcare*, 15(1), 46–54. https://doi.org/10.1097/SIH.0000000000000411.

Freire, P. (1970). *Pedagogy of the Oppressed*. Herder and Herder.

International Council of Nurses (2021a). *Global Nursing Leadership: ICN Policy Brief*. Geneva: ICN.

International Council of Nurses (2021b). *ICN calls for investment in nursing education, jobs, and leadership*. https://www.icn.ch

Kolb, D. A. (1984). *Experiential Learning: Experience as the Source of Learning and Development*. Prentice-Hall.

Koplan, J. P., Bond, T. C., Merson, M. H., Reddy, K. S., Rodriguez, M. H., Sewankambo, N. K., & Wasserheit, J. N. (2009). Towards a common definition of global health. *The Lancet*, 373(9679), 1993–1995. https://doi.org/10.1016/S0140-6736(09)60332-9.

McInally, W., Metcalfe, S., & Garner, B. (2015). Enriching the student experience through a collaborative cultural learning model. *Creative Nursing*, 21(3), 161–166. https://doi.org/10.1891/1078-4535.21.3.161.

Mezirow, J. (1991). *Transformative Dimensions of Adult Learning*. Jossey-Bass.

Nursing and Midwifery Council (NMC) (2018). *Future Nurse: Standards of Proficiency for Registered Nurses*. London: NMC. https://www.nmc.org.uk

Nursing and Midwifery Council (NMC) (2020). *Emergency standards for education and training programmes*. https://www.nmc.org.uk/globalassets/sitedocuments/education-standards/current-recovery-programme-standards.pdf

Our World in Data (2021). Map of the WHO Regions. https://ourworldindata.org/world-region-map-definitions

Richardson, J., Grose, J., Bradbury, M. & Kelsey, J., (2017). Developing awareness of sustainability in nursing and midwifery using a scenario-based approach: Evidence from a pre and post educational intervention study. *Nurse Education Today*, 54, pp. 51–55.

Romanello, M., McGushin, A., Di Napoli, C., Drummond, P., Hughes, N., Jamart, L., Kennard, H., Lampard, P., Rodriguez, B. S., Arnell, N., & Ayeb-Karlsson, S., (2021). The 2021 report of the Lancet Countdown on health and climate change: code red for a healthy future. *The Lancet*, 398(10311), pp. 1619–1662.

Salm, M., Ali, M., Minihane, M., & Conrad, P. (2021). Defining global health: findings from a systematic review and thematic analysis of the literature. *BMJ Global Health*, 6(6), e005292. https://doi.org/10.1136/bmjgh-2021-005292.

Sims, B. (2016). Sending our professionals overseas is one of the best things we can do. *Health Service Journal*. http://tinyurl.com/h9z9xz4

UNESCO (2015). *Global citizenship education: topics and learning objectives*. https://unesdoc.unesco.org/ark:/48223/pf0000232993

United Nations (2015). *The 17 Sustainable Development Goals*. United Nations.

Watermeyer, R., Crick, T., Knight, C., & Goodall, J. (2021). COVID-19 and digital disruption in UK universities: afflictions and affordances of emergency online migration. *Higher Education*, 81, 623–641. https://doi.org/10.1007/s10734-020-00561-y

World Health Organization (WHO) (2010). *Framework for Action on Interprofessional Education and Collaborative Practice*. Geneva: WHO.

World Health Organization (WHO) (2020). Naming the coronavirus (COVID-19) and the virus that causes it. https://www.who.int/emergencies/diseases/novel-coronavirus-2019/technical-guidance

World Health Organization (WHO) (2021). *Global Strategic Directions for Nursing and Midwifery 2021–2025*. Geneva: WHO.

World Health Organization (WHO) (2023). *WHO report on global health worker mobility*. World Health Organization.

World Health Organization (WHO) (2025). Where we work: WHO organisational structure. https://www.who.int/about/structure

Sustainability

CHAPTER 9

Melanie Madison

Florence Nightingale Faculty of Nursing, Midwifery and Palliative Care, Department of Adult Nursing, King's College London, UK

AIM

To explore how transformative nursing education can empower nurses to lead sustainable, inclusive, and ethical healthcare by embedding the principles of environmental stewardship, social justice, and interprofessional leadership across curricula and practice.

LEARNING OUTCOMES

By the end of this chapter, readers will be able to:

1. Describe the impact of healthcare and nursing education on sustainability and global resource consumption.

2. Discuss the integration of the Sustainable Development Goals (SDGs) and Social Determinants of Health (SDH) in nursing curricula.

3. Evaluate practical educational strategies to promote carbon literacy, sustainable practice, and community resilience.

4. Reflect on how leadership, well-being, and interprofessional collaboration underpin sustainability in nursing education and healthcare systems.

CHAPTER INTRODUCTION

Sustainability is no longer a peripheral concern in healthcare education; it is central to preparing nurses for the realities of modern clinical practice. As the climate crisis intensifies and health systems face growing resource constraints, there is an urgent need to equip nurses with the knowledge, values, and skills to deliver care that is environmentally responsible, socially just, and economically viable. This chapter explores how transformative nursing education can address these challenges by embedding the principles of sustainability, global citizenship, and interprofessional leadership into curricula and teaching practices. It draws on recent evidence, policy frameworks, and educational innovation to illustrate how nurses can be empowered to become agents of change, supporting health equity, protecting planetary resources, and promoting well-being for all.

PRACTICES OF SUSTAINABLE HEALTHCARE IN NURSING

Planetary health is inextricably bound to human health, and the climate crisis represents one of the largest global threats to both (Watts et al., 2019). Extreme weather events are affecting populations globally, leading to an increase in water-borne diseases, malnutrition, and respiratory diseases linked to air pollution. It is often the most vulnerable communities that suffer the most and have the least resources to survive. Possibly a more shocking fact

Transformative Nursing Education, First Edition. Edited by Aby Mitchell and Barry Hill.

is that healthcare delivery is also responsible for a large global carbon footprint due to a continued dependence on unsustainable resources, gas emissions, and fossil fuels (Healthcare without Harm (HWH), 2019). The human population is predicted to increase to 10 billion by 2050 (United Nations, 2016), with implications for the planet's natural resources and an imperative for sustainable healthcare. If the NHS were a country, it would be the fourth largest emitter of greenhouse gases in the world (NHSE, 2022). This stark fact lies behind the drive to reduce the carbon footprint of healthcare delivery.

These environmental impacts can be considered across Scope 1, Scope 2 and Scope 3 emissions, which are explained in Table 9.1.

Identified as an urgent problem in the Health and Care Act 2022, the United Kingdom's Government became the first in Europe to commit to reaching Net Zero in the NHS by 2040 (National Health Service England [NHSE], 2022). It is important to note that Net Zero is not the same as becoming carbon neutral, as the health service will always produce GHG but refers instead to ensuring that the GHG produced by the NHS is equal to or less than those emissions removed from the environment (NHSE, 2022) with the impact being on a cleaner environment and better health for future generations. This means that current practice must strive to reduce emissions where possible as well as contribute to emissions removal through activities such as tree planting on NHS sites (NHS Forest).

It has been widely observed that whilst health professionals care about the climate and the planet, they often lack the confidence, skills, attitudes, and knowledge required to address it (Leffers et al., 2017; López-Medina et al., 2019; Neal-Boylan et al., 2019). A recent literature review of the nursing role in hospital-based emissions reduction identified that the nursing profession is in a unique and powerful position to make change, but this was only possible through transformative education and research (Ward et al., 2022).

Healthcare in the UK is facing the impact of decades of unsustainable resourcing that is adversely affecting the care being delivered and those delivering it (Issa et al., 2024). Cost versus benefit is a familiar management dilemma and touches the working lives of every health professional. Calls to 'lean up' and restructure the NHS in the face of growing populations and dwindling global resources using quality improvement and innovation to change processes are not new (NHSE, 2014). For healthcare professionals and educators, the burning question is how to apply the principles of sustainability in a safe way that will balance the books, serve the population, and keep the planet's resources safe from extinction. Education must hold the answers and have the agility to facilitate that learning.

Environmental sustainability has been included in the revised Nursing and Midwifery (NMC) education standards (NMC, 2023) but still requires a more explicit place in the professional Code (NMC, 2018a). The General

Table 9.1 Explanation of Scope 1, 2, and 3 GHG Emissions in the NHS

Scope 1 emissions—these are direct emissions controlled by the NHS	Use of fossil fuels
	Anesthetic gases
	NHS Fleet of Vehicles
	Facilities and sites
Scope 2 emissions—indirectly controlled by the NHS arising from the activities required of the service	Electricity
Scope 3 emissions—all the emissions that the company is indirectly responsible for e.g procurement	Metered dose inhalers, medical devices, Medicines
	Water and sanitation, waste disposal, food and catering
	Business travel, staff commuting, logistics
	Construction, energy
	Commissioned external services
	Information Technology and AI
	Manufacturing

Source: Adapted from NHSE (2022).

Medical Council has already mandated learning on the climate crisis for all graduate programmes, developing a curriculum that will produce global citizens (Tun & Martin, 2022). The Nursing & Midwifery Council have recently produced their consensus on the environmental sustainability of the profession's governing body as an institution (NMC, 2023), and it is hoped that the next review of the Code has a visionary and resilient plan to address sustainability as a core value. There also needs to be a commitment from the Government and the NHS as employers to allow higher education to continue to embed knowledge and agency into post qualification programmes such as the Advanced Nurse practitioner courses, where a direct impact on patient care can be seen whilst also supporting continuous professional development.

The detrimental impact that healthcare has on the environment has made the need to teach about sustainable practice an imperative (NHSE, 2022). Educators need to have an awareness that wicked problems, such as the climate catastrophe, can cause anxiety and overwhelm in some students or a sense of hopelessness that leads to passive acceptance that they cannot change the problem (Álvarez-Nieto et al., 2022). In a pre-registration nursing curriculum that is largely competency based and driven by prescribed learning outcomes, values-based teaching can be a challenge. It is important to gauge how much students already know about the climate crisis from a personal perspective and then link it to their professional lives. Goodman (2011) suggested that teaching should foster interconnectedness and inspire change that improves the students' lives. Students need to feel safe enough to say that they are unaware or not informed (Chicca & Shellenbarger, 2020).

Ice breakers can be used to open the discussion at the start of a session and provide a safe and supportive environment to discuss this wicked problem. Sustainability Bingo was designed to encourage social interaction and disclosure to peers about what students were already doing to reduce their carbon footprint in their daily lives and their clinical practice. The competitive element of the game made it more desirable to be environmentally aware and led to the participants pledging to do more of the activities on the score card (Figure 9.1).

The bingo card was designed with specific activities listed, these included personal choices such as cycling or walking whenever possible, composting food, holidaying in the UK, avoiding eating meat as well as professional actions such as understanding when to use gloves in practice, only using sharps boxes for sharps, advising patients to return unwanted medication to the pharmacy and considering if new bed linen is required every day. Each group is given a scorecard with the sections in different orders. Each activity was then called out, and the first team to complete a line of answers shouted 'WASTE'. The rest of the activities were then called out, and the group completing the whole card called out 'Sustainability'. Lively group discussions can take place about what each member is already doing.

The aim of the game was to start a difficult conversation that might lead to an increased awareness of solutions and an intention to action. The interactive nature of the game gave participants a sense of shared responsibility to complete the card with their combined efforts. It was also fun, inclusive and safe.

Another essential part of education for sustainable development (ESD) is to empower students and educators with carbon literacy (Sawyer, 2020). Having a working knowledge of key concepts and a vocabulary to be eco-literate and fit for the future is an essential skill. Levett-Jones et al. (2024) have produced a comprehensive list of common terms with definitions from reputable sources as part of their study to achieve consensus on the essential skills and knowledge for sustainable education. Talking about the impact of the climate crisis on health in an informed way could enrich patient interactions, as it is likely that some patients will also care about the environment but may not realise the impact of some of their care has, from the inhalers they use to the number of trips to the hospital. More support for professionals who need to talk to their patients about the impact of the climate on health has been recognised by the World Health Organisation (WHO), which has designed a communication tool kit for health professionals (WHO, 2024).

A glossary of terms should be available alongside any teaching to enhance understanding and provide consistency (Table 9.2). There are also useful introductory resources, such as the e-learning for Health (eLfH) modules: Environmentally Sustainable Healthcare and Carbon Literacy for Healthcare (eLfH, 2023) that could be used as self-directed learning prior to the teaching.

Without sustainable competence and the confidence to lead change, the profession will be unable to promote planetary and human health and slow the crisis down. It is an imperative for education to give students and educators the foundational knowledge and communication skills to discuss environmental sustainability. This requires collaboration with external experts, access to

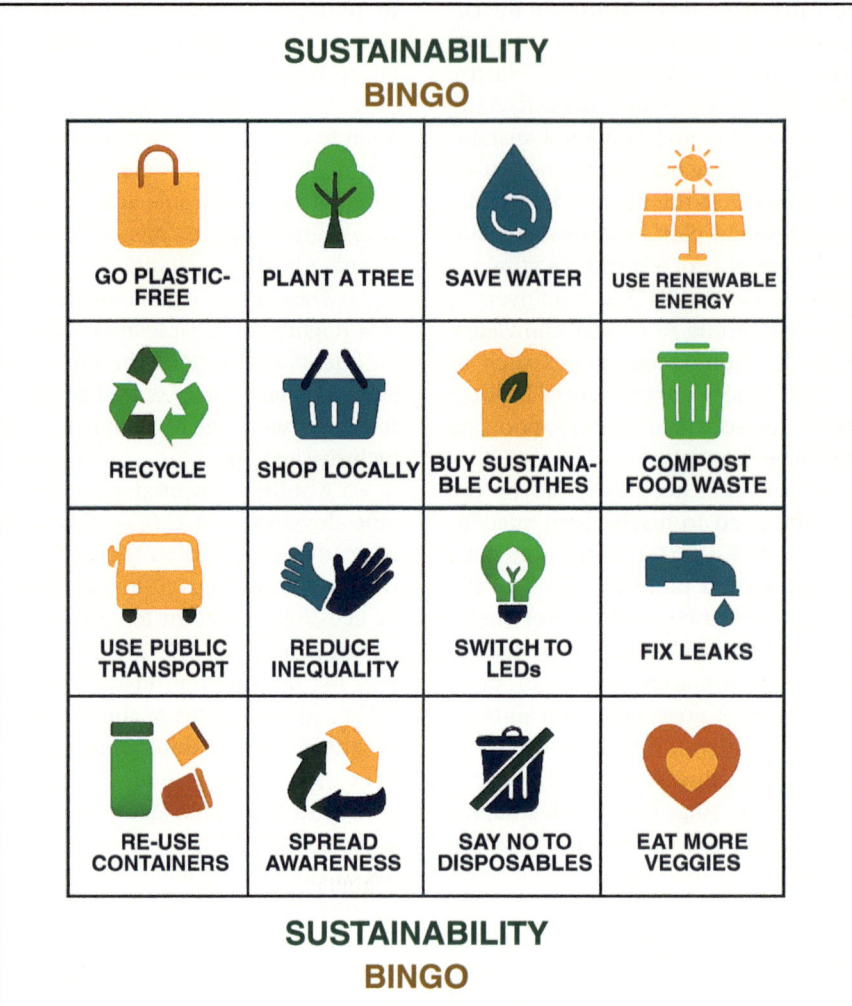

FIGURE 9.1 Sustainability bingo instructions and card

Table 9.2 Examples of Glossary of Terms

Glossary of terms—some examples	
Carbon dioxide equivalent eCO_2	The measurement used to compare greenhouse gas emissions (GGEs) of anything by conversion to an equivalent amount of carbon dioxide with the same impact on warming. GHG gases include
Net Zero	The reduction of GGEs to the lowest possible point and the offsetting of unavoidable emissions.
Eco-anxiety	Refers to severe mental distress suffered in relation to the impending threat of the climate crisis and often accompanied by a sense of helplessness.
Environmental Stewardship	Like antibiotic stewardship, this refers to the role of health professionals as guardians or caretakers of the environmental impact of healthcare on humans and the planet.
Carbon Hotspots	This refers to activities that create the majority of GHG either as an organisation e.g. waste disposal or at a local level e.g. inefficient care pathways.

reputable training resources and a commitment from Higher Education institutes to continuing professional development (CPD) for educators.

The faculty of one London-based nursing school has successfully embedded sustainability across a range of undergraduate and postgraduate programmes in collaboration with the Centre for Sustainable Healthcare (CSH). A group of educators from a range of nursing disciplines and programmes, including Adult, Child, Mental Health, Midwifery and Specialist Community Public Health Nurses (SCPHN), attended a one-day sustainability workshop developed by the CSH for educators. Attendance included free access to a range of materials, including a library of case studies from practice and a Creative Commons free set of slides with a lesson plan to deliver a sustainability workshop that could be adapted for each speciality. The workshop has been successfully delivered across all programmes with a positive response from students. Educators were also given the opportunity to assess their confidence in delivering the workshop via a yearly evaluation form that identified confidence levels and areas where more information and development were required. This opportunity was supported by the Faculty Staff Development funding and required protected time for CPD in attending the course, and then time for design and redesign of curricula. This strategy for embedding sustainability into teaching addresses the imbalance that is sometimes felt by educators when delivering a current or wicked problem, who may feel that their students know more than they do and that they have no time to reflect on this (Aronsson et al., 2024). It is therefore a pre-requisite that educators can keep up to date with such a dynamic field of enquiry, and this needs to be acknowledged by Universities and Faculties by embracing CPD and further training.

One approach to teaching sustainable practice allows students to consider the environmental, financial and social determinants of healthcare. This concept forms a key part of any sustainability teaching (Mortimer et al., 2018; Stanford, 2023). It is also known as the triple bottom line and can be applied by students to any patient intervention or care pathway to determine the value of that patient care.

Students can estimate the environmental impact of an intervention using a simple non mathematical framework that considers three elements. Resource use such as medical equipment, transport, lighting and heating. The financial cost of delivering the intervention. The potential negative impact on the patient, for example frequent admissions or missed appointments.

Post-qualification students already in practice could be asked to consider whether habitual practices such as unnecessary cannulations or blood tests in the Emergency room could be challenged, and the subsequent social, financial and environmental benefits presented using quality improvement methodology in their final dissertations (Cornish, 2021).

Having identified a problem in their own practice, using the triple bottom line, students can choose one of the four sustainable clinical strategies shown in Table 9.3 to identify how a problem in their practice could be tackled using sustainable quality improvement methodology and submit a proposal as their final dissertation or capstone assessment.

Table 9.3 Adapted from the Centre for Sustainable Healthcare 'Principles of Sustainable Clinical Practice'

Leaning up service delivery	**Sourcing low-carbon alternatives**
Services that fit the needs of the users	Making intentional choices in procurement, using effective and sustainable treatments and care pathways.
Minimising waste, duplication and low value processes	Using medical technology to reduce the carbon impact.
Providing joined up, streamlined care.	Minimising waste from consumables, pharmaceuticals and energy.
Prevention	**Patient empowerment and self-care**
Health promotion	Helping patients to take a central role in their own health and care
Disease prevention	
Reduced the burden of disease on healthcare resource	

Source: Adapted from Mortimer (2010).

LICENSING | CENTRE FOR SUSTAINABLE HEALTHCARE

Teaching environmentally sustainable practices could include students studying resource consumption and waste disposal in their own hospitals through access to individual Trust Green Plans and an awareness of the Government's commitment (NHSE, 2022). The learning outcomes would be for nurses to consider how the health service can reduce the use of single-use plastics and personal protective equipment and still maintain patient safety standards. It would also require an understanding of environmental stewardship over correct waste segregation by using the right bins, as well as considering energy-efficient practices, such as turning off lights and computers when not in use and a commitment to eco-friendly procurement that moves away from single-use plastics and items like tourniquets.

Students might also be asked to consider the working environment of hospitals themselves, with the environmental implications of old buildings and energy reliance on fossil fuels. Promoting healthier environments could positively impact the sustainability of the profession by addressing retention and burnout (Boudreau & Rheaume, 2024). Classroom discussions do not need to remain on the negative impacts of the climate on health and vice versa, as this may cause a sense of hopelessness but can include showcasing impactful initiatives such as the electric ambulance fleet and the removal of desflurane in anaesthetics found on the Greener NHS website.

Nominating sustainability leads or champions in faculties as well as hosting climate cafes or events that showcase the best sustainable practices are other ways to engage with educators and students about their beliefs. The social element of a climate café encourages collaborations and co-design for solutions, informal and informative; they provide a space where the problems can be discussed, and solutions proposed in a collective and safe manner.

SUSTAINABLE DEVELOPMENT GOALS AND NURSING EDUCATION

Sustainability requires inclusivity and cultural competence from nurses so that the results of more sustainable practice can be felt by individuals from all backgrounds. To ensure this, nursing education should address social injustice and promote equity using sustainable principles in line with the Sustainable Development Goals.

In 2016, the United Nations (UN) enacted the 2030 Agenda for Sustainable Development (UN, 2016), which is a globally agreed set of 17 Sustainable Development Goals (SDGs) and 169 targets with the overarching aim of ensuring a healthy, safe, and sustainable world (Figure 9.2). The agenda identified 17 key areas that cover access to education, health, clean water, and equality. The goals are further divided into five themes essential to the sustainability of planetary well-being and survival known as the 5Ps: People, Planet, Peace, Prosperity, and Partnership (Table 9.4).

Since then, there has been a global health pandemic, an increase in severe weather events and natural disasters, alongside wars and increasing global poverty. The need for transformative actions and empowerment in line with these goals is more needed than ever. Nursing as a front-line profession with the presence and influence to profoundly impact global communities through actions is vital to the success of the UN SDG goals. Nursing education is crucial to creating a sustainable future for the profession and needs to inform and empower healthcare professionals to understand the problems and integrate sustainable practices into their everyday work. Sustainability is not just about survival, it is about long-term and robust resilience in the way healthcare is delivered, acknowledging that resources are finite and that depleting them without regard will jeopardise the future of healthcare and the planet.

Healthcare is embedded into all aspects of the SDGs, and nursing as the largest professional body in healthcare organisations, is central to achieving these global goals. Nurses are critical in addressing inequalities, the impact of resource scarcity and climate change. Nursing education must therefore provide the profession not only with an understanding of the principles of sustainable healthcare but also empower nurses to be agents of change through policy change, activism, and action (Rafferty, 2018).

The relevance of the SDGs to nursing practice lies in the details of each goal and can offer educators the opportunity to use them as a lens for discussion (Upvall & Luzincourt, 2019). Of relevance to health and the nursing profession are Goals 3, 4, 8, 11, 12, 13, and 17 (Table 9.5).

It has been argued that progress towards the goals has not been dynamic enough since the enactment of the Agenda (Independent Group of Scientists appointed by the Secretary-General, 2023), driving a sense of urgency and highlighting the importance of acting on the evidence

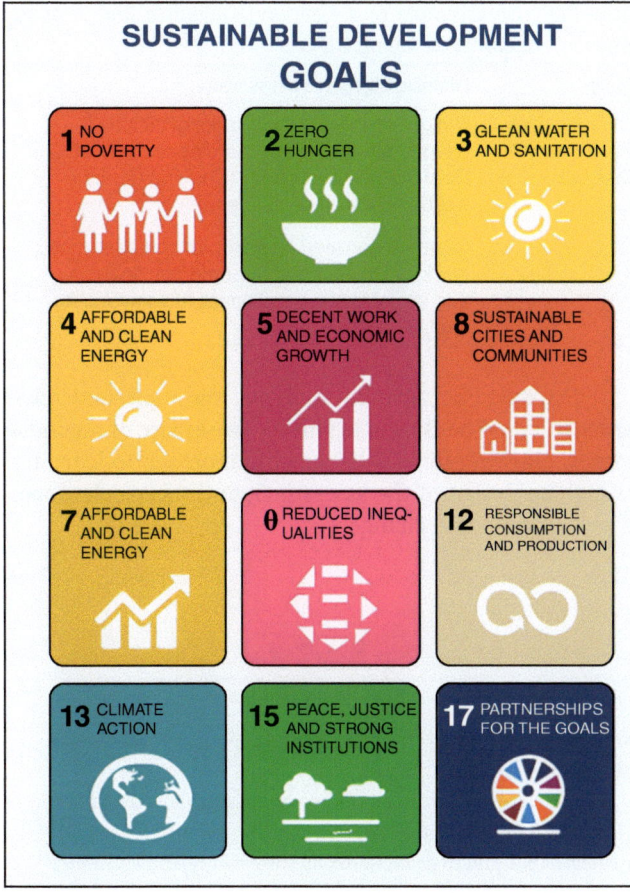

FIGURE 9.2 The United Nations Sustainable Development Goals (UN, 2016). *Source*: https://www.un.org/sustainable development. The content of this publication has not been approved by the United Nations and does not reflect the views of the United Nations or its officials or Member States

Table 9.4   The 5Ps

People	Ensuring healthy lives and promoting well-being for all at all ages.
Planet	Protecting the planet from degradation, ensuring sustainable use of natural resources.
Prosperity	Ensuring that all people can enjoy prosperous and fulfilling lives, in harmony with nature.
Peace	Promoting peaceful, just, and inclusive societies, free from fear and violence.
Partnership	Strengthening the means of implementation and revitalising global partnerships for sustainable development.

Source: Adapted from UN SDG (2016).

Table 9.5   The Sustainable Development Goals (UN, 2016)

Goal 3	Support health and wellbeing for people of all ages.
Goal 4	Provide inclusive, high-quality education and foster lifelong learning opportunities.
Goal 8	Encourage sustainable economic growth, productive employment, and decent work for everyone.
Goal 11	Develop inclusive, safe, resilient, and sustainable cities and communities.
Goal 12	Promote responsible consumption and production practices.
Goal 13	Take immediate measures to address climate change and its effects.
Goal 17	Enhance implementation strategies and renew global partnerships for sustainable development.

behind the goals. Nursing is a global profession with a reach that is both diverse and without boundaries. From front-line bedside care to policy makers and innovators, nurses have the power through their sheer numbers to be the change makers and pioneers of more sustainable practices in healthcare. Sustainable development through intentional practice is required and should be reflected in nursing education.

Global healthcare already contributes to harmful emissions that affect the growing population, and it is predicted that this may increase with further pandemics. The environmental impact of the COVID-19 pandemic can be seen in one recent study that identified Personal Protective Equipment (PPE) used by health professionals in the first six months of the COVID-19 pandemic alone created 106, 478 tonnes of carbon dioxide equivalents (eCO2) which equates to emissions from 244 return flights between London and New York (Rizan et al., 2019). Disposal of PPE by health professionals meant that the items were incinerated, causing an increase in greenhouse gas emissions (GHG); the public disposal of the same items resulted in oceans being contaminated by masks and gloves (The Ocean Conservancy, 2021).

Where sustainable advancements in practice occur, it is essential to reflect these in the classroom. Many Trusts have committed to the Royal College of Nursing's (RCN) 'gloves off' campaign (RCN, 2019) which has been endorsed by infection control teams and has proven that intentional use of personal protective equipment results in better patient outcomes, reduced financial cost and less environmental waste. Skills sessions that involve students assessing if they need to use gloves to carry out a procedure or intervention will not only allow students to reflect on their evidence-based practice but also provide authentic alignment with what is going on in healthcare settings.

Using backwards classroom design (Wiggins & McTighe, 2005)., educators can use the SDGs to frame any learning by constructing learning objectives that link to individual SDGs, or the climate crisis itself. One example would be to use the lens of sustainability (Goodman & East, 2014) and the SDGs when teaching the epidemiology of large-scale diseases such as cardiovascular disease (CVD) or cancer, conveying the interrelated nature of human and planetary health (Table 9.6).

Table 9.6 An Example of a Learning Objective and Aligned Assessment Question Using SDG 3

Topic	Learning objective/assessment
CVD, Cancer, Respiratory Disease	Critically evaluate the impact of climate change on cardiovascular disease and SDG Goal 3—Ensure healthy lives and promote wellbeing for all at all ages.
	Create a narrated PowerPoint/poster/portfolio demonstrating the environmental, financial and social impact and possible solutions for quality improvement

For post-qualification students, the topic and relevant SDG could be chosen to suit the workplace of the individuals, allowing for a collaborative approach to learning through co-design of the assessment and social relevance, as well as impactful change.

ACTIVITY

Prepare an activity to integrate sustainability into clinical teaching by encouraging students to identify and reflect on environmentally sustainable practices within a simulated hospital ward scenario.

- Identify these learning outcomes for the session. These may include:
- Recognise the environmental impact of healthcare practices.
- Identify opportunities for sustainable action in clinical environments.
- Reflect on the nurse's role in promoting environmental sustainability in practice.

Identify an appropriate learning environment for your session. Include common elements such as PPE, medication packaging, food waste, documentation systems, single-use plastics, and energy-consuming equipment.

Divide students into small groups. Ask them to conduct a 'Sustainable Ward Round', where they identify as many unsustainable practices or items as they can in the simulated environment.

Encourage each group to create a list of sustainable alternatives or actions that could be taken by nurses to improve the sustainability of care (e.g., reprocessing equipment, digital documentation, waste segregation, turning off unused equipment).

Facilitate a discussion on the proposed ideas. Encourage critical thinking about feasibility, patient safety, cost-effectiveness, and organisational culture.

Ask students to write a short reflection: *'How can I be a sustainability advocate in my future clinical practice'?*

PROMOTING SOCIAL EQUITY AND WELL-BEING IN HEALTHCARE

Nurses often work with the most vulnerable and marginalised communities and are key pioneers and leaders compared to other professions due to the trust that is placed in them and their proximity to vulnerable and marginalised communities that need their activism and advocacy (Butterfield et al., 2021). Fields et al. (2023) identified the urgent need for transformative nursing education in the face of severe global challenges to health and well-being, advocating for teaching methodology that raises critical awareness and thinking rather than the traditional transfer of information. It has therefore become a non-negotiable truth that nurses need to be empowered through education to explore their responsibility as global citizens to social, economic and environmental sustainability. Educators can use the SDGs along with the Social Determinants of Health (SDH), which are defined as the daily lived non-medical circumstances that affect population health (Upvall & Luzincourt, 2019). They refer to socioeconomic and environmental factors that impact on humans over their lifespan including age, ethnicity, religion, income and employment. The SDH are inextricably linked to the SDG targets and require an understanding of the importance of collaboration and partnerships between global health care organisations to drive policy and practice towards a more equitable world (Figure 9.3).

Nurses have an ethical responsibility to reduce health inequalities in marginalised groups. Teaching that includes the use of case studies about communities affected by extreme weather events, war or famine can be used to allow students to explore their beliefs and values. Awareness of

social inequalities at a local, national or international level could be explored using virtual placements or simulation, avoiding the need for environmentally and financially costly travel. Students could meet digitally from around the world and use reflective engagement in discussions with health care professionals and indigenous populations to cultivate their cultural awareness and competency to provide inclusive care.

Mitchell (2020) recommends the use of virtual learning platforms such as short films showcasing simulated patients to bridge the gap between exposure to real patients and theory-based sessions. Using an experiential learning approach, short videos can be created using actors to show real life sustainability issues, such

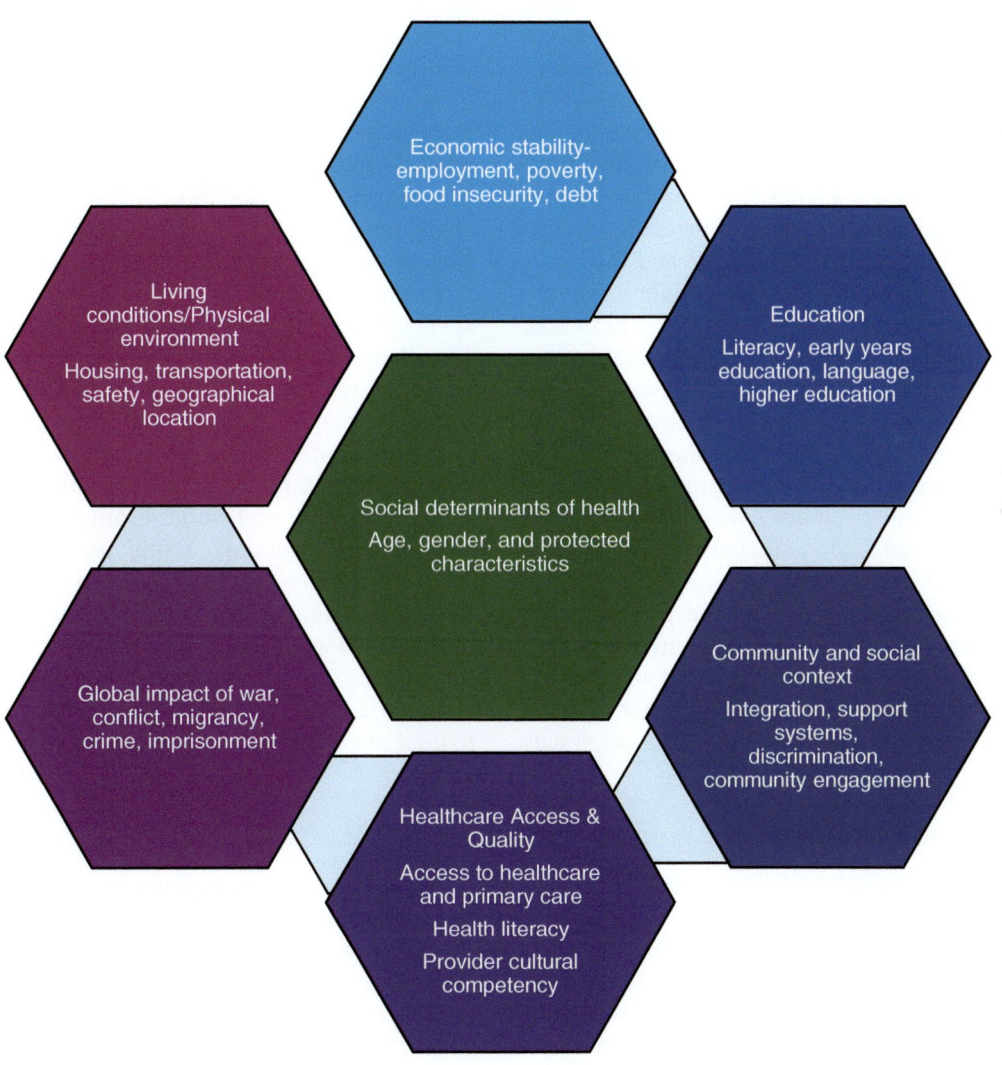

FIGURE 9.3 Social determinants of health

as understaffing, poor waste management, or the clinical effects of pollution on patients and staff. The thought of environmental and social harm requires educators to use scaffolding and carefully constructed activities to prevent a negative learning experience and demotivation. Educational innovation, such as exposure to simulated patient journeys or emergency planning situations, can enhance the acquisition of this skill set with the careful construction of psychological safety in the classroom (Daniels et al., 2021; De Rezendes et al., 2022)

The pre-registration nursing curriculum is prescribed and already densely packed, so it is sometimes hard to see where emerging topics can be addressed. Instead of stand-alone sustainability modules, it can be more helpful to view core nursing topics through the lens of sustainability (Goodman & East, 2014). Teaching clinical skills through a sustainable lens can bring an awareness of sustainable products and practices that do not harm human or planetary health. This may be by considering the lifecycle of an oxygen mask or syringe, or more considerate disposal of PPE or schemes for repurposing of single use plastics. Through analysis and enquiry, students could gain an understanding of how to critically evaluate the sustainability of clinical items used in healthcare and their part in promoting or lobbying to find sustainable alternatives.

Using the principles of sustainable practice (Table 9.2), these strategies can be applied to almost any disease process or condition. For example, cardiovascular disease (CVD) is one of the leading disease processes affected by climate change (Peters & Schneider, 2021). Mediterranean diets are known to be beneficial for the prevention of CVD but also have a demonstrably smaller environmental impact than the ultra-processed foods that contribute to the disease (Shrestha et al., 2024). Evidence-based health promotion around plant-based diets and the prevention of diabetes and heart disease considers the environmental, social and financial impact of keeping patients well and out of hospital and can enable nurses to confidently promote human and planetary health. Educators and professionals

alike should be confident that what is good for the planet will be good for patients. There is growing evidence base for the benefits of green spaces in improving health outcomes by reducing stress as a risk factor for many of the global diseases. (Markevych et al., 2017). Nurses themselves can reduce the impact of stress from their workplaces by connecting with nature more often (Middleton & Astell-Burt, 2023). Examples such as these can be used to give students the confidence to advocate for care pathways and green prescribing that improve health outcomes and reduce environmental impact, and to reflect on their own need to connect with nature. The integration of green spaces into nursing education itself is something to consider, as it is linked to improved student learning (Browning & Rigolon, 2019) and could improve the well-being of both educators and students.

Well-being and how it relates to patients and healthcare providers is a core value that education needs to address. Integrating well-being into nursing practice through self-care, disease prevention, health promotion, mental health first aid, and holistic care models is essential in preparing professionals to be resilient in an increasingly challenging world. Huss et al. (2020) argue for a humanistic approach to learning that is learner-centred and relies on reflection for growing self-awareness and change agency. Integration, rather than seeing sustainability as an adjunct, can begin in pre-registration training when students are first exploring their professional values and beliefs. To acquire foundational knowledge that includes an understanding of the global imperative and interplay between planetary and human health, students can consider local and real-world examples of unsustainable or iniquitous practices. Using problem-based learning, learners should be encouraged to be creative and collaborative about finding solutions. This could mean working in interprofessional teams from other disciplines. The focus on complex, multifactorial problems will require thinking critically and using problem solving skills that are relevant to their professional and personal beliefs.

INTERPROFESSIONAL LEADERSHIP

As the largest group of health professionals covering every aspect of clinical and public health provision, nursing leadership is essential to improving patient outcomes. The World Health Organisation recently recognised the need for investment into nurse education and the development of nurse leaders (WHO, 2020). The glass ceiling and barriers to nursing in leadership need to be broken down by

empowering nursing students to understand their own agency and potential to make sustainable changes through political mobilisation and advocacy.

Embedding sustainability as a core leadership skill is essential to curriculum design that fit well with contemporary leadership styles such as transformative, adaptive and compassionate leadership. McKimm &

Maclean (2020) make the argument for both health professionals and educators to adopt an 'eco-ethical leadership' style where the focus is on sustainability, justice and collaborative action.

Leadership modules need to equip students with the skills, knowledge and attitudes of future leaders in healthcare. Learning outcomes should reflect current issues such as global citizenship, environmental sustainability, digital literacy, wellbeing and resilience and nurse advocacy, which are core to modern nursing practice. Halverson (2021) notes that nursing education should be steered by modern events such as the pandemic, AI use and climate change. However, it can be argued that even early nursing leadership under Florence Nightingale was mindful of the link between planetary health and human health in her treatise on the need for good ventilation and light to promote health (Nightingale, 1859, cited in Butterfield et al., 2021). It is essential for nurses to know that they have influence over individuals and policy makers and that they are represented in consultative roles in many global institutions and groups, e.g. Health Care Without Harm, WHO International Council of Nurses. This need for nurses to realise their potential as change agents is clearly linked to better patient care (Rafferty, 2018).

Sustainability was identified by this author as a core leadership quality in a final year module and reflected in the learning outcomes, course content and assessment. The aim of the module was to support students in developing the skills, knowledge and understanding required to be future leaders in healthcare (NMC, 2018b). Outcomes that ask students to consider the political, social, financial and environmental impact of healthcare on patient and health outcomes would address the educational requirement to understand healthcare legislation and policy in the context of the climate crisis. Another important outcome would be translating this understanding into agency so that students could contribute to innovation in care through the application of quality improvement and sustainable practice. The way to do this would be for the students to participate in activities that help them build confidence, resilience and self-awareness in working with others and give them opportunities to develop insight into real-world problems affecting the profession (Table 9.7). Using backwards design (Wiggins & McTighe, 2005) activities can be mapped to these outcomes. It is important, however, to move beyond outcomes and aims and be able to evaluate the impact on students. Assessment for learning needs to be constructively aligned with the objectives, but include the ability for students to gain self-awareness through reflection and stated intention. The NMC states that nurses must provide leadership through an awareness of their own behaviours and values (NMC, 2018a). Reflective practice is mandated by the NMC in the revalidation process to retain professional registration. Tsimane & Downing (2020) identify self-reflection as a core tool in transformative learning, which should be student-centred, encouraging them to question the status quo and reach a deeper understanding of their own values and beliefs that will guide their practice. The Describe, Interpret, Evaluate, and Plan (DIEP) academic reflection framework (Boud et al., 1985) was used by this author to frame an assessment that asked students to reflect on a leadership topic from the course. Students could choose from more traditional leadership attributes as well as more current

Table 9.7 Constructive Alignment Between Learning Outcomes, Activities, and Assessment

Learning outcome	Activity	Assessment topic
Demonstrate a critical understanding of the environmental, economic and financial impact of health care and its impact on patient and health outcomes.	Case study of a patient journey using the triple bottom line to evaluate impact in all three domains on the patient and resources used.	Sustainable leadership and improving health outcomes through quality improvement.
Demonstrate confidence, resilience, and self-awareness in working with others, and develop a critical insight and strategy for meeting own ongoing professional development needs.	Co-design a motivational talk about a wicked problem that affects nursing and present as a group to peers.	Sustainable lives: maintaining wellbeing and resilience in the workplace.
Contribute to the leadership of change in clinical practice to promote innovation in care with an understanding of quality improvement models and sustainable practice in healthcare.	Consider the excess use of personal protective equipment and single use plastics in clinical skills teaching using quality improvement methodology to find solutions that can be tested in the classroom and in practice.	Environmental sustainability in healthcare: becoming an agent of change.

considerations, such as wellbeing and resilience and environmental sustainability in healthcare.

Economic sustainability requires the delivery of cost-effective healthcare and should involve budget management and an awareness of resource scarcity. Nurse leaders can feel ill-equipped in this aspect of their role and require financial literacy skills to be sustainable (Ismail et al., 2025). An education that addresses the need for financial sustainability will ultimately empower nurses to use those resources more efficiently, reducing unnecessary costs and practising sustainable budgeting. The use of case studies that compare the costs of interventions and healthcare episodes such as bed days and prolonged hospital stays, with more integrated care in the community, would provide the students real life examples of the savings that could be made when sustainable practice is applied to their practice. The Centre for Sustainable Healthcare provides many examples of quality improvement initiatives from practice that have cut the cost of care provided in a range of settings from the ED to community care. Using what is termed the sustainable quality improvement model (SusQI), students could study a particular care pathway and look for carbon hotspots such as multiple trips to hospital or wasted medications. Having identified the problems and causes e.g. inefficient appointment systems, they can apply the principles of sustainability and measure the resulting cost savings after the intervention. Each case study should also address social sustainability issues, such as equity of access and addressing healthcare disparities. Effective leadership can drive sustainable practices as nurse leaders should advocate for sustainability and social responsibility. This requires interprofessional collaboration of diverse teams that could be led by nurses with an understanding of diversity and inclusion.

BUILDING AND SUSTAINING COMMUNITY PARTNERSHIPS

Education for sustainable development (ESD) (United Nations Educational, Scientific and Cultural Organisation [UNESCO], 2020) has identified three essential areas for improvement that align with the acquisition of sustainable competencies. These are ways of thinking, practising and being. Recent consensus papers on ESD from the Council of Deans (2023) and the Association for Medical Education in Europe (Shaw et al., 2021) have begun to shape some sector agreed principles and practices for education providers that demonstrate a commitment to sustainability and the SDGs with the aim that all learners can acquire the knowledge and skill sets needed to promote sustainable development as global citizens and protect the future of the planet. The Quality Assurance Agency for Higher Education (2024) suggests that educators consider the inclusivity and environmental sustainability in the creation and development of learning resources as well as the learning environment itself.

Translated into educational practice, this would mean empowering students with the ability to think critically about the future and the resilience of healthcare. It goes beyond aims and objectives and needs to be operationalised in a way that has an impact on patient outcomes and practitioner behaviours. Much like the NHS, it will require interdisciplinary collaborations between disciplines not normally associated with healthcare education. This could involve nursing students working with engineering students or geographers, or it could also see educational institutes forge links with industries that produce the items used in practice. To be transformative, Education for Sustainable Learning (ESL) may need to be disruptive and use problem-based, pedagogical approaches to tackle real world and 'wicked' problems that stimulate a sense of justice in students and a belief in their own agency.

Part of the nursing role will be to help build resilient communities with shared care planning, and this will require the acquisition of sustainable competencies based on sustainable principles in practice. Awareness of the paradox of a health system that should promote health and prevent harm yet contributes to the environmental risk in such a significant way should be embedded into nursing education to prepare the profession with the skills to practice sustainably and create a resilient health service for future generations.

This requires knowledge of what is known as a circular economy, which is a sustainable healthcare model driven by increasing the life cycle of products through recycling, reducing and repurposing (Figure 9.4).

By raising awareness of the circular economy as well as treating the effects of this on populations, the nursing profession can have a profound and sustainable impact on the future of the planet and the survival of humanity. Teaching sessions where students consider the life cycle of commonly used clinical items in the face of future resource scarcity have been shown to be impactful (Richardson et al., 2014) and have the potential to include interprofessional collaboration with other disciplines, such as engineers and design students. Clinical skills and simulation contribute to a large amount of waste, and there are some small-scale areas of best practice where attempts are already being

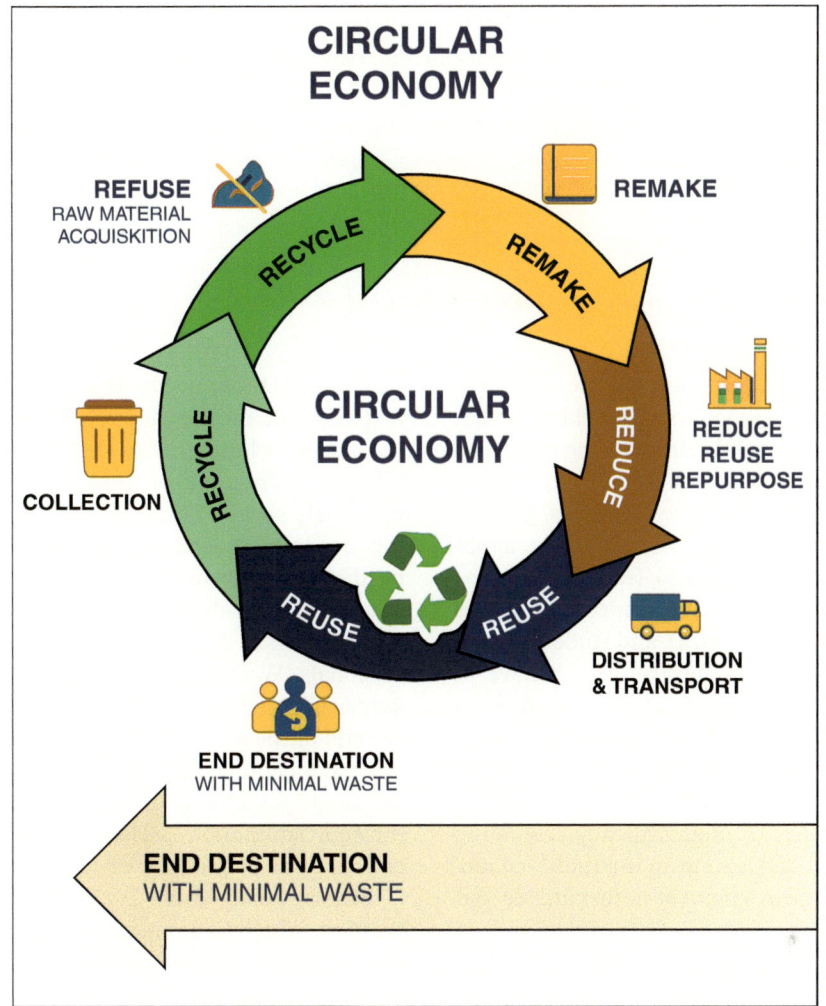

FIGURE 9.4   Circular economy and life cycle assessment

made to reduce the carbon footprint of this type of teaching (Alyeddin et al., 2022).

Leading by example, this author has seen firsthand the environmental impact of clinical skills teaching in the contents of the waste bins after each teaching session. The waste created in clinical skills centres is usually sent for incineration as if it were contaminated, a significant contribution to air pollution and greenhouse gas emissions. This has led to the formation of the Clinical Skills Sustainability Project Group (CSSPG). A collaborative project between students, educators, professional services, Trust partners and the Estates Team at a university. Final year nursing students and educators were asked to consider waste produced by clinical skills sessions and the environmental, financial and social impact of disposal by

using sustainable quality improvement methodology and the four-step approach seen in Table 9.8.

The contents of the yellow clinical waste bins in the classrooms were identified through audit as including:

- items that could be repurposed/ reused e.g. syringes, and suction catheters.

- items that could be recycled e.g. paper packaging.

- items that were incorrectly disposed of e.g. sharps, coffee cups, domestic waste.

- items that had not been used at all.

Students used root cause analysis to understand why this happens, identifying human habits, lack of sanctions

Table 9.8 The Four Stages of Sustainable Quality Improvement (SuSQI)

Step one: setting the goals	What will be the environmental, financial and social benefits of reducing the waste produced in teaching sessions?
Step two: studying the system	Identify the causes of the problem and the carbon hotspots that occur
Step three: design the improvement	Use focus groups, climate cafes and evidence-based inquiry to determine what will drive change and what small acts of change are feasible.
Step four: measure the impact	Measure the impact of the changes in terms of the eCO_2, financial cost savings and social benefits.

Source: Adapted from Stanford et al., (2023) and the Centre for Sustainable Healthcare Model.

and the time constraints during sessions as some of the reasons for the unsustainable behaviours. They then considered possible solutions that would drive change, such as induction training, rationing of items, smarter equipment lists and improved access to paper recycling bins. Raising awareness of the correct disposal of items and the application of the sustainable principles to teaching sessions would mean that the educational setting reflects the values of the Net Zero mandate (NHSE, 2022), and students could make informed decisions about the way they behave in classrooms. Co-creation and collaboration with students are essential for the success of education for sustainable development. Other student-led initiatives, such as the Planetary Health Report Card (PHRC), can give students a sense of their own agency through critically evaluating the learning environment and lead to an international recognition that the learning environment is sustainable and future-proof.

The delivery of sustainable education needs alignment with the wider University's strategic visions of sustainability and requires collaboration with a variety of teams outside of academia. Educators and students can collaborate with estates and procurement teams to ensure that these processes become more streamlined and sustainable. Something as simple as an equipment list with intentional use of items and the principle of rationing could result in financial and environmental savings whilst benefiting the students' awareness of resource scarcity. Connections with other faculties, business schools and industry could be forged to optimise the potential of digital technologies and AI and industry innovation and advancements that reduce the environmental impact of teaching and encourage shared learning. This requires consideration of the economy of scale and the impact of these ideas on staff time and resources.

Nurses are central to building community partnerships with their patients that promote sustainability in healthcare. Through an understanding of the health needs of the communities they serve, they can foster collaborations

that address those needs. This is known as service learning and requires meaningful reflection on global citizenship (Brown & Schmidt, 2016). Exposure to diverse communities in simulation and AI-driven education can facilitate a safe space to explore inequity in care provision and the need to understand the diverse and specific social needs. The construction of simulated scenarios using live simulated patients representing marginalised groups has been proven to enhance the understanding of health professionals (Walkowska et al., 2023), but also requires facilitated reflection in the form of debriefing and synthesis at the end of the session (Ryoo & Ha, 2015).

Educational initiatives that use experiential learning, allowing students to visit diverse communities, whether through simulation, virtual or elective placements, can enhance the acquisition of identifying as a global citizen (Morrison-Beedy et al., 2021). See previous Chapter 8 by Boulton, which illustrates a low carbon and highly impactful teaching environment where the learner is a global citizen and nursing has no boundaries. The use of activities using reflective writing, social events and walking tours can be used to expand students' understanding of the use of resources in different locations and experience of diverse cultures. This type of creative education outside the classroom and in green spaces can be replicated locally and nationally without the need for excessive travel and cost.

Developing the skills to use social prescribing, where health professionals refer patients to non-clinical services in the community that support health and wellbeing and reduce the burden on clinical services, is an essential requirement of sustainable modern practice. The Government has proposed a new approach in the Neighbourhood Health Guidelines (NHSE, 2025) that aims to address the problem of a population that suffers from complex and long-term ill health in their own homes (Darzi, 2024). The King's Fund highlights that the impact of social prescribing on marginalised or disadvantaged communities is amplified, particularly for those with long-term conditions (Chikwira & Arobi, 2025). Raising awareness of the evidence base for initiatives such as green spaces and community groups lies within the gift of educators and presents an alternative to relying on traditional medical pathways that carry larger carbon footprints.

Nurses are the largest healthcare occupation and trusted sources of information for the public and policymakers. They work with diverse population groups and provide safe, therapeutic environments, especially amongst disadvantaged communities. Using evidence-based practice to inform their work and translating the science into actions, nurses can communicate the rationale for patient interventions and practices in an understandable way. Research nurses and advanced clinical practitioners may be engaged in inquiry about the link between health and the environment. The Code (NMC, 2018a) requires that the profession reduce harm, and this must include exposure to environmental health hazards caused by healthcare and climate change. Through transformative education that uses sustainable pedagogies, nurses can be empowered with the agency to change to sustainable practice in their homes, workplaces, communities and the wider world.

KEY TAKE-HOME POINTS

- Nurses are central to climate-resilient healthcare and must be equipped through transformative education to advocate for environmental, social, and economic sustainability.

- Embedding sustainability into nursing curricula supports global health goals, reduces healthcare's carbon footprint, and enhances future workforce readiness.

- Interprofessional collaboration, reflective practice, and inclusive teaching methods are essential to addressing eco-anxiety, inequity, and real-world health system challenges.

CPD REFLECTIVE QUESTIONS

1. How does my current teaching or practice prepare nurses to act on the sustainability challenges facing health systems today?

2. In what ways can I use the Sustainable Development Goals to enhance critical thinking and global awareness in nursing students?

3. What role can I play in modelling sustainable leadership and fostering resilience among students and colleagues?

4. How can I integrate experiential, inclusive, and values-based activities that build sustainable thinking into my own teaching or curriculum design?

REFERENCES

Álvarez-Nieto, C., Álvarez-García, C., Parra-Anguita, L., Sanz-Martos, S., & López-Medina, I. M. (2022). Effectiveness of scenario-based learning and augmented reality for nursing students' attitudes and awareness toward climate change and sustainability. *BMC Nursing*, 21(1), 1–245. https://pmc.ncbi.nlm.nih.gov/articles/PMC9439938.

Alyeddin, W., Peters, S., Zembrzycka, A. A., Hudson, L., & Tun, S. (2022). Bleeding green: sustainability in practice in a clinical skills teaching laboratory. *The Journal of Climate Change and Health*, 8, 100149.

Boud, D., Keogh, R., & Walker, D. (eds.) (1985). *Reflection: Turning Experience into Learning*. Oxford: Taylor & Francis Group, ProQuest Ebook Central.

Boudreau, C., & Rhéaume, A. (2024). Impact of the work environment on nurse outcomes: a mediation analysis. *Western Journal of Nursing Research*, 46(3), 210–218. https://doi.org/10.1177/01939459241230369.

Brown, J. M., & Schmidt, N. A. (2016). Service–learning in undergraduate nursing education: where is the reflection? *Journal of Professional Nursing*, 32(1), 48–53. https://doi.org/10.1016/j.profnurs.2015.05.001.

Browning, M. H. E. M., & Rigolon, A. (2019). School green space and its impact on academic performance: a systematic literature review. *International Journal of Environmental Research and Public Health*, 16(3), 429. https://www.proquest.com/scholarly-journals/school-green-space-impact-on-academic-performance/docview/2328965891/se-2?accountid=11862.

Butterfield, P., Leffers, J., & Vásquez, M. D. (2021). Nursing's pivotal role in global climate action. *BMJ*, 373, n1049. https://librarysearch.kcl.ac.uk/permalink/44KCL_INST/jp52pk/cdi_pubmedcentral_primary_oai_pubmedcentral_nih_gov_8201521.

Chicca, J., & Shallenbarger, T. (2020). Fostering inclusive clinical learning environments using a psychological safety lens. *Teaching and Learning in Nursing*, 15, 226–232. https://doi.org/10.1016/j.teln.2020.03.002.

Chikwira, L., & Arobi, N. A. (2025). Shared leadership is crucial to integrating and maximising social prescribing in neighbourhood health. *The King's Fund*, https://www.kingsfund.org.uk/insight-and-analysis/blogs/shared-leadership-integrating-maximising-social-prescribing-neighbourhood-health.

Cornish, J. (2023). Learning about sustainability in class can lead to improvements in care. *Nursing Times*. https://www.nursingtimes.net/opinion/learning-about-sustainability-in-class-can-lead-to-improvements-in-care-02-08-2023/. Accessed: (1 April 2025).

Council of Deans (2023). Education for sustainable healthcare within UK pre-registration curricula for allied health professions. Council of Deans. https://www.councilofdeans.org.uk/wp-content/uploads/2023/12/ES-curricula-guidance-CoDH-version_SM-final-no-links.pdf. Accessed: (3 April 2025).

Daniels, A. L., Morse, C., & Breman, R. (2021). Psychological safety in simulation-based prelicensure nursing education: a narrative review. *Nurse Educator*, 46(5), E99–E102. https://doi.org/10.1097/NNE.0000000000001057.

Darzi, A. (2024). *Independent Investigation of the National Health Service in England*. Department of Health and Social Care. https://www.gov.uk/government/publications/independent-investigation-of-the-nhs-in-england.

De Rezende, H., Vitorio, A. M. F., Morais, A. S., Garzin, A. C. A., Nicole, A. G., Quadrado, E. R. S., de Andrade Lourencao, D. C., & Martins, M. S. (2022). Effectiveness of educational interventions to develop patient safety knowledge, skills, behaviours and attitudes in undergraduate nursing students: a systematic review protocol. *BMJ Open*, 12(3), e058888. https://www.proquest.com/scholarly-journals/effectiveness-educational-interventions-develop/docview/2637328492/se-2?accountid=11862.

Fields, L., Moroney, T., Perkiss, S., & Dean, B.A., (2023). Enlightening and empowering students to take action: embedding sustainability into nursing curriculum. *Journal of Professional Nursing*, 49, 57–63. https://doi.org/10.1016/j.profnurs.2023.09.001.

Goodman, B. (2011). The need for a 'sustainability curriculum' in nurse education. *Nurse Education Today*, 31(8), 733–737. https://doi.org/10.1016/j.nedt.2010.12.010.

Goodman, B., & East, L. (2014). The 'sustainability lens': a framework for nurse education that is 'fit for the future'. *Nurse Education Today*, 34(1), 100–103. https://doi.org/10.1016/j.nedt.2013.02.010.

Greener NHS (n.d.). Reducing unnecessary cannulation at Charing Cross Hospital. https://www.england.nhs.uk/greenernhs/whats-already-happening/reducing-unnecessary-cannulation-at-charing-cross-hospital/. Accessed: (1 April 2025).

Halverson, K. L. (2021). Sailing in the winds of change: navigating the future of nursing education. *The Journal of Nursing Education*, 60(12), 661–667. https://doi.org/10.3928/01484834-20211102-02.

Healthcare Without Harm (HWH) (2019). Health Care's Climate Footprint: How the health sector contributes to the global climate crisis and opportunities for action. HWH & ARUP. https://global.noharm.org/resources/health-care-climate-footprint-report. Accessed: (2 April 2025).

Huss, N., Ikiugu, M. N., Hackett, F., Sheffield, P. E., Palipane, N., & Groome, J. (2020). Education for sustainable health care: from learning to professional practice. *Medical Teacher*, 42(10), 1097–1101. https://doi.org/10.1080/0142159X.2020.1797998.

Independent Group of Scientists appointed by the Secretary-General (2023). Global Sustainable Development Report 2023: Times of crisis, times of change: Science for accelerating transformations to sustainable development (United Nations). https://sdgs.un.org/gsdr/gsdr2023. Accessed: (1 April 2025).

Ismail, H. A., Kotp, M. H., Basyouny, H. A. A., Abd Elmoaty, A. E. E., Hendy, A., Ibrahim, R. K., Abdelaliem, S. M. F., Hendy, A., & Aly, M. A. (2025). Empowering nurse leaders: leveraging financial management practices to foster sustainable healthcare – a mixed-methods study. *BMC Nursing*, 24, 335. https://doi.org/10.1186/s12912-025-02981-6.

Issa, R., Forbes, C., Baker, C., Morgan, M., Womersley, K., Klaber, B., Mulcahy, E., & Stancliffe, R. (2024). Sustainability is critical for future proofing the NHS. *BMJ*, 385, e079259. https://www.proquest.com/scholarly-journals/sustainability-is-critical-future-proofing-nhs/docview/3041593349/se-2?accountid=11862.

Leffers, J., Levy, R. M., Nicholas, P. K., & Sweeney, C. F. (2017). Mandate for the nursing profession to address climate change through nursing education. *Journal of Nursing Scholarship*, 49(6), 679–687. https://www.proquest.com/scholarly-journals/mandate-nursing-profession-address-climate-change/docview/1957086554/se-2?accountid=11862.

Levett-Jones, T., Catling, C., Cheer, S., Fields, L., Foster, A., Maguire, J., Mcintyre, E., Moroney OAM, T., Pich, J., Pitt, V., & Whiteing, N. (2024). Achieving consensus on the essential knowledge and skills needed by nursing students to promote planetary health and sustainable healthcare: a Delphi study. *Journal of Advanced Nursing*, 00, 1–19. https://doi.org/10.1111/jan.16229.

López-Medina, I. M., Álvarez-Nieto, C., Grose, J., Elsbernd, A., Huss, N., Huynen, M., & Richardson, J. (2019). Competencies on environmental health and pedagogical approaches in the nursing curriculum: a systematic review of the literature. *Nurse Education in Practice*, 37, 1–8. https://www.proquest.com/scholarly-journals/competencies-on-environmental-health-pedagogical/docview/2239608571/se-2?accountid=11862.

Markevych, I., Schoierer, J., Hartig, T., Chudnovsky, A., Hystad, P., Dzhambov, A. M., De Vries, S., Triguero-Mas, M., Brauer, M., Nieuwenhuijsen, M. J., & Lupp, G. (2017). Exploring pathways linking greenspace to health: theoretical and methodological guidance. *Environmental Research*, 158, 301–317. https://doi.org/10.1016/j.envres.2017.06.028.

McKimm, J., & McLean, M. (2020). Rethinking health professions' education leadership: developing 'eco-ethical' leaders for a more sustainable world and future. *Medical Teacher*, 42(8), 855–860. https://doi.org/10.1080/0142159X.2020.1748877.

Middleton, R., & Astell-Burt, T. (2023). Nurses and nature; does green space make a difference? *Journal of Clinical Nursing*, 32(15–16), 4214–4216. https://onlinelibrary.wiley.com/share/ZHIVNN8DDCCCI2TBKDJY?target=10.1111/jocn.16697.

Mitchell, A. (2020). Pandemic inspires innovative use of virtual simulation to teach practical skills. *British Journal of Nursing (Mark Allen Publishing)*, 29(20), 1214–1214. https://doi.org/10.12968/bjon.2020.29.20.1214.

Morrison-Beedy, D., Jenssen, U., Bochenek, J., Bowles, W., King, T. S., & Mathisen, L. (2021). Building global nursing citizens through curricular integration of sustainable development goals within an international clinical experience. *Nurse Educator*. 46(1), 10–12. https://dx.doi.org/10.1097/NNE.0000000000000831.

Mortimer, F. (2010). The sustainable physician. *Clinical Medicine*, 10(2), 110–111. https://www.proquest.com/scholarly-journals/sustainable-physician/docview/500884559/se-2?accountid=11862.

Mortimer, F., Isherwood, J., Wilkinson, A., & Vaux, E. (2018). Sustainability in quality improvement: redefining value. *Future Healthcare Journal*, 5(2), 88–93. https://pmc.ncbi.nlm.nih.gov/articles/PMC6502556.

National Health Service England (NHSE) (2014). Bringing lean to life: making processes flow in healthcare. NHSE. https://www.england.nhs.uk/improvement-hub/wp-content/uploads/sites/44/2017/11/Bringing-Lean-to-Life.pdf. Accessed: (3 April 2025).

National Health Service England (NHSE) (2022). Delivering a NetZero National Health Service 2022. NHSE/NHSI. https://www.england.nhs.uk/greenernhs/wp-content/uploads/sites/51/2022/07/B1728-delivering-a-net-zero-nhs-july-2022.pdf. Accessed: (2 April 2025).

National Health Service England (NHSE) (2025). Neighbourhood health guidelines 2025/26. NHSE. https://www.england.nhs.uk/long-read/neighbourhood-health-guidelines-2025/26/. Accessed: (2 April 2025).

Neal-Boylan, L., Breakey, S., & Nicholas, P. K. (2019). Integrating climate change topics into nursing curricula. *The Journal of Nursing Education*, 58(6), 364–368. https://www.proquest.com/scholarly-journals/integrating-climate-change-topics-into-nursing/docview/2233828569/se-2?accountid=11862.

Nursing and Midwifery Council (NMC) (2018a). The Code: Professional Standards of practice and behaviour for nurses, midwives and nursing associates. NMC. [Online]. https://www.nmc.org.uk/globalassests/sitedocument/nmc-publications/nmc-code.pdf Accessed: (2 April 2025).

Nursing and Midwifery Council (NMC) (2018b). *Standards of proficiency for registered nurses*. London: NMC. https://www.nmc.org.uk/standards/standards-for-nurses/standards-of-proficiency-for-registered-nurses/. Accessed: (10 December 2025).

Nursing and Midwifery Council (NMC) (April 2023). Standards for education and training: Standards framework for nursing and midwifery education. NMC. https://www.nmc.org/standards-for-education-and-training/standards-framework-for-nursing-and-midwifery-education/ Accessed: (2 April 2025).

Ocean Conservancy. (March 2021). Pandemic Pollution: the rising tide of plastic PPE. Ocean Conservancy. https://oceanconservancy.org/wp-content/uploads/2021/03/FINAL-Ocean-Conservancy-PPE-Report-March-2021.pdf. Accessed: (3 April 2025).

Peters, A., & Schneider, A. (2021). Cardiovascular risks of climate change. *Nature Reviews Cardiology*, 18(1), 1–2. https://www.proquest.com/scholarly-journals/cardiovascular-risks-climate-change/docview/2473191850/se-2?accountid=11862.

Rafferty, A. M. (2018). Nurses as change agents for a better future in health care: the politics of drift and dilution. *Health Economics, Policy and Law*, 13(3–4), 475–491. https://www.proquest.com/scholarly-journals/nurses-as-change-agents-better-future-health-care/docview/2055229588/se-2?accountid=11862.

Richardson, J., Grose, J., Jackson, B., Gill, J. L., Sadeghian, H. B., Hertel, J., & Kelsey, J. (2014). Effect of climate change and resource scarcity on health care. *Nursing Standard*, 28(45), 44–49. https://journals.rcni.com//doi/abs/10.7748/ns.28.45.44.e8415.

Rizan, C., Reed, M., & Bhutta, M. F. (2021). Environmental impact of personal protective equipment distributed for use by health and social care services in England in the first six months of the COVID-19 pandemic. *Journal of the Royal Society of Medicine*, 114(5), 250–263. https://doi.org/10.1177/01410768211001583.

Royal College of Nursing (RCN) (2019). How to reduce glove use. RCN. https://www.rcn.org.uk/magazines/Action/2022/Jan/How-to-reduce-glove-use-170122. Accessed: (2 April 2025).

RYOO, E. N., & HA, E.-H. (2015). The importance of debriefing in simulation-based learning: comparison between debriefing and no debriefing. *Computers, Informatics, Nursing*, 33(12), 538–545. https://doi.org/10.1097/CIN.0000000000000194.

Sawyer, M. (2020). Why all health professionals should be carbon literate and practise sustainably. *BMJ Opinion*, 20 Nov. https://seesustainability.co.uk/blog/f/why-should-all-health-professionals-be-carbon-literate. Accessed: [2 April 2025].

Shaw, E., Walpole, S., McLean, M., Alvarez-Nieto, C., Barna, S., Bazin, K., Behrens, G., Chase, H., Duane, B., El Omrani, O., & Elf, M. (2021). AMEE consensus statement: planetary health and education for sustainable healthcare. *Medical Teacher*, 43(3), 272–286. https://doi.org/10.1080/0142159X.2020.1860207.

Shrestha, P., Nukala, S. K., Islam, F., Badgery-Parker, T., & Foo, F. (2024). The co-benefits of climate change mitigation strategies on cardiovascular health: a systematic review. *The Lancet Regional Health. Western Pacific*, 48, 101098. https://pmc.ncbi.nlm.nih.gov/articles/PMC11458989/.

Stanford, V., Barna, S., Gupta, D., & Mortimer, F. (2023). Teaching skills for sustainable health care. *The Lancet. Planetary Health*, 7(1), e64–e67. https://www.thelancet.com/journals/lanplh/article/PIIS2542-5196(22)00330-8/fulltext.

The Quality assurance Agency for Higher Education (2024). UK Quality Code for Higher Education. [Online] UK Quality Code for Higher Education 2024. Accessed: (2 April 2025).

Tsimane, T. A., & Downing, C. (2020). Transformative learning in nursing education: a concept analysis. *International Journal of Nursing Sciences*, 7(1), 91–98. https://doi.org/10.1016/j.ijnss.2019.12.006.

Tun, S., & Martin. T. (2022). *Education for Sustainable Healthcare – A Curriculum for the UK*. London, UK: Medical Schools Council.

United Nations (2016). *Transforming Our World: The 2030 Agenda for Sustainable Development*. United Nations. https://sdgs.un.org/publications/transforming-our-world-2030-agenda-sustainable-development-17981.

United Nations Educational, Scientific and Cultural Organisation (UNESCO) (2020). *Education for Sustainable Development: A Roadmap*. UNESCO. https://doi.org/10.54675/YFRE1448.

Upvall, M. J., & Luzincourt, G. (2019). Global citizens, healthy communities: integrating the sustainable development goals into the nursing curriculum. *Nursing Outlook*, 67(6): 649–657. https://doi.org/10.1016/j.outlook.2019.04.004.

Walkowska, A., Przymuszała, P., Marciniak-Stępak, P., Nowosadko, M., & Baum, E. (2023). Enhancing cross-cultural competence of medical and healthcare students with the use of simulated patients–a systematic review. *International Journal of Environmental Research and Public Health*, 20(3), 2505. https://www.proquest.com/scholarly-journals/enhancing-cross-cultural-competence-medical/docview/2774908197/se-2?accountid=11862.

Ward, A., Heart, D., Richards, C., Bayliss, L. T., Holmes, M., Keogh, S., & Best, O. (2022). Reimagining the role of nursing education in emissions reduction. *Teaching and Learning in Nursing*, 17(4), 410–416. https://doi.org/10.1016/j.teln.2022.02.003.

Watts, N., Amann, M., Arnell, N., Ayeb-Karlsson, S., Belesova, K., Boykoff, M., Byass, P., Cai, W., Campbell-Lendrum, D., Capstick, S., & Chambers, J. (2019). The 2019 report of the lancet countdown on health and climate change: ensuring that the health of a child born today is not defined by a changing climate. *The Lancet (British Edition)*, 394(10211), 1836–1878. https://doi.org/10.1016/S0140-6736(19)32596-6.

Wiggins, G. P., & McTighe, J. (2005). Understanding by design. Association for Supervision & Curriculum Development. https://files.ascd.org/staticfiles/ascd/pdf/siteASCD/publications/UbD_WhitePaper0312.pdf. Accessed: (2 April 2025).

World Health Organisation (WHO) (2020). *State of the World's Nursing 2020: Investing in Education, Jobs and Leadership*. WHO https://iris.who.int/bitstream/handle/10665/331677/9789240003279-eng.pdf?sequence=1.

World Health Organisation (WHO) (2024). *Communicating on Climate Change and Health: Toolkit for Health Professionals*. WHO. https://www.who.int/publications/i/item/9789240090224.

Future Directions in Transformative Nursing Education

Barry Hill[1] and Aby Mitchell[2]

[1] *School of Healthcare and Nursing Sciences (HNS), Faculty of Health and Wellbeing, Northumbria University, UK*
[2] *Florence Nightingale Faculty for Nursing, Midwifery and Palliative care, King's College London, UK*

AIM

To explore the future directions of transformative nursing education, focusing on emerging innovations, sector-wide challenges, and strategic opportunities that shape the development of future-ready nursing professionals.

LEARNING OUTCOMES

By the end of this chapter, readers will be able to:

1. Identify and critically appraise emerging trends and innovations that influence nursing education globally.

2. Analyse current and future challenges affecting the design and delivery of transformative nursing curricula.

3. Explore strategic opportunities to advance educational equity, sustainability, and technological integration in nursing.

4. Formulate forward-thinking, practice-based actions to support continued transformation in nursing education.

CHAPTER INTRODUCTION

Transformative nursing education continues to develop in response to global health priorities, technological advancement, demographic change, and growing workforce expectations. As nurse educators and practice leaders, we face a future shaped by complexity and uncertainty, but also one that offers unparalleled potential to strengthen the preparation and ongoing development of nurses.

This chapter brings together the core ideas explored throughout the book and looks forward, anticipating how the next decade may reshape the landscape of nursing education. It considers how educational innovation, national and global policy priorities, digital transformation, and the evolving expectations of society will continue to influence how nurses are educated and supported. With growing pressures on health systems and rapid technological change, nurse educators must not only adapt but also lead change, ensuring that curricula, pedagogy, and professional values remain aligned with the demands of future healthcare.

The chapter is structured to examine key emerging trends and innovations that are already beginning to redefine pedagogical approaches, assessment, and student engagement. It also addresses the practical and strategic challenges that educators, institutions, and regulatory bodies must confront in delivering sustainable and equitable nursing education. The final section offers a reflective call to action, emphasising the shared responsibility of educators, leaders, and learners to ensure that nursing education remains inclusive, future-focused, and grounded in the values of compassion, accountability, and justice.

EMERGING TRENDS AND INNOVATIONS

The future of nursing education is characterised by profound shifts in pedagogy, technology, and expectations of the profession. As the health and education sectors confront the challenges of increasing demand, complexity, and inequality, nurse educators are being called upon to take a more adaptive and transformative role. No longer is it sufficient to prepare students for static roles within healthcare; instead, we must educate nurses for future-readiness, roles that are collaborative, digitally fluent, ethically aware, and socially engaged.

ARTIFICIAL INTELLIGENCE (AI) IN EDUCATION

AI continues to gain traction in higher education, including nursing, by enabling responsive, data-driven, and personalised learning experiences. Adaptive learning platforms, such as intelligent tutoring systems, dynamically adjust content difficulty and pacing based on a student's individual performance. For example, systems like Carnegie Learning or Squirrel AI have demonstrated improved student outcomes by delivering tailored problem-solving scenarios (Aleven et al., 2016). Predictive analytics are increasingly being used to flag early signs of disengagement or academic risk, allowing for earlier, targeted intervention.

However, AI adoption in nurse education must be approached critically. Concerns remain around algorithmic bias, the dehumanisation of learning, and the potential erosion of the student–educator relationship. Moreover, reliance on AI may widen inequalities if digital literacy and access are not prioritised. Nurse educators must therefore act as facilitators who integrate AI judiciously, upholding human-centred values and professional judgement (Topol, 2019).

IMMERSIVE TECHNOLOGIES: VR, AR, AND MR

Immersive technologies are becoming essential tools for creating realistic and emotionally resonant learning experiences. VR, AR, and MR allow students to 'step into' complex clinical scenarios without the risks associated with live patient care. These technologies are especially effective in bridging the gap between theory and practice by enabling learners to rehearse, reflect, and repeat situations in a safe environment.

For instance, VR platforms such as Body Interact allow learners to manage virtual trauma patients in real time, making critical decisions under pressure. MR applications like HoloPatient simulate ward environments, offering opportunities to practice prioritisation, escalation, and team leadership. AR, on the other hand, overlays real-time information on physical settings, such as anatomical visualisations using Microsoft HoloLens, enhancing memory retention and clinical reasoning (Padilha et al., 2019). Table 10.1 summarises a few examples of technology, their application, and proposed benefits.

These technologies also support remote learning, making them highly valuable in a post-pandemic educational landscape. However, issues of cost, access, and faculty preparedness must be addressed to ensure equitable implementation.

COMPETENCY-BASED EDUCATION

Competency-based education (CBE) represents a significant departure from traditional time-based curricula. It allows learners to progress once they demonstrate mastery, rather than simply completing a set number of clinical hours or attending a fixed sequence of modules (Frank et al., 2010). This model promotes learner agency and recognises prior learning, which is particularly relevant for return-to-practice nurses, internationally educated nurses, and those entering advanced roles.

CBE aligns well with the Nursing and Midwifery Council's emphasis on proficiency-based outcomes, enabling alignment between university education and practice requirements. Digital portfolios, clinical dashboards, and mobile competency tracking apps are increasingly used to streamline assessment and reflection.

Table 10.1 Examples of Technology, Their Application, and Proposed Benefits

Technology	Application	Educational benefit
VR (e.g. Body Interact)	Trauma simulation	Enhances decision-making and teamwork
AR (e.g. HoloLens)	Anatomy overlay	Aids spatial understanding and retention
MR (e.g. HoloPatient)	Virtual ward rounds	Supports communication and leadership

GAMIFICATION AND SCENARIO-BASED LEARNING

Gamification applies game design elements, points, levels, and feedback loops to enhance student motivation and engagement. In healthcare, it is used to reinforce infection control, pharmacology, communication skills, and ethical reasoning. Game-based simulations offer emotionally engaging, goal-oriented scenarios that prompt students to think critically under timed or high-pressure conditions (Schmidt-Kraepelin et al., 2019).

Interactive tools such as Kahoot! and branching scenario software like Twine or SimX provide safe opportunities for students to make mistakes, receive immediate feedback, and reflect. These approaches also align with principles of adult learning and experiential learning theory, both of which prioritise engagement, relevance, and reflection.

SUSTAINABLE AND EQUITABLE APPROACHES

Cloud-based and hybrid learning platforms have environmental, economic, and pedagogical benefits. They reduce reliance on printed materials and physical commuting, while expanding access for students with caregiving responsibilities, disabilities, or those living in remote areas. The World Health Organization (2021) highlights digital-first strategies as key to achieving equity and global workforce development.

Nurse educators have a responsibility to model and embed sustainability as part of curriculum content and delivery. This includes examining the environmental impact of simulation equipment, advocating for greener placements, and encouraging students to engage in sustainable health advocacy.

AI-SUPPORTED CLINICAL REASONING

Clinical decision-making tools powered by AI are becoming more commonplace. Platforms like IBM Watson and Isabel Diagnostic Assist simulate complex reasoning processes, offering students opportunities to test and refine their thinking without compromising patient safety (Chen et al., 2021). Used ethically, these tools can improve diagnostic confidence but must never replace the development of sound clinical judgement rooted in critical reflection and professional values.

INTERPROFESSIONAL DIGITAL COLLABORATION

Collaborative virtual learning platforms, such as Microsoft Teams, Moodle forums, or bespoke simulation software, are facilitating interprofessional education (IPE). These platforms support real-time collaboration between nursing students and peers from pharmacy, medicine, and social care. Shared learning on subjects such as end-of-life care, mental health, and health inequalities enables the development of mutual respect, communication, and collaborative problem-solving (Reeves et al., 2016).

MODULAR, STACKABLE, AND FLEXIBLE PATHWAYS

Flexible learning pathways support lifelong learning by allowing nurses to accumulate academic credit in smaller blocks, or 'micro-credentials'. These can later be built into full degrees or specialist certifications. For example, a nurse may complete a digital health CPD course and later stack this toward an MSc in Advanced Clinical Practice (Dede, 2020). This approach supports widening participation, especially among those who may be balancing work, care, and financial constraints.

RESPONSIBLE USE OF GENERATIVE AI TOOLS

Students are increasingly using AI writing aids such as Grammarly, Quillbot, and ChatGPT. While these tools can support efficiency, their misuse raises academic integrity concerns. Educators must provide explicit guidance on the responsible, critical use of such technologies, integrating academic writing support, digital literacy, and ethical reflection into modules (Huang et al., 2020).

RELATIONAL PEDAGOGY AND EMOTIONAL INTELLIGENCE

In the midst of technological advancement, the importance of human connection in education must not be lost. Emotional intelligence, compassion, and cultural humility remain central to the identity of the nurse educator. Narrative pedagogy, guided reflection, and dialogic teaching foster trust, vulnerability, and empathy (Benner et al., 2010). These approaches support students to develop not only professional knowledge, but also the moral and emotional grounding necessary for ethical practice.

CHALLENGES AND STRATEGIC PRIORITIES

While emerging innovations offer exciting potential, the future of transformative nursing education must also be viewed through a critical lens that acknowledges ongoing and new challenges. These span structural, pedagogical, policy, and professional domains, each of which shapes the ability of educators to deliver meaningful, equitable, and sustainable learning experiences. Nurse educators must be equipped not only to recognise these issues but to lead strategic responses that uphold the integrity and future-readiness of the profession. See Table 10.2 for a summary of key challenges in transformative nursing education, and examples of strategic responses available to educators and institutions.

CURRICULUM OVERLOAD AND COMPETING DEMANDS

One persistent challenge in nursing education is curriculum overcrowding. As new topics and competencies, such as genomics, digital health, sustainability, trauma-informed care, and planetary health, are added, there is rarely a corresponding removal or integration of outdated content. This often results in fragmented or superficial coverage of essential areas, reducing opportunities for depth, reflection, and critical engagement.

The pressure to include both national regulatory requirements and employer-led priorities can also lead to tension between compliance and creativity. Nurse educators often find themselves navigating a curriculum shaped more by policy and risk management than by pedagogical principles. Transformative education requires time and space for inquiry, values clarification, and identity formation—elements which may be squeezed out by procedural or heavily assessed programmes.

REGULATORY AND QUALITY ASSURANCE PRESSURES

In the UK, nurse education is regulated by the Nursing and Midwifery Council (NMC), alongside oversight from the Office for Students (OfS) and university-specific quality assurance mechanisms. While regulation ensures safety and standards, it can also constrain innovation. For example, novel assessment approaches, such as student-led viva examinations, creative outputs, or portfolio-based assessment, may be difficult to implement within rigid institutional templates or external examiner expectations.

Moreover, metrics-based cultures, such as those driven by the Teaching Excellence Framework (TEF), often reward surface indicators (e.g. progression, satisfaction) over deeper outcomes such as critical consciousness, resilience, or graduate impact in underserved areas. Strategic leadership is needed to balance accountability with pedagogical freedom, ensuring transformative ambitions are not eclipsed by performative measures.

WIDENING PARTICIPATION AND STRUCTURAL INEQUITY

Efforts to widen access to nursing programmes have led to greater diversity among student populations. However, equity of outcome has not always followed. Students from underrepresented groups, whether based on ethnicity, disability, socioeconomic background, or neurodiversity, continue to face systemic barriers. Differential attainment remains a major concern, as does the risk of deficit-based thinking that places responsibility for 'success' solely on the student.

Transformative education requires a reorientation towards inclusion as a collective and institutional responsibility. Nurse educators must examine hidden curricula, biased assessment practices, and teaching styles that may inadvertently marginalise learners. Intersectional approaches, co-designed curricula, and culturally sustaining pedagogies are essential in tackling these enduring disparities.

Table 10.2   A Summary of Key Challenges in Transformative Nursing Education, and Examples of Strategic Opportunities

Challenge	Strategic opportunity
Curriculum Overcrowding	Integrate overlapping themes (e.g. digital health with ethics); use spiral curriculum design
Regulatory Constraints	Pilot flexible assessment within regulatory frameworks; showcase innovation in TEF narratives
Differential Attainment	Adopt inclusive pedagogy; co-create content with diverse student reps
Academic Burnout	Redistribute workload; value scholarship of teaching and mentoring
Clinical-Academic Gap	Create joint educator roles; align university and placement expectations
Digital Exclusion	Embed digital literacy; provide tech bursaries and scaffolded induction
Climate Crisis	Integrate planetary health themes; run sustainability-focused simulations

Reflect on your current educational provision. What can you change to reduce hidden curricula, biased assessment practices, and teaching styles that may inadvertently marginalise learners and ensure your session fosters inclusion and equity by embedding intersectional and culturally sustaining approaches into your teaching.

Think about a particular topic you teach. Consider how hidden curricula (unspoken norms or values), assessment bias, or dominant teaching styles may affect learners from diverse backgrounds. Ask yourself:

- Whose voices are centred?
- Whose perspectives might be excluded or marginalised?
- Are there cultural assumptions embedded in how the topic is taught or assessed?

Describe how you will create a safe space for open discussion and critical thinking. How will you address power dynamics in the classroom?

ACADEMIC WORKLOAD AND BURNOUT

There is growing concern about the sustainability of the nurse educator role itself. Many academic staff juggle teaching, research, practice engagement, mentorship, and governance, often without adequate time or resources. The emotional labour of supporting students, many of whom may be in crisis, adds further complexity.

High workloads, combined with rigid systems and unclear promotion pathways, risk undermining staff well-being and retention. As the Council of Deans of Health has noted, academic careers in nursing are under strain, with fewer clinicians choosing to transition into education roles. Investment in educator development, leadership pipelines, and workload reform is therefore a strategic imperative for the future.

Beyond the UK, concerns about the sustainability of the nurse educator workforce are echoed internationally. The ICN (2023) highlights a global shortage of nursing faculty, noting that many countries face a depleted supply of nurse educators due to retirement, migration, and insufficient institutional investment—trends that threaten the sustainability of nursing education worldwide.

CLINICAL ACADEMIC GAP

The persistent divide between academic learning and clinical practice continues to challenge the transformative ambitions of nursing education. Placement shortages, inconsistent supervision quality, and competing placement demands (especially during times of workforce crisis) can result in variable student experiences.

Bridging the clinical-academic gap requires stronger partnerships between universities and practice providers. Collaborative curriculum design, embedded clinical educators, and joint appointments can help foster alignment and relevance. Furthermore, clinical educators need access to the same pedagogical development as academic staff to ensure consistency and coherence in the student journey.

TECHNOLOGICAL AND DIGITAL EXCLUSION

While digital innovations are celebrated for their potential, the digital divide must not be overlooked. Not all students, and not all educators, have reliable access to devices, Wi-Fi, or digital confidence. Digital poverty is a significant equity issue and disproportionately affects mature students, carers, and those from lower-income households.

Furthermore, the overuse of digital platforms can contribute to disengagement and cognitive overload, particularly when poorly designed or overly transactional. The challenge is not simply one of access but of digital pedagogy—ensuring that technologies are used to enhance, not replace, human connection, reflection, and purpose in learning.

Another cross-cutting challenge for the future is student mental health and well-being. Nursing students often balance academic demands, clinical placements, and personal responsibilities, placing them at heightened risk of stress and burnout. Digital intensification, financial strain, and societal pressures can amplify these risks. Future-ready curricula must therefore embed proactive well-being strategies, including access to mental health support, reflective practice, and approaches that normalise conversations about resilience and self-care. Protecting student well-being is essential to retention, equity, and the formation of sustainable professional identities.

POLITICAL AND ECONOMIC PRESSURES ON NURSING EDUCATION IN THE UK

Recent shifts in UK higher education (HE) policy and funding are placing increased strain on the delivery and sustainability of nursing programmes. In early 2025, the Royal College of Nursing (RCN) published data showing that 65% of universities in England had reduced their number of nurse lecturers between August 2024 and February 2025 (RCN, 2025). These cuts occurred during a period when government priorities highlighted the need to expand the domestic nursing workforce, creating a stark contradiction between policy ambition and resource allocation.

The reduction in nurse educator posts directly affects student experience, placement support, and the ability to deliver innovative curricula. Where staffing levels fall below a safe threshold, the workload burden on remaining academics intensifies, threatening both retention and well-being. These trends challenge the long-term viability of transformative nursing education models, particularly those that rely on relational pedagogy and personalised learning.

This pressure is part of a wider funding crisis in UK higher education. Recent analysis found that one in four leading UK universities is engaged in staff redundancies due to escalating costs, frozen tuition fees, and reduced income from international students following changes to visa regulations (Adams, 2025). These challenges have had a disproportionate impact on healthcare education, where costs are higher due to simulation, placement management, and regulatory compliance. Some institutions have begun reviewing the scope of their nursing and midwifery provision, which may further affect student access, regional workforce supply, and educational equity.

In this context, political decisions about immigration policy, tuition fees, and domestic workforce planning have immediate consequences for nursing education. It is essential that nurse educators and academic leaders actively engage with policymakers, professional bodies, and regulatory agencies to advocate for sustainable investment and to protect the future pipeline of nurse educators and students. Without strategic reform and sustained financial support, the progress made in inclusive, technologically integrated, and values-led nurse education may be compromised.

ADVOCACY AND STRATEGIC LEADERSHIP

Policy decisions, funding constraints, and sector leadership shape the environment in which they teach, assess, and support students. The Council of Deans of Health (CoDH) plays a key strategic role in shaping the direction of nursing and healthcare education across the UK, particularly in response to current pressures on the higher education sector.

Following the RCN's 2025 report highlighting a 65% reduction in nurse educator roles across English universities (Royal College of Nursing, 2025), CoDH publicly emphasised the need to protect and strengthen the academic nursing workforce. Ed Hughes, CEO of CoDH, noted that these staffing reductions often stem from financial challenges within universities, leading to growing pressure to deliver larger cohorts with fewer staff, a situation that is unsustainable for both educators and students (Council of Deans of Health, 2025a).

For clinical or academic educators undertaking the PGCAP, this context is more than background noise; it directly influences workload, student support, and the potential for innovation. Understanding CoDH's advocacy work can help educators locate their own professional experience during times of acute pressure. This awareness can inform reflective practice, influence curriculum design, and support constructive engagement with institutional strategy.

CoDH also provides practical leadership on emerging areas of importance for nurse educators. Through its Clinical Academic Roles Implementation Network (CARIN), it supports the development of roles that bridge education, practice, and research. For educators navigating dual roles or considering clinical academic careers, such frameworks are essential in supporting role clarity, identity formation, and sustainable professional development.

Additionally, CoDH's Innovation and Pedagogy Strategic Policy Group has begun to explore the ethical and pedagogical use of generative AI in healthcare education. This includes efforts to develop guidance on how technologies such as ChatGPT and machine learning tools might be responsibly integrated into learning and assessment (Council of Deans of Health, 2025b). For educators developing new teaching strategies or supporting students' digital literacy, such national leadership offers a helpful reference point for aligning practice with wider sector expectations.

For those undertaking formal training in nurse education, whether through the PGCAP or clinical educator roles, engaging with the work of CoDH provides a way to move from local reflection to national contribution. It reinforces the idea that nurse educators are not merely delivering curricula but are essential contributors to the strategic direction of the profession.

INNOVATION BOX

Assessment Title: Clinical Decision-making and Reflection Using AI Support (ChatGPT)

This assessment is designed to encourage responsible and critical use of ChatGPT as a tool to enhance clinical reasoning, information synthesis, and reflective thinking in nursing education. It promotes AI literacy, academic integrity, and evidence-informed practice.

Task

Students will complete a structured clinical case study, using ChatGPT as a support tool. The assignment will have three parts:

Part 1: Clinical Scenario Analysis (Written Report— 1,000 words)

- Students are provided with a realistic patient scenario (e.g. an older adult admitted with a suspected pressure ulcer and multiple comorbidities).
- They must:
  - Identify and prioritise nursing problems
  - Propose a nursing care plan
  - Justify decisions using evidence-based guidelines (referenced)
- Students are encouraged to use ChatGPT to:
  - Clarify concepts
  - Generate care plan ideas
  - Explore evidence-based interventions

- Students must document how they used ChatGPT, including:
  - Prompts used
  - A summary of responses
  - Critical evaluation of usefulness, accuracy, and any errors or gaps

Part 2: Critical Reflection on AI Use (500 words)

- Students reflect on:
  - How ChatGPT influenced their thinking
  - What they learned through verifying and triangulating AI-generated content with academic sources
  - Ethical considerations in using AI in clinical and academic settings

Part 3: Oral Viva or Group Discussion (10 minutes)

- Students participate in a brief discussion or viva:
  - To articulate and defend their clinical reasoning
  - To discuss how ChatGPT supported or challenged their decision-making
  - To demonstrate understanding beyond AI-generated suggestions with evidence of fact checking

GLOBAL WORKFORCE MOBILITY AND ETHICAL RESPONSIBILITY

The international mobility of nurses, particularly from lower-income to higher-income countries, raises ethical and educational questions. Programmes that prepare students for global employment must also address issues of language, power, cultural safety, and sustainability. For example, UK-based education that recruits from countries with nursing shortages must be designed with mutual benefit and ethical recruitment practices in mind.

The WHO's Global Strategic Directions for Nursing and Midwifery (2021–2025) call for education that strengthens local systems, builds indigenous leadership, and resists extractive approaches to workforce development. Nurse educators, therefore, have a responsibility to critically appraise the global implications of their curricula and partnerships.

Looking ahead, global solidarity in nursing education must extend beyond recruitment pipelines to the design of curricula that support mutual benefit and justice. Partnerships between institutions in higher- and lower-income countries should prioritise reciprocity, capacity building, and culturally sustaining approaches rather than extractive models of workforce supply. Embedding ethical responsibility at the heart of curriculum design ensures that mobility initiatives contribute to stronger health systems globally, rather than deepening inequities between them.

CLIMATE CRISIS AND PLANETARY HEALTH

The climate emergency is arguably the defining health challenge of this century, yet it remains underrepresented in many nursing curricula. Future-ready education must embed planetary health not only as content, but as a framework that connects environmental justice with health equity, social responsibility, and sustainable practice.

This includes developing students' capacity to advocate for greener healthcare systems, understand the health impacts of climate change, and practice sustainably. It also requires institutions to lead by example through sustainable campuses, carbon-conscious placements, and climate-responsive policies.

PRESERVING PROFESSIONAL IDENTITY AND CORE VALUES

In a fast-moving and often technocentric context, there is a risk that the moral and relational foundations of nursing may be diluted. Transformative education must centre professional identity formation as an explicit outcome, encouraging students to articulate their values, reflect on their purpose, and navigate tensions between institutional pressures and patient-centred care.

Narrative pedagogy, ethics-based simulation, and longitudinal mentorship are among the approaches that can support this development. Educators must also model the behaviours and dispositions they seek to nurture, including humility, integrity, and critical openness.

A SHARED RESPONSIBILITY

Transformative nursing education demands more than individual innovation; it requires a collective, sustained, and critically reflective effort to reshape systems and pedagogies in ways that are inclusive, future-facing, and values-driven. As health and education systems face increasing uncertainty, nurse educators must embrace their role not just as teachers, but as leaders, facilitators, and advocates of structural and cultural change.

REFRAMING THE EDUCATOR ROLE

Educators are increasingly expected to shift from the traditional 'knowledge authority' to co-creators of learning, guiding students to develop critical, reflective, and socially aware professional identities (Freire, 1970; Brookfield, 2017). This role transformation is echoed in Mezirow's (1997) theory of transformative learning, which emphasises the need for disorienting dilemmas, critical reflection, and dialogue as catalysts for deep change in learners' frames of reference.

In nursing education, this means supporting students not only to pass assessments, but to examine power, bias, and ethics in clinical care. It also involves modelling professional behaviours, integrity, and the capacity to navigate ambiguity (Taylor & Cranton, 2013). Nurse educators must encourage a learning environment that values voice, vulnerability, and social justice. See Box 10.1 for action priorities for nurse educators.

COLLABORATIVE LEADERSHIP IN CURRICULUM DESIGN

Curricula that reflect the lived realities of contemporary nursing must be built collaboratively. Service users, students, clinical partners, and educators should co-design

---

BOX 10.1   ACTION PRIORITIES FOR NURSE EDUCATORS

- **Reclaim Pedagogical Time:** Prioritise space for reflective, relational teaching amidst regulatory demands.
- **Strengthen Digital Confidence:** Undertake CPD on immersive technologies, AI, and online facilitation.
- **Co-create with Learners:** Embed partnership in module and assessment design.

- **Model Inclusive Practice:** Actively embed anti-racism, accessibility, and decolonised content in curriculum delivery.
- **Advocate Systemically:** Use your platform to influence institutional policies on workload, equity, and educator development.

learning that is culturally safe, locally relevant, and globally aware. Research shows that collaborative curriculum development enhances authenticity and encourages ownership among all stakeholders (Bovill et al., 2011). It also improves curricular flexibility, a key priority in post-pandemic recovery and resilience planning (OECD, 2020).

LEARNER AGENCY AND PARTNERSHIP

Transformative education requires not only inclusive curriculum design but also a shift in power relations between educators and students. Learner agency—the capacity of students to take an active role in shaping their learning experience—is a key pillar of contemporary pedagogy (Bovill et al., 2011). This includes co-creating assessment tasks, contributing to programme development, and engaging in peer-led initiatives.

Student partnership enhances engagement, retention, and relevance. For nurse educators, it provides critical insight into lived student realities and supports a culture of respect and collaboration. Practical applications include student representation on curriculum boards, co-authored teaching resources, and learner-led teaching evaluation. These approaches align with sector-wide calls for inclusive and democratic education.

EMBEDDING FUTURE-READY PRINCIPLES

Future-oriented nursing curricula must equip students to navigate complexity, ambiguity, and rapid technological change. This includes integrating principles such as systems thinking (Arnold & Wade, 2015), digital fluency (Health Education England [HEE], 2021), and sustainability literacy (Annan-Diab & Molinari, 2017).

For example, HEE's Digital Capabilities Framework (2021) outlines essential knowledge, skills, and behaviours required for digital healthcare practice, advocating integration of these competencies across all nursing education. Likewise, the planetary health movement urges embedding climate science, environmental justice, and ecological determinants of health within health curricula.

Distributed leadership models, where responsibility and decision-making are shared, can support this work by breaking down hierarchies and empowering educators to lead change from within (Bolden et al., 2009). Institutional support for this approach is essential and must include time for staff development, recognition of teaching excellence, and space for scholarship.

These forward-looking elements must be thoughtfully embedded, rather than treated as bolt-ons. Table 10.3 highlights features of future-ready curricula and their practical application in nurse education.

MAINTAINING COMPASSION AND CONNECTION

The relational foundation of nursing education must be protected amid increasing digitalisation and performance pressures. Studies have consistently shown that authentic educator–student relationships improve engagement, belonging, and academic performance (Hagenauer & Volet, 2014). Relational pedagogy, informed by the work of Noddings (2005) and Hooks (1994), prioritises care, trust, and mutual respect, key in cultivating the emotional intelligence and reflective capacity central to compassionate nursing practice (Freshwater & Stickley, 2004).

Compassionate pedagogy also means acknowledging the emotional labour of healthcare education. This includes supporting students to process clinical experiences, make sense of moral distress, and explore the often-unspoken dimensions of professional development (Jack & Wibberley, 2014).

ADVOCACY FOR STRUCTURAL CHANGE

Educators play a critical role in highlighting and challenging inequities within nursing education. Whether it be digital poverty, differential attainment, or institutional bias, nurse educators are uniquely placed to advocate for reform at the curriculum, faculty, and policy levels (Bhopal, 2018).

Table 10.3 Features of Future-ready Curricula and Their Practical Application in Nurse Education

Curriculum feature	Educational benefit	Example
Systems thinking	Encourages holistic care and policy awareness	Teaching about care transitions across services
Digital fluency	Prepares nurses for EHRs, AI, and telehealth	Embedding NHS Digital tools and AI workshops
Sustainability literacy	Promotes environmentally conscious practice	Assignments on carbon footprints in care
Relational pedagogy	Enhances belonging, identity, and empathy	Use of life story interviews in simulation
Co-production with students	Increases engagement and inclusivity	Student-designed OSCEs or feedback tools

Advocacy may involve resisting deficit narratives, centring marginalised voices in teaching content, or influencing strategic decisions around widening participation and staff development.

Engaging in this work requires a blend of critical pedagogy (Freire, 1970), scholarly activism (Mountz et al., 2015), and professional responsibility. It also aligns with the values promoted by international frameworks such as the WHO's Global Strategic Directions for Nursing and Midwifery (2021–2025), which call for inclusive, rights-based education to strengthen global healthcare systems. See box 10.2 for Future Directions.

BOX 10.2 FUTURE DIRECTIONS

The next decade of nurse education will require innovation underpinned by relational values. Based on the trends, challenges, and reflections explored in this chapter, future directions for transformative nursing education include:

- **Curriculum Evolution:** Embedding sustainability, systems thinking, and digital fluency as core content.
- **Pedagogical Innovation:** Expanding the use of immersive and AI-supported learning while protecting time for dialogue, compassion, and critical thinking.

- **Inclusive Design:** Ensuring accessibility, equity, and co-creation with students and service users across all programmes.
- **Educator Empowerment:** Developing nurse educators through structured CPD, workload reform, and leadership opportunities.
- **Strategic Partnerships:** Strengthening collaboration with clinical partners and global organisations to deliver contextually responsive and ethically informed curricula.

CONCLUSION

The future of transformative nursing education will be shaped by rapid technological change, complex workforce demands, and evolving societal expectations. Yet innovation alone will not guarantee success. The challenge for nurse educators is to ensure that advances in pedagogy, digital integration, and curriculum design are grounded in values of compassion, justice, and sustainability.

This chapter has outlined how trends such as immersive technologies, competency-based assessment, and flexible learning pathways are reshaping possibilities for nursing education. It has also highlighted structural challenges including workload, regulatory pressures, equity gaps, and political constraints that risk undermining progress. Responding to these tensions requires strategic leadership, advocacy, and collaborative approaches that position educators as both facilitators of learning and agents of change.

Ultimately, the strength of future nursing education will rest on its ability to balance innovation with humanity. Future-ready nurses must be digitally fluent and clinically competent, but also reflective, resilient, and ethically attuned. For educators, this means protecting time and space for dialogue, modelling inclusivity, and working in partnership with students, service users, and policymakers. If these responsibilities are embraced collectively, transformative nursing education can contribute not only to the preparation of future professionals but also to the creation of more equitable, sustainable, and compassionate health systems.

TAKE-HOME POINTS

1. Transformative nursing education requires ongoing adaptation to technological, societal, and environmental changes, while staying rooted in the profession's humanistic values.

2. Educators must lead with critical reflection, collaboration, and inclusivity to ensure that curricula remain relevant, equitable, and future-focused.

3. Real transformation occurs when educators, students, and institutions work together to challenge norms, embrace innovation, and advocate for just and sustainable educational systems.

CPD REFLECTIVE QUESTIONS

1. How do your current teaching practices reflect the principles of transformative education, and where might there be opportunities to evolve?

2. In what ways do you engage students in shaping their learning experiences, and how might co-creation enhance inclusivity and relevance?

3. What role do you play—or could you play— in advocating for equity, sustainability, or digital inclusion within your institution or professional networks?

REFERENCES

Adams, R. (2025). *Quarter of Leading UK Universities Cutting Staff Due to Budget Shortfalls*. The Guardian. https://www.theguardian.com/education/2025/feb/01/quarter-of-leading-uk-universities-cutting-staff-due-to-budget-shortfalls.

Aleven, V., Roll, I., McLaren, B. M., & Koedinger, K. R. (2016). Help helps, but only so much: research on help seeking with intelligent tutoring systems. *International Journal of Artificial Intelligence in Education*, 26(1), 205–223.

Annan-Diab, F., & Molinari, C. (2017). Interdisciplinarity: practical approach to advancing education for sustainability and for the sustainable development goals. *The International Journal of Management Education*, 15(2), 73–83.

Arnold, R. D., & Wade, J. P. (2015). A definition of systems thinking: a systems approach. *Procedia Computer Science*, 44, 669–678.

Benner, P., Sutphen, M., Leonard, V., & Day, L. (2010). *Educating Nurses: A Call for Radical Transformation*. Jossey-Bass.

Bhopal, K. (2018). *White Privilege: The Myth of a Post-Racial Society*. Policy Press.

Bolden, R., Petrov, G., & Gosling, J. (2009). Distributed leadership in higher education: rhetoric and reality. *Educational Management Administration & Leadership*, 37(2), 257–277.

Bovill, C., Cook-Sather, A., & Felten, P. (2011). Students as co-creators of teaching approaches, course design, and curricula. *International Journal for Academic Development*, 16(2), 133–145.

Brookfield, S. D. (2017). *Becoming a Critically Reflective Teacher* (2nd ed.). Jossey-Bass.

Chen, X., Xie, H., Hwang, G. J., & Chen, W. (2021). A multi-perspective study on artificial intelligence in education: grants, conferences, journals, software tools, institutions, and researchers. *Computers & Education: Artificial Intelligence, 2*, 100012.

Council of Deans of Health (2025a, May 15). *Council response to RCN's report on the nurse educator workforce in higher education in England*. https://www.councilofdeans.org.uk/2025/05/council-response-to-rcns-report-on-the-nurse-educator-workforce-in-higher-education-in-england/

Council of Deans of Health (2025b, February 28). *Briefing: Looking ahead to establish principles of generative AI in healthcare education – Innovation Month 2025*. https://www.councilofdeans.org.uk/2025/02/briefing-looking-ahead-to-establish-principles-of-generative-ai-in-healthcare-education-innovation-month-2025/

Dede, C. (2020). *The 60-Year Curriculum: New Models for Lifelong Learning in the Digital Economy*. Routledge.

Frank, J. R., Snell, L. S., & ten Cate, O. (2010). Competency-based medical education: theory to practice. *Medical Teacher, 32*(8), 638–645.

Freire, P. (1970). *Pedagogy of the Oppressed*. Continuum.

Freshwater, D., & Stickley, T. (2004). The heart of the art: emotional intelligence in nurse education. *Nursing Inquiry*, 11(2), 91–98.

Hagenauer, G., & Volet, S. E. (2014). 'I don't think I could, you know, just teach without any emotion': exploring the nature and origin of university teachers' emotions. *Research Papers in Education*, 29(2), 240–262.

HEE (2021). *Digital capabilities framework*. Accessed: (10 December 2025).

Hooks, B. (1994). *Teaching to Transgress: Education as the Practice of Freedom*. Routledge.

Huang, R., Spector, J. M., & Yang, J. (2020). *Educational Technology: A Primer for the 21st Century*. Springer.

International Council of Nurses (2023). *Policy brief: nursing education and workforce sustainability*. Geneva: ICN. https://www.icn.ch/system/files/2023-04/ICN%20Policy%20Brief_Nursing%20Education.pdf. Accessed: (10 December 2025).

Jack, K., & Wibberley, C. (2014). The meaning of emotion work to student nurses: a Heideggerian analysis. *International Journal of Nursing Studies*, 51(6), 900–907.

Mezirow, J. (1997). Transformative learning: theory to practice. *New Directions for Adult and Continuing Education*, 74, 5–12.

Mountz, A., Bonds, A., Mansfield, B., Loyd, J., Hyndman, J., Walton-Roberts, M., Basu, R., Whitson, R., Hawkins, R., Hamilton, T., & Curran, W. (2015). For slow scholarship: a feminist politics of resistance through collective action in the neoliberal university. *ACME: An International Journal for Critical Geographies*, 14(4), 1235–1259.

Noddings, N. (2005). *The Challenge to Care in Schools: An Alternative Approach to Education* (2nd ed.). Teachers College Press.

Organisation for Economic Co-operation and Development (OECD) (2020). *The impact of COVID-19 on education: Insights from education at a glance 2020*. https://www.oecd.org/education/

Padilha, J. M., Machado, P. P., Ribeiro, A., Ramos, J., & Costa, P. (2019). Clinical virtual simulation in nursing education: randomized controlled trial. *Journal of Medical Internet Research*, 21(3), e11529.

Reeves, S., Fletcher, S., Barr, H., Birch, I., Boet, S., Davies, N., & Kitto, S. (2016). A BEME systematic review of the effects of interprofessional education: BEME guide No. 39. *Medical Teacher*, 38(7), 656–668.

Royal College of Nursing (RCN) (2025). *Nurse lecturer cuts explode as domestic workforce plans put at risk: New report shows.* https://www.rcn.org.uk/news-and-events/Press-Releases/nurse-lecturer-cuts-explode-as-domestic-workforce-plans-put-at-risk-new-report-shows.

Schmidt-Kraepelin, M., Thiebes, S., Tran, M., & Sunyaev, A. (2019). What's in the game? Developing a taxonomy of gamification concepts for health apps. *Proceedings of the 52nd Hawaii International Conference on System Sciences.*

Taylor, E. W., & Cranton, P. (2013). *The Handbook of Transformative Learning: Theory, Research, and Practice.* Jossey-Bass.

Topol, E. (2019). *Deep Medicine: How Artificial Intelligence Can Make Healthcare Human Again.* Basic Books.

World Health Organization (WHO) (2021). *Global strategic directions for nursing and midwifery 2021–2025.* https://www.who.int/publications/i/item/9789240033863

Index

Note: Page numbers in *italics* and **bold** refers to figures and tables respectively.

A

adapted learning, 127
Advanced Clinical Practice (ACP) programmes, 7
AI-assisted clinical decision-making, 74
analytical thinking, 16
artificial intelligence (AI)
  formative and summative assessments, 73
  virtual patients and simulation training, 72–73
  and translation tools, 126
Association for Simulated Practice in Healthcare
    (ASPiH), 103
augmented reality (AR), 105, 125–126
autocratic leadership
  benefits and challenges, 42
  clinical simulation setting, 42
  curriculum enforcement, 41–42
  definition and features, 41
  vs. democratic leadership, **42**
  emergency protocol training, 42

B

balancing theory, 61
bingo card, 139
blended learning, 69–70
book club, 124

C

Campinha-Bacote's model of cultural competence, 118
carbon footprint of digital education, 80
case-based discussions, 20
case-based learning (CBL), 23
Centre for Sustainable Healthcare (CSH), 141
ceremony and meaning, 123
challenges and strategic priorities
  academic workload and burnout, 159
  clinical academic gap, 159
  competing demands, 158
  curriculum overload, 158
  regulatory and quality assurance, 158
  structural inequity, 158
  technological and digital exclusion, 159
  widening participation, 158
ChatGPT, 161
chronic obstructive pulmonary disease (COPD), 22
citizenship, 119
Clinical Skills Sustainability Project Group (CSSPG), 149
co-design and authenticity, 95, **96**
cognitive cultural intelligence (COGCQ), 93
Community of Inquiry (CoI) framework, 103
community partnerships, 148–151, *149*
competency-based education (CBE), 79
concept mapping, 20, 23
constructivist theories, 9
COVID-19 pandemic, 143
critical thinking
  analytical thinking, 20
  assessment of, 24–25, **25**
  characteristics of, 16–17, **16**
  in clinical practice, 16
  clinical questioning, 16
  clinical reasoning, 16, 17, 20, **21**
  cognitive process, 15
  in curricula, 20
  debrief sessions, 16
  defining, 19
  educators and practice partners, 20–21
  educators' capacity, 25–27
  evidence-based practice (EBP), 17
  inquisitiveness, 20
  interprofessional perspectives, 23
  journalling and portfolios, 16
  judgement, 17
  open-mindedness, 20
  psychological safety, 22

critical thinking (*Cont.*)
  recommendations, 29–30
  and reflective practice, 17, 27–29
  scenario-based learning, 16
  simulation, 24
  structured transition programmes, 22–23
  systematic thinking, 20
  teaching, 23
cultural competence, 62, 117–118
cultural expression and diversity, 121–122
curiosity, 16
curriculum, 134
  assessment strategies, 28
  design considerations, 27, **28**
  design and contemporary education, 78–79
  evolution, 164
  mapping, 28, **29**
  module learning outcomes (MLOs), 27–28
  programme review, 29
  quality assurance, 29
  teaching strategies, 28

D
debates and ethical dilemmas, 20
debriefing
  description, 88–89
  diamond debrief, 89–90
  gas model, 90
  with good judgement, 89
  plus delta, 89, **90**, 91
  promoting excellence and reflective learning, 90
  science of, **89**
decolonising education, 134
decolonising global health, 132
democratic leadership
  vs. autocratic leadership, **42**
  benefits and challenges, 40–41
  classroom environment, 40
  curriculum development, 40
  leadership development, 40
  overview, 39–40
dialogic teaching, 23
diamond debrief, 89–90
digital and immersive technologies
  artificial intelligence (AI), 105
  augmented reality (AR), 105
  curriculum design, 111
  in education, 112
  ethical considerations, 109

future aspects, 113
gamification in, 110
implementation, 110–111
integration strategies, 106
pedagogical foundations, 103–104
principles of, 109
professional development and cultural change, 111–112
reflective practice, 112
student voice and co-creation, 109
360-degree video, 106–107
trends and challenges, 108
virtual teaching and practice environments, 104–105
digital feedback, 78
digital equity
  sustainability and, 134–135
  open educational resources (OERS) and, 72
digital interventions efficacy, 75–77, **76**
digital platforms, 75
digital technologies, 43
digital tools, competency assessment, 79–80

E
Education for sustainable development (ESD), 148
Education for Sustainable Learning (ESL), 148
educators
  AI-driven nursing education, 74
  collaborative feedback, 26
  communities of practice (CoPs), 26–27
  empowerment, 164
  mentorship and leadership, 27
  peer observation schemes, 26
  practice partners, 19
  preparedness, 92–93
  reflective practice, 26
  self-assessment and reflection tools, 26
  structured reflection tools, 26, **26**
  toolkit, 133
e-learning
  online modules, 64
  global health equity, 80–81
emerging trends and innovations
  AI in education, 156
  clinical decision-making, 157
  competency-based education (CBE), 156
  emotional intelligence, 157
  gamification, 157
  generative AI tools, 157
  immersive technologies, 156

interprofessional digital collaboration, 157
    modular, stackable, and flexible pathway, 157
    scenario-based learning, 157
    sustainable and equitable approaches, 157
emotional intelligence, 93–94
equality, diversity, and inclusion, 58, **58**
ethical and cultural competence
    balancing theory, 61
    barriers to, 60
    classroom, 55–56
    defining cultural competence, 62
    development, delivery, and education, 60
    diversity in nursing, 57–58
    e-learning and online modules, 64
    equality, diversity, and inclusion, 58, **58**
    experiential learning, 56–57, *56*
    faculty preparedness and institutional support, 60–61
    implicit bias and structural inequality, 59
    inclusive learning environment, 59–60
    measuring, 63
    nursing ethics education, 54
    overview, 52–53
    personal and professional growth, 57
    professional standards and guidelines, 54–55
    promoting equality and diversity, 57
    technology, 63–65
    theoretical foundations, 53–54
    training strategies, 62
experiential learning, 3, 56–57, *56*, 85, *86*, *87*, 117

F
faculty development, 92–93
faculty preparedness, 60–61
flexible and accessible learning resources, 69, **69**
Freire's critical pedagogy, 118

G
gamification, 43, 126
gas model, 90
global citizenship education, 118
global health
    across curriculum, 134
    adapted learning, 127
    artificial intelligence and translation tools, 126
    book club, 124
    building research capacity, 135
    Campinha-Bacote's model of cultural competence, 118
    case study, 120–121
    ceremony and meaning, 123

challenges, 126
citizenship in nursing education, 119
climate change and health, 132
cohesion and community, 124
cost-effectiveness of virtual models, 131
critical pedagogy, 118
cultural competence, 117–118, 122–123
cultural expression and diversity, 121–122
decolonising education, 134
decolonising global health, 132
educator toolkit, 133
electives and exchanges, 119–120
embracing technology, 125
equality, diversity, and inclusion, 126–127
equity and access, 130
equity and economic justice, 131
ethical dimensions, 129
experiential learning theory, 117
Freire's critical pedagogy, 118
funding models and sustainability, 131
future aspects, 126, 132
games and gamification, 126
global citizenship education, 118
global health policy context, 116
global pandemics and cross-border collaboration, 132
health systems strengthening and workforce capacity, 132
influence nurse education, 129
institutional and system-level costs, 131
International Council of Nurses (ICN), 117
interprofessional learning, 128
Kolb's experiential learning cycle, 118
language and communication, 121
leadership, 129
learning through film, 124
massive open online courses (MOOCS), 126
Mezirow's transformative learning, 118
migration, displacement, and refugee health, 132
nursing curricula, 119
open access learning, 126
overview, 115–116
policy and workforce alignment, 134
policy context, 116
professional responsibility, 130
reciprocity, 127
reciprocity and partnership, 130
representation and cultural sensitivity, 130
student feedback, 122

global health (*Cont.*)
  student voice and co-creation, 124–125
  sustainability, 125
  sustainability and digital equity, 134–135
  synchronised experiences, 121
  theoretical perspectives, 119
  traditional electives, 131
  transformative learning theory, 117
  UK policy context, 117
  United Nations Sustainable Development Goals,
    116–117
  verifying practice hours, 123
  virtual and augmented reality, 125–126
  World Health Organization, 116
global pandemics and cross-border collaboration,
  132

H
Health and Care Act 2022, 138
Hill and Wamburu model, 29, *29*

I
improvement simulation, 94–95
inclusive design, 164
inclusive learning environment, 59–60
innovation and practical application
  AI-assisted clinical decision-making, 74
  AI-driven formative and summative assessments, 73
  AI-driven virtual patients and simulation
    training, 72–73
  artificial intelligence (AI), 72–73
  blended learning and hybrid models, 69–70
  carbon footprint of digital education, 80
  challenges, 70–71, **71**
  collaborative digital platforms, 75
  competency-based education (CBE), 79
  curriculum design and contemporary education, 78–79
  digital and mobile learning innovations, 71
  digital feedback, 78
  digital interventions efficacy, 75–77, **76**
  digital tools in competency assessment, 79–80
  educators role, AI-driven nursing education, 74
  e-learning for global health equity, 80–81
  ethical considerations and challenges of, 73–74, **74**
  flexible and accessible learning resources, 69, **69**
  future aspects, 81–82
  learners diverse needs, 69
  lifelong learning and professional development, 70
  microlearning and just-in-time learning, 71–72

  open educational resources (OERS) and digital equity, 72
  overview, 68
  personalised learning, 72–73
  simulation-based team training, 75
  sustainability, in digital learning and nursing
    education, 80
  sustainable development goals (SDGS), 81
innovative leadership, 42
institutional and system-level costs, 131
institutional support, 60–61
International Council of Nurses (ICN), 117
interprofessional leadership, 146–148, **147**
interprofessional learning, 43, 88, 128
intervention simulation, 95
involvement simulation, 95

J
just-in-time learning, 71–72

K
Kolb's Experiential Learning Cycle, *86*, **86**, 118

L
leadership and innovation
  autocratic leadership. *see* autocratic leadership
  continuous quality improvement, 48
  definition and importance, 44
  democratic leadership. *see* democratic leadership
  developing culture, 45–46
  digital technologies, 43
  gamification, 43
  innovative leadership, 42
  interprofessional learning, 43
  overview, 32–33
  performance review, 47
  post-registration direct entry, 44–45
  pre-registration direct entry, 44
  quality assurance, 46
  regulatory and accreditation requirements, 46–47
  servant leadership. *see* servant leadership
  simulation-based learning, 43
  stakeholder coproduction, 47
  strategies, 43
  transformational leadership. *see* transformational
    leadership
  UK nursing education, 44–45
learner agency and partnership
  compassionate pedagogy, 163
  structural change, 163–164

learner's diverse needs, 69
licensing, 142
lifelong learning and professional development, 70

M
massive open online courses (MOOCS), 126
metacognitive cultural intelligence (METACQ), 93
Mezirow's transformative learning, 118
microlearning, 71–72

N
Neighbourhood Health Guidelines, 150
NMC code domains, 22, **22**
Nursing and Midwifery Council (NMC), 2, 16, 123
nursing curricula, 119
nursing education
    academic skills and research literacy, 5
    advanced and specialist roles, 7
    advocacy and strategic leadership, 160
    artificial intelligence (AI), 105
    augmented reality (AR) in, 105
    Bologna process, 7
    Briggs report, 7
    career readiness, 6
    challenges and considerations, 4
    climate crisis and planetary health, 162
    complexity and uncertainty, 4
    curriculum and pedagogy, 8
    digital and technological agenda, 5
    early models of, 6
    emotional awareness, 4
    European influence, 7
    flexible and sustainable education models, 6
    historical perspectives and evolution of, 6–8
    implications for practice, 13
    integration strategies, 106
    interprofessional learning, 5
    learner agency and partnership, 163–164
    learning environment, 3
    mobility and ethical responsibility, 161
    NHS and workforce transformation, 2
    ongoing tensions, 8
    overview, 1
    person-centred and inclusive practice, 4–5
    political and economic pressures, 160
    professional formation, 4
    professional identity, 6, 162
    project 2000 and university integration, 7
    push reform, 7

reflection in, 17, **17**
    regulation and quality assurance, 8
    regulatory and institutional expectations, 2–3
    shared responsibility, 162–163
    simulation, reflection, and placement learning, 3–4, 103
    student diversity, 3
    sustainable development goals and, 142–144
    team-based care, 5
    360-degree video, 106–107
    transformative education, 2, 8–12
    trends and challenges, 108
    twentieth century, 6–7
    well-being and retention, 5–6
nursing ethics education, 54

O
online nursing education, 108, **108**
open access learning, 126
open educational resources (OERS), 72
open-mindedness, 16

P
pedagogical innovation, 164
personalised learning, 72–73
Personal Protective Equipment (PPE), 143
Planetary Health Report Card (PHRC), 150
plus delta, 89, **90**, 91
policy and workforce alignment, 134
post-registration direct entry, 44–45
practice hours verification, 123
pre-registration direct entry, 44
problem-based learning (PBL), 20, 23
professional responsibility, 130
psychological safety, 88

Q
quality assurance, 46

R
reflective environment
    aligning reflection, 18, **19**
    novice reflectors, 19
    reflective dialogue, 18
    reflective writing, 18
    simulation-based education, 18
reflective practice
    assessment of, 24–25, **25**
    constructive feedback, 24
    curriculum, 27–29

reflective practice (*Cont.*)
  educators' capacity, 25–27
  end-of-life decision-making, 21–22
  NMC standards and regulatory expectations, 22
  person-centred care, 21
  professional identity, 21
  recommendations, 29–30
  simulation, 24
  structured transition programmes, 22–23
  teaching, 24
Royal College of Nursing's (RCN) 'gloves off'
    campaign, 143–144

S
'SafeStart VR,' 97
self-reflection, 16
The Servant as Leader (Greenleaf), 36
servant leadership
  across team stages, 37–38, **38**
  application, 38–39
  benefits and challenges, 39
  characteristics, 35–36, **36**
  humility, 37, *37*
  in nursing education, 36–37
simulation-based education, 87–88
simulation-based learning, 43
simulation-based team training, 75
Social Determinants of Health (SDH), 144–145, *145*
social equity and well-being, 144–146
Society in Europe for Simulation Applied to Medicine
    (SESAM), 103
Socratic questioning, 23
Specialist Community Public Health Nurses
    (SCPHN), 141
Stages of Sustainable Quality Improvement (SuSQI), **150**
stakeholder coproduction, 47
strategic partnerships, 164
student feedback, 122
student voice and co-creation, 124–125
sustainability, 125
  and digital equity, 134–135
  in digital learning and nursing education, 80
Sustainable Development Goals (SDGs), 81, 142–144
sustainable healthcare
  building and sustaining community partnerships,
      148–151, *149*
  interprofessional leadership, 146–148, **147**
  licensing, 142
  in nursing, 137–141

  overview, 137
  social equity and well-being, 144–146
  sustainable development goals and nursing
      education, 142–144
synchronised experiences, 121
systematic thinking, 16

T
traditional electives, 131
transformational leadership
  addressing incivility and enhancing teamwork, 34–35
  definition and principles, 33–34
  development and mentorship, 35
  education satisfaction, 34
  nursing education, 34–35
  positive workplace culture, 34, *35*
  reducing burnout, 34
transformative education
  adult learning theory, 9
  affective learning, 10
  communities of practice, 10
  constructivism, 9
  critical pedagogy, 9
  emotional intelligence, 10
  experiential learning, 9
  Hill and Mitchell model, 11–12, *12*
  integrating theories into practice, 10
  learning environment, 12
  pedagogical theory, 11–12
  professional identity, 12
  reflective practice, 10
  reimagining, 11–12
  theoretical frameworks, 10, **11**
  threshold concepts, 10
  vs traditional education, 2, **2**
  transformative learning theory, 8–9
transformative learning theory, 8–9, 117
transformative simulation
  case studies, 97, **98**
  co-design and authenticity, 95, **96**
  contemporary issues, healthcare simulation, 97
  debriefing, 88–90
  educator preparedness, 92–93
  emotional, social, and cultural intelligence, 93–94
  experiential learning, 85, *86*, 87
  faculty development, 92–93
  gap analysis, 95
  improvement simulation, 94–95
  influence and inform nursing practice, 96

interprofessional learning through simulation, 88
intervention simulation, 95
involvement simulation, 95
overview, 84
practice assessors and supervisors, 92
psychological safety, 88
'SafeStart VR,' 97
simulation-based education, 87–88
simulation governance, ethics and consent, 92
simulation modalities and fidelity, 88
simulation scenario, 93
skills sessions from simulation sessions, 85
standards and frameworks guiding simulation, 85

U
UK nursing education, 44–45
UK policy context, 117
United Nations Sustainable Development Goals, 116–117

V
Virtual International Elective (VIE), 123
virtual reality (VR), 68, 125–126

W
World Health Organisation (WHO), 116, 139